Anti-Herpesvirus Drugs and Vaccines

Anti-Herpesvirus Drugs and Vaccines

Editor

Barry J. Margulies

MDPI • Basel • Beijing • Wuhan • Barcelona • Belgrade • Manchester • Tokyo • Cluj • Tianjin

Editor
Barry J. Margulies
Towson University
USA

Editorial Office
MDPI
St. Alban-Anlage 66
4052 Basel, Switzerland

This is a reprint of articles from the Special Issue published online in the open access journal *Viruses* (ISSN 1999-4915) (available at: https://www.mdpi.com/journal/viruses/special_issues/anti_herpetic_drugs).

For citation purposes, cite each article independently as indicated on the article page online and as indicated below:

LastName, A.A.; LastName, B.B.; LastName, C.C. Article Title. *Journal Name* **Year**, *Volume Number*, Page Range.

ISBN 978-3-0365-4037-5 (Hbk)
ISBN 978-3-0365-4038-2 (PDF)

Contents

About the Editor ix

Barry J. Margulies
The World of Antiherpetic Vaccines and Drugs, 2022
Reprinted from: *Viruses* **2022**, *14*, 850, doi:10.3390/v14050850 1

Lauren A. Sadowski, Rista Upadhyay, Zachary W. Greeley and Barry J. Margulies
Current Drugs to Treat Infections with Herpes Simplex Viruses-1 and -2
Reprinted from: *Viruses* **2021**, *13*, 1228, doi:10.3390/v13071228 3

Kimiyasu Shiraki, Shinichiro Yasumoto, Nozomu Toyama and Hiroaki Fukuda
Amenamevir, a Helicase-Primase Inhibitor, for the Optimal Treatment of Herpes Zoster
Reprinted from: *Viruses* **2021**, *13*, 1547, doi:10.3390/v13081547 . . . . **15**

Eleonora Naimo, Jasmin Zischke and Thomas F. Schulz
Recent Advances in Developing Treatments of Kaposi's Sarcoma Herpesvirus-Related Diseases
Reprinted from: *Viruses* **2021**, *13*, 1797, doi:10.3390/v13091797 . . . . **37**

Maimoona S. Bhutta, Daniel G. Sausen, Kirstin M. Reed, Elisa S. Gallo, Pamela S. Hair, Brittany P. Lassiter, Neel K. Krishna, Kenji M. Cunnion and Ronen Borenstein
Peptide Inhibitor of Complement C1, RLS-0071, Reduces Zosteriform Spread of Herpes Simplex Virus Type 1 Skin Infection and Promotes Survival in Infected Mice
Reprinted from: *Viruses* **2021**, *13*, 1422, doi:10.3390/v13081422 . . . . **53**

Jaeyeun Lee, Jennifer Stone, Prashant Desai, John G. Kosowicz, Jun O. Liu and Richard F. Ambinder
Arsenicals, the Integrated Stress Response, and Epstein–Barr Virus Lytic Gene Expression
Reprinted from: *Viruses* **2021**, *13*, 812, doi:10.3390/v13050812 . . . . **65**

Xin Guo, Ayan Kumar Ghosh, Robert F. Keyes, Francis Peterson, Michael Forman, David J. Meyers and Ravit Arav-Boger
The Synthesis and Anti-Cytomegalovirus Activity of Piperidine-4-Carboxamides
Reprinted from: *Viruses* **2022**, *14*, 234, doi:10.3390/v14020234 . . . . **79**

Lauren M. Hook, Sita Awasthi, Tina M. Cairns, Mohamad-Gabriel Alameh, Bernard T. Fowler, Kevin P. Egan, Molly M. H. Sung, Drew Weissman, Gary H. Cohen and Harvey M. Friedman
Antibodies to Crucial Epitopes on HSV-2 Glycoprotein D as a Guide to Dosing an mRNA Genital Herpes Vaccine
Reprinted from: *Viruses* **2022**, *14*, 540, doi:10.3390/v14030540 . . . . **95**

Brent A. Stanfield, Konstantin G. Kousoulas, Agustin Fernandez and Edward Gershburg
Rational Design of Live-Attenuated Vaccines against Herpes Simplex Viruses
Reprinted from: *Viruses* **2021**, *13*, 1637, doi:10.3390/v13081637 . . . . **107**

Maria Luisa Visciano, Aakash Mahant Mahant, Carl Pierce, Richard Hunte and Betsy C. Herold
Antibodies Elicited in Response to a Single Cycle Glycoprotein D Deletion Viral Vaccine Candidate Bind C1q and Activate Complement Mediated Neutralization and Cytolysis
Reprinted from: *Viruses* **2021**, *13*, 1284, doi:10.3390/v13071284 . . . . **121**

K. Yeon Choi, Nadia S. El-Hamdi and Alistair McGregor
Cross Strain Protection against Cytomegalovirus Reduces DISC Vaccine Efficacy against CMV in the Guinea Pig Model
Reprinted from: *Viruses* **2022**, *14*, 760, doi:10.3390/v14040760 . . . . **133**

Lukas van de Sand, Maren Bormann, Yasmin Schmitz, Christiane Silke Heilingloh, Oliver Witzke and Adalbert Krawczyk
Antiviral Active Compounds Derived from Natural Sources against Herpes Simplex Viruses
Reprinted from: *Viruses* **2021**, *13*, 1386, doi:10.3390/v13071386 . . . . **151**

About the Editor

Barry J. Margulies received B.S. at MIT in Applied Biological Sciences and researched controlled release technology under Drs. Eyal Ron and Robert Langer. He earned his Ph.D. at the Johns Hopkins University School of Medicine in the field of Biochemistry, Cellular, and Molecular Biology under Dr. Wade Gibson, during which he studied the G protein-coupled receptors encoded by human cytomegalovirus. He also completed his post-doctoral studies at the Hopkins School of Medicine (Division of Comparative Medicine), with Dr. Janice Clements, studying CD4-independent entry of human and simian immunodeficiency viruses. From 2001–2021, he was a faculty member at Towson University, where he established the Towson University Herpes Virus Lab. His research encompassed the molecular biology of human cytomegalovirus and new methods for the long-term prevention of recurrent outbreaks of HSV-1 and -2, VZV, and feline herpes virus-1. He is currently a Scientific Review Officer with the NIH.

viruses

MDPI

Editorial

The World of Antiherpetic Vaccines and Drugs, 2022

Barry J. Margulies †

Towson University Herpes Virus Lab, Department of Biological Sciences, Towson University, Towson, MD 21252, USA; bjmarg@alum.mit.edu; Tel.: +1-(410)-704-5019; Fax: +1-(410)-704-2405

† Current address: NIH/NIAID/SRP, AIDS Review Branch, 5601 Fishers Lane, Rockville, MD 20852, USA.

Citation: Margulies, B.J. The World of Antiherpetic Vaccines and Drugs, 2022. *Viruses* **2022**, *14*, 850. https://doi.org/10.3390/v14050850

Received: 18 April 2022

Accepted: 19 April 2022

Published: 20 April 2022

The world of antiherpetics has grown by leaps and bounds since the discovery of what would become the first antiherpetic drug in 1964 [1]. We now have licensed vaccines to prevent veterinary diseases associated with equine herpesvirus-1 [2,3], pseudorabies virus [4,5], bovine herpesvirus-1 [6], feline herpesvirus-1 [7], infectious laryngotracheitis virus/gallid herpesvirus-1 [8], Marek's Disease Virus [9,10], and cyprinid herpesvirus-3 [8], all herpesviruses that cause significant morbidity and mortality. We also have excellent vaccines, Varivax/Zostavax [11,12] and Shingrix [13], to prevent chicken pox and shingles in humans. There are many licensed drugs, e.g., letermovir [14] and acyclovir [15,16], to prevent herpesvirus outbreaks. However, we are constantly discovering new ways to attack herpesviruses, including novel methods aiming at prophylactic and therapeutic approaches.

In this Special Issue, we begin with the mundane, the currently applicable anti-herpes simplex drug market [17,18]; these articles cover the pharmaceutical armaments available today to deal with recurrent HSV outbreaks. Current treatments for Kaposi's sarcoma are addressed, especially drugs that combat the cancer itself [19]. We also present information on the search for novel antiherpetics [20–22] to combat infection with other human herpesviruses. However, none of the chemotherapeutic interventions discussed deal with preventing a herpes infection.

Novel work in herpesvirus vaccines is extending the original work of anti-VZV work. As was seen with current anti-SARS-CoV-2 approaches, vaccines to combat HSV-2 based on recombinant protein subunits or mRNAs are discussed [23]. This exciting research may be a major step forward in preventing primary infection. Similarly, live, attenuated herpesviruses can be used to elicit durable, lasting, immune responses to diminish the number and severity of reactivations [24,25]. A fourth paper in this issue [26] addresses limitations that may be encountered when working with live, attenuated herpesviruses.

While the established pharmacopeia typically uses synthetic molecules that have been discovered through direct design or high-throughout screens, a number of researchers have taken the path of exploring natural compounds. This Special Issue describes multiple natural products used to prevent primary infection in vitro and in vivo [27]. Furthermore, and of greater consequence, they demonstrate the incredible safety of these compounds in animal models, an important step towards testing these compounds in Phase I safety trials.

It is with great pleasure that we provide this Special Issue, presenting both current and forward-looking concepts in antiviral intervention, and we welcome your feedback.

Conflicts of Interest: The authors declare no conflict of interest.

References

1. Engle, C.G.; Stewart, R.C. Anti-Herpetic Activity of 5-Iodo-2'-Deoxyuridine in Presence of Its Degradation Products. *Proc. Soc. Exp. Biol. Med.* **1964**, *115*, 43–45. [CrossRef] [PubMed]
2. Goehring, L.S.; Wagner, B.; Bigbie, R.; Hussey, S.B.; Rao, S.; Morley, P.S.; Lunn, D.P. Control of EHV-1 viremia and nasal shedding by commercial vaccines. *Vaccine* **2010**, *28*, 5203–5211. [CrossRef] [PubMed]
3. Minke, J.M.; Audonnet, J.C.; Fischer, L. Equine viral vaccines: The past, present and future. *Vet. Res.* **2004**, *35*, 425–443. [CrossRef] [PubMed]
4. Ferrari, M.; Brack, A.; Romanelli, M.G.; Mettenleiter, T.C.; Corradi, A.; Dal Mas, N.; Losio, M.N.; Silini, R.; Pinoni, C.; Pratelli, A. A study of the ability of a TK-negative and gI/gE-negative pseudorabies virus (PRV) mutant inoculated by different routes to protect pigs against PRV infection. *J. Vet. Med. B Infect. Dis. Vet. Public Health* **2000**, *47*, 753–762. [CrossRef]
5. Freuling, C.M.; Muller, T.F.; Mettenleiter, T.C. Vaccines against pseudorabies virus (PrV). *Vet. Microbiol.* **2017**, *206*, 3–9. [CrossRef]
6. Van Oirschot, J.T.; Kaashoek, M.J.; Rijsewijk, F.A. Advances in the development and evaluation of bovine herpesvirus 1 vaccines. *Vet. Microbiol.* **1996**, *53*, 43–54. [CrossRef]
7. Day, M.J.; Horzinek, M.C.; Schultz, R.D.; Squires, R.A.; Group of the World Small Animal Veterinary Assotiation WSAVA. Guidelines for the vaccination of dogs and cats. *J. Small Anim. Pract.* **2016**, *57*, E1–E45. [CrossRef]
8. Tizard, I.R. *Vaccines for Veterinarians*; Elsevier: Amsterdam, The Netherlands, 2020.
9. Darteil, R.; Bublot, M.; Laplace, E.; Bouquet, J.F.; Audonnet, J.C.; Riviere, M. Herpesvirus of turkey recombinant viruses expressing infectious bursal disease virus (IBDV) VP2 immunogen induce protection against an IBDV virulent challenge in chickens. *Virology* **1995**, *211*, 481–490. [CrossRef]
10. Okazaki, W.; Purchase, H.G.; Burmester, B.R. Protection against Marek's disease by vaccination with a herpesvirus of turkeys. *Avian Dis.* **1970**, *14*, 413–429. [CrossRef]
11. Gershon, A.A. Varicella-zoster virus: Prospects for control. *Adv. Pediatr. Infect. Dis.* **1995**, *10*, 93–124.
12. Robinson, D.M.; Perry, C.M. Zoster vaccine live (Oka/Merck). *Drugs Aging* **2006**, *23*, 525–531. [CrossRef]
13. Shingrix—An Adjuvanted, Recombinant Herpes Zoster Vaccine. Available online: https://secure.medicalletter.org/article-share?a=1535a&p=tml&title=Shingrix%20-%20An%20Adjuvanted,%20Recombinant%20Herpes%20Zoster%20Vaccine&cannotaccesstitle=1 (accessed on 4 December 2017).
14. Kim, E.S. Letermovir: First Global Approval. *Drugs* **2018**, *78*, 147–152. [CrossRef]
15. Hopkins, S.J. Zovirax: Fighting a sore problem. *Nurs. Mirror* **1982**, *154*, 38.
16. Liu, C. Antiviral drugs. *Med. Clin. N. Am.* **1982**, *66*, 235–244. [CrossRef]
17. Sadowski, L.A.; Upadhyay, R.; Greeley, Z.W.; Margulies, B.J. Current Drugs to Treat Infections with Herpes Simplex Viruses-1 and -2. *Viruses* **2021**, *13*, 1228. [CrossRef]
18. Shiraki, K.; Yasumoto, S.; Toyama, N.; Fukuda, H. Amenamevir, a Helicase-Primase Inhibitor, for the Optimal Treatment of Herpes Zoster. *Viruses* **2021**, *13*, 1547. [CrossRef]
19. Naimo, E.; Zischke, J.; Schulz, T.F. Recent Advances in Developing Treatments of Kaposi's Sarcoma Herpesvirus-Related Diseases. *Viruses* **2021**, *13*, 1797. [CrossRef]
20. Bhutta, M.S.; Sausen, D.G.; Reed, K.M.; Gallo, E.S.; Hair, P.S.; Lassiter, B.P.; Krishna, N.K.; Cunnion, K.M.; Borenstein, R. Peptide Inhibitor of Complement C1, RLS-0071, Reduces Zosteriform Spread of Herpes Simplex Virus Type 1 Skin Infection and Promotes Survival in Infected Mice. *Viruses* **2021**, *13*, 1422. [CrossRef]
21. Lee, J.; Stone, J.; Desai, P.; Kosowicz, J.G.; Liu, J.O.; Ambinder, R.F. Arsenicals, the Integrated Stress Response, and Epstein-Barr Virus Lytic Gene Expression. *Viruses* **2021**, *13*, 812. [CrossRef]
22. Guo, X.; Ghosh, A.K.; Keyes, R.F.; Peterson, F.; Forman, M.; Meyers, D.J.; Arav-Boger, R. The Synthesis and Anti-Cytomegalovirus Activity of Piperidine-4-Carboxamides. *Viruses* **2022**, *14*, 234. [CrossRef]
23. Hook, L.M.; Awasthi, S.; Cairns, T.M.; Alameh, M.G.; Fowler, B.T.; Egan, K.P.; Sung, M.M.H.; Weissman, D.; Cohen, G.H.; Friedman, H.M. Antibodies to Crucial Epitopes on HSV-2 Glycoprotein D as a Guide to Dosing an mRNA Genital Herpes Vaccine. *Viruses* **2022**, *14*, 540. [CrossRef]
24. Stanfield, B.A.; Kousoulas, K.G.; Fernandez, A.; Gershburg, E. Rational Design of Live-Attenuated Vaccines against Herpes Simplex Viruses. *Viruses* **2021**, *13*, 1637. [CrossRef]
25. Visciano, M.L.; Mahant, A.M.; Pierce, C.; Hunte, R.; Herold, B.C. Antibodies Elicited in Response to a Single Cycle Glycoprotein D Deletion Viral Vaccine Candidate Bind C1q and Activate Complement Mediated Neutralization and Cytolysis. *Viruses* **2021**, *13*, 1284. [CrossRef]
26. Choi, K.; El-Hamdi, N.; McGregor, A. Cross Strain Protection against Cytomegalovirus Reduces DISC Vaccine Efficacy against CMV in the Guinea Pig Model. *Viruses* **2022**, *14*, 760. [CrossRef]
27. Van de Sand, L.; Bormann, M.; Schmitz, Y.; Heilingloh, C.S.; Witzke, O.; Krawczyk, A. Antiviral Active Compounds Derived from Natural Sources against Herpes Simplex Viruses. *Viruses* **2021**, *13*, 1386. [CrossRef]

viruses MDPI

Review

Current Drugs to Treat Infections with Herpes Simplex Viruses-1 and -2

Lauren A. Sadowski [1,†], Rista Upadhyay [1,2,†], Zachary W. Greeley [1,‡] and Barry J. Margulies [1,3,*]

1 Towson University Herpes Virus Lab, Department of Biological Sciences, Towson University, Towson, MD 21252, USA; lsadow2@students.towson.edu (L.A.S.); rupadh1@students.towson.edu (R.U.); zgreel1@gmail.com (Z.W.G.)
2 Towson University Department of Chemistry, Towson, MD 21252, USA
3 Molecular Biology, Biochemistry, and Bioinformatics Program, Towson University, Towson, MD 21252, USA
* Correspondence: bjmarg@alum.mit.edu
† Authors contributed equally to this manuscript.
‡ Current address: Becton-Dickinson, Sparks, MD 21152, USA.

Abstract: Herpes simplex viruses-1 and -2 (HSV-1 and -2) are two of the three human alphaherpesviruses that cause infections worldwide. Since both viruses can be acquired in the absence of visible signs and symptoms, yet still result in lifelong infection, it is imperative that we provide interventions to keep them at bay, especially in immunocompromised patients. While numerous experimental vaccines are under consideration, current intervention consists solely of antiviral chemotherapeutic agents. This review explores all of the clinically approved drugs used to prevent the worst sequelae of recurrent outbreaks by these viruses.

Keywords: acyclovir; ganciclovir; cidofovir; vidarabine; foscarnet; amenamevir; docosanol; nelfinavir; HSV-1; HSV-2

Citation: Sadowski, L.A.; Upadhyay, R.; Greeley, Z.W.; Margulies, B.J. Current Drugs to Treat Infections with Herpes Simplex Viruses-1 and -2. *Viruses* **2021**, *13*, 1228. https://doi.org/10.3390/v13071228

Academic Editor: Graciela Andrei

Received: 24 May 2021
Accepted: 21 June 2021
Published: 25 June 2021

1. Introduction

The world of anti-herpes simplex (anti-HSV) agents took flight in 1962 with the FDA approval of idoxuridine [1,2]. Since then, advances in understanding the genetics of herpes simplex viruses-1 and -2 (HSV-1 and -2) and their enzymology have opened the doors to many new, approved, and active pharmaceuticals, all provided as completely synthetic entities, to treat herpes simplex infections.

2. HSV-1 and -2 Infection

The human herpesviruses HSV-1 and HSV-2 (HSVs) are major human pathogens in the simplexvirus family [3]. Both viruses infect people of all ages, with HSV-1 being more prevalent than HSV-2 [3]; the seroprevalence of the latter tends to increase in different populations as they age [4]. Once primary infection occurs, these viruses tend to retreat to local ganglia, where they remain latent for an indeterminant amount of time [3]. Nonetheless, at various times during the life of the host, the latent genomes of these viruses may reactivate and cause productive, lytic infections that may result in clinical signs and symptoms, such as skin lesions, genital sores, keratitis, whitlow, or other mucocutaneous pathologies [3]. In the most extreme cases, HSVs can cause fatal systemic infections or encephalitis, problems typically most associated with immune naïve or immunocompromised patients [3]. Therefore, providing antiviral intervention for those most severely affected by these viruses is necessary.

3. Nucleoside Analogs

The majority of anti-HSV drugs are nucleoside analogs that directly target the viral DNA polymerase when in their active form. The virally encoded DNA polymerase provides an essential function, and interfering with this enzyme results in inhibition of viral

DNA replication, therefore preventing the production of infectious virions. Although this mechanism is effective, a potential issue is that these agents could also target the host DNA polymerase and lead to higher toxicity. All nucleoside analogs require tri-phosphorylation before binding to and inhibiting the viral DNA polymerase at its active site [5].

The first phosphorylation of antiviral nucleoside analogs typically occurs via a viral enzyme, thymidine kinase (TK); the subsequent di- and tri-phosphorylations are enacted through cellular kinases [6]. One benefit of this pathway is that host toxicity is limited because these drugs require the presence of said viral TK, which only appears during the early phase of an active, lytic HSV infection. Without the viral TK, these anti-HSV drugs tend not to become activated and therefore cannot inhibit any DNA polymerase. Nonetheless, the host's own TK could potentially phosphorylate the drug first, but after cellular kinases tri-phosphorylate it, the drug will still have a higher affinity toward inhibiting the virus' DNA synthesis over that of the host [7].

The main basis for resistance to nucleoside analogs resides in mutations in TK. Hence, some antiherpetic drugs that utilize a TK-directed pathway and may be less useful in the face of such resistance include acyclovir, valacyclovir, penciclovir, famciclovir, trifluridine, idoxuridine, vidarabine, sorivudine, brivudine, ganciclovir, and valganciclovir.

4. Acyclovir, the First in Its Class of Antiherpetic Drugs

Many of the antiherpetic nucleoside analogs primarily in clinical use are based on the core structure of deoxyguanosine (Figure 1A). Acyclovir (ACV; Figure 1B) is one of the most commonly used of these; it is activated by TK and inhibits both TK and DNA polymerase activities. ACV itself is a competitive inhibitor of the viral TK [8], whereas ACV-triphosphate (ACV-TP) acts as a competitive suicide inhibitor for the viral DNA polymerase [9]. Although ACV is known as a chain terminator, the nucleotide after ACV can be added to the growing DNA chain, but this forms a suicide inhibitor complex [10] in which the exonuclease activity of the DNA polymerase cannot excise ACV to restore activity; HSV DNA polymerase then gets caught in an ever-cycling trap of adding a few nucleotides, excising those nucleotides back towards the ACV, and repeating the cycle. Thus, the inactivation of the viral DNA polymerase prevents the complete replication of the viral genome and subsequently the formation of mature virions [11].

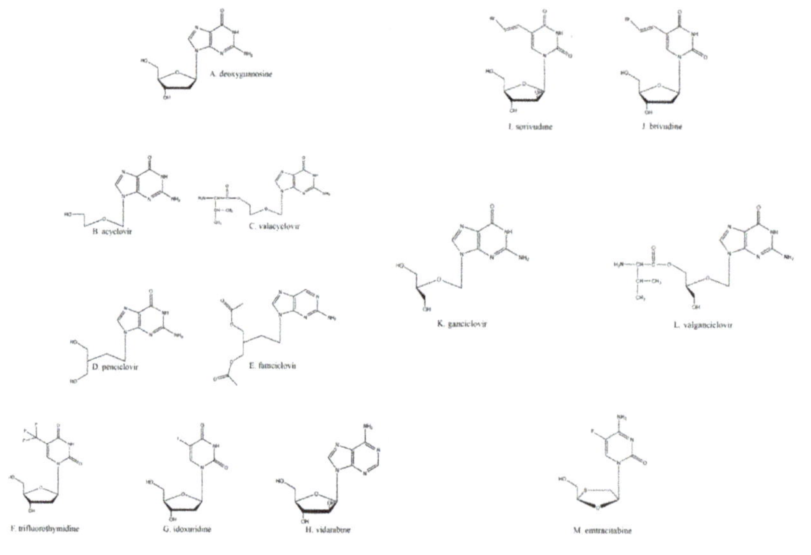

Figure 1. Nucleoside analogs.

ACV toxicity in the host is generally low because of the requirement of viral TK for the first phosphorylation. Nonetheless, host TKs are able to perform the first phosphorylation of ACV at an extremely low level; typically, ACV-TP is found at a 40–100× greater concentration in infected cells than in uninfected cells [8], reflective of a measured selectivity index of 869 [12]. Furthermore, the toxicity of ACV is also abrogated because ACV-TP is a poor inhibitor of host DNA polymerase [13].

Viral resistance to ACV can be achieved through two different mechanisms: mutations to the DNA polymerase or mutations to the viral TK. Mutations to the DNA polymerase would disrupt the active site. However, the most common mutations that affect ACV-TP's activity against viral DNA polymerase usually result in weak inhibition of DNA synthesis because they only slightly diminish the affinity for the ACV-TP in the active site [14]. More important are the more prevalent mutant TKs, which are not able to phosphorylate ACV. Strains of HSV that have ACV-resistant TKs lower drug activation and prevent the subsequent host enzyme phosphorylation of ACV [14,15]. Moreover, single and multiple mutations are more commonly found in the TK gene than in the DNA polymerase gene [14].

One other potentially problematic issue with ACV is its low oral bioavailability, which may be obviated by intravenous dosing [16,17]. This problem has been obviated with the introduction of valacyclovir (VaCV; Figure 1C), a prodrug of ACV created by the esterification of valine to ACV [18]; VaCV has a much higher absorption rate in the gut, resulting in less wasted drug with every oral dose [18]. As a prodrug, VaCV is converted through metabolism in the liver and kidney into ACV and valine by biphenyl hydrolase-like protein, which cleaves the esterified amino acid from the molecule [19,20]. Once VaCV is converted into ACV, all the properties and mechanisms of action as stated previously for ACV are the same.

5. Other Nucleoside Analogs

Another anti-HSV guanosine analog is penciclovir (PCV; Figure 1D). Although PCV and ACV are both analogs of the same nucleoside, the slight differences in structure between the drugs (Figure 1B,D) have led to minor differences in their pharmacology. PCV has about a 100× higher affinity for HSV TK compared to that of ACV [21]. This leads to much higher levels of PCV-TP than ACV-TP in vivo. Alternatively, ACV-TP shows about a 100× greater affinity for viral DNA polymerase than PCV-TP [21].

The differences between ACV's and PCV's molecular structures also result in PCV having oral absorption significantly lower than that of ACV; PCV's oral bioavailability is 1.5%, and its in vivo half-life is 2–2.5 h [22–24]. As a potential solution to this issue, PCV has been acetylated, resulting in its prodrug famciclovir (FamCV; Figure 1E) [24], which has a much higher oral uptake (up to 73% of the dose) [25]. FamCV is rapidly converted to PCV by aldehyde oxidase in the liver, after which the PCV enters general circulation as the active drug [26]. VaCV and FamCV are some of the most widely available antivirals because of their high oral bioavailability and rapid metabolism into their active forms, although once converted into active drugs, their in vivo half-lives are not improved over those of the parent compounds.

Trifluridine (TFT; Figure 1F) and idoxuridine (IDU; Figure 1G), while still in use, are much less commonly employed antiherpetic drugs due to their toxicity. Both TFT and IDU are used optically to limit systemic toxicity [27], such as dermatitis and local burning [28] and bone marrow suppression [29]. TFT and IDU are both deoxyuridine analogs and utilize the same activation and antiviral schemes as the drugs previously described.

Vidarabine (Figure 1H), a general polymerase inhibitor, was first synthesized as an anti-cancer drug [30]. The drug is an adenosine analog that retains activity against IDU- and ACV-resistant HSVs. However, because vidarabine acts indiscriminately on all polymerases, the drug can also impact host cell activities such as ribonucleoside reduction (by ribonucleoside reductase) and RNA polyadenylation [31]. Therefore, vidarabine suffers from much more limited clinical utility because of its mutagenic and oncogenic potential [32]. Hence, despite vidarabine being the first clinically approved antiviral drug, it is no longer available in the United States [33]. It should also be noted that vidarabine is less effective than other available antiherpetic drugs for treating HSV keratoconjunctivitis [34], so it suffers from poorer clinical reliability except in extreme cases.

Sorivudine (Figure 1I) and brivudine (Figure 1J) are thymidine analogs that inhibit DNA replication in the same fashion as described above. Brivudine ([(E)-5-(2-bromovinyl)-2′-deoxyuridine]) has greater potency than ACV against the varicella-zoster virus (VZV), another human alphaherpesvirus [35,36]; the drug appears to be not nearly as effective against HSV-1 because of the higher rates of HSVs that are resistant to these two medications [35,37].

Ganciclovir (GCV; Figure 1K), a guanosine analog like ACV, has an extra hydroxyl group on the ostensible 3′ carbon when compared to ACV. Ganciclovir is used primarily for cytomegalovirus (CMV) infections since most clinical CMV strains are still sensitive to it [38]. Although GCV's anti-CMV activity can be attributed to its activation with the first phosphate being added via the UL97 kinase encoded by CMV [39], the HSV TK can also activate GCV via primary phosphorylation [40,41]. Similar to ACV, GCV exhibits poor oral bioavailability; subsequent work resulted in the creation of the VaCV analog valganciclovir (VGCV; Figure 1L) by esterifying valine to GCV [42]. As with VaCV, once inside the body, VGCV is converted into its active form, GCV [43].

6. Nucleotide Analogs: Cidofovir, Adefovir, and Brincidofovir

Resistance to the drugs previously described is primarily acquired through mutations to the TK [44]. As previously noted, all the nucleoside analogs require TK for phosphorylation to initiate their antiviral activity, and TK mutants can no longer activate those drugs. Hence, without phosphorylation, none of the nucleoside analogs are active against herpesviruses. One way to overcome this requirement for TK is to use a nucleotide analog that already has a monophosphate attached, such as ones based on deoxycytosine monophosphate (Figure 2A), like cidofovir (CDV; Figure 2B). None of these nucleotide analogs require activation by TK.

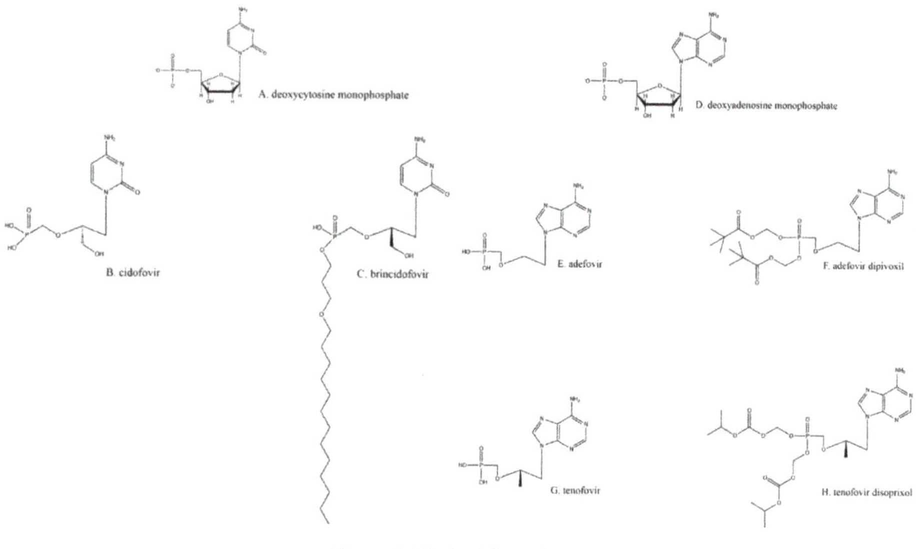

Figure 2. Nucleotide analogs.

CDV is di- and tri-phosphorylated by cellular kinases, much like nucleoside analogs [45]. The resulting cidofovir–triphosphate binds to the HSV DNA polymerase and is incorporated into the growing viral DNA chain, which reduces the speed of elongation. Furthermore, if two cidofovirs are incorporated adjacently in a growing HSV DNA chain, elongation is terminated [11]. Resistance to CDV occurs through mutations in the HSV DNA polymerase, typically with substitutions of amino acids that occur in less conserved regions of the enzyme [46,47]. Likewise, these mutations may allow the virus to become resistant to other drugs that are nucleoside analogs. A major drawback to the use of CDV is higher host toxicity, primarily in the kidneys [48].

Due to the limited bioavailability of CDV, the lipidated precursor brincidofovir (Figure 2C) has been created and is currently in clinical trials [49,50]. The increased biological distribution of the latter drug leads to greater virus inhibition at a lower overall dose [51]. The difference in brincidofovir metabolism also makes it a less toxic drug overall [48].

An analog of deoxyadenosine monophosphate (Figure 2D), adefovir (Figure 2E), is a drug already licensed as an anti-hepatitis B virus agent [52]. Adefovir also inhibits HSV replication [53,54]. Because of its similarity to CDV and tenofovir (Figure 2G), adefovir does not require activation by TK. Adefovir is primarily administered orally as a prodrug, adefovir dipivoxil (Figure 2F; [55]), with diesterified pivalic acids on its primary phosphate group [56]; this chemical alteration improves bioavailability, oral absorption, and other pharmacologic characteristics [56]. The pivalic acids adducts are removed through first-pass metabolism to create the active drug [56]. Adefovir treatment of HSV infections is not a common practice, partly because its use against any virus has been shown to cause nephrotoxicity [55,57] and partly because it can even help select for multidrug-resistant strains. Therefore, this option is best reserved for a minority of cases.

7. Non-Nucleoside/Nucleotide Inhibition of Herpes DNA Polymerase

Foscarnet (Figure 3) is a pyrophosphate analog that reversibly binds to the viral DNA polymerase and hence does not require activation by TK. Unlike other antiherpetic drugs that bind to the viral DNA polymerase, the binding of foscarnet does not result in chain termination; the drug binds at the pyrophosphate binding site, within the active site of the herpesvirus DNA polymerase, preventing nucleotides from binding to the active site and from being incorporated into the growing DNA strand [58]. Foscarnet also differs from nucleoside-based drugs because it exists in its active form and requires no further modifications to inhibit herpesviruses. Since foscarnet does not require phosphorylation by the viral TK, it can also be used to inhibit ACV-resistant herpesviruses [46]. However, foscarnet is poorly selective. Since this drug does not get activated by viral enzymes and it binds to the active site of all polymerases, it has a higher potential to bind to and inhibit host DNA polymerases. While foscarnet shows 100× greater affinity for viral DNA polymerases than it does for human DNA polymerases [59], this level of difference may not be high enough for patients who are sensitive to the drug's side effects, including acute nephrotoxicity [60,61], hypocalcemia [62], electrolyte disturbances, nausea, penile ulcerations, seizures, and metabolic disturbances [61,63]. On a cellular level, as the dosage of foscarnet increases, cell division slows by 50%; all phases of mitosis are impacted in some capacity as the G1, G2, and S phases are all greatly shortened [64]. Although foscarnet may inhibit host DNA replication, the greater inhibitory effects on viral DNA replication dictate that foscarnet can still be used therapeutically for ACV-resistant HSVs. Nonetheless, patients who have neurological or cardiovascular abnormalities while taking calcium-foscarnet must stop taking it [62]. Resistance to foscarnet typically appears in mutations at the pyrophosphate binding site of virus DNA polymerases.

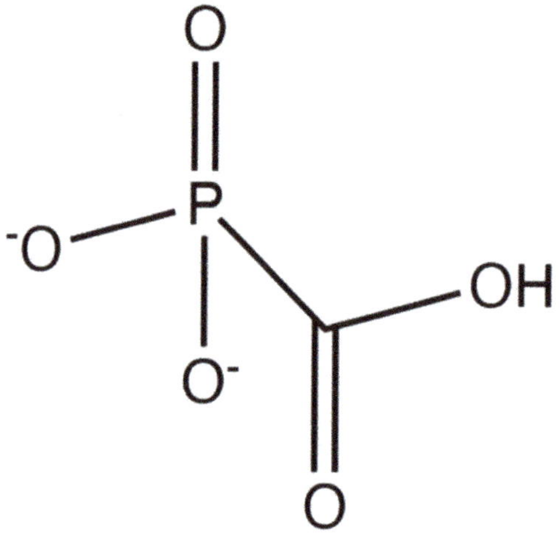

Figure 3. Foscarnet.

8. Helicase/Primase Inhibitors

All the drugs discussed above typically target viral DNA replication at the elongation step, which means that individual mutations in only one gene (e.g., the TK or the DNA polymerase) could result in resistance to multiple drugs. Therefore, targeting other viral processes, at other loci, would prevent cross-resistance from appearing by such single mutations. One of these newer classes of antiherpetics is the helicase–primase inhibitors (HPIs; Figure 4), which also do not require preliminary phosphorylation by TK.

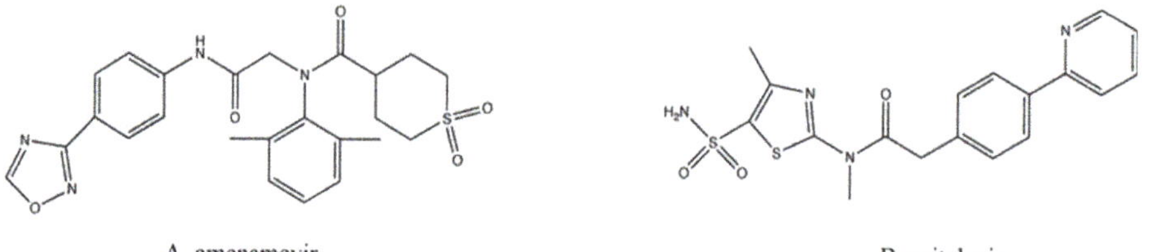

Figure 4. Helicase–primase inhibitors.

During replication of viral DNA, the helicase and primase enzymes (encoded by HSV-1 UL5 and UL52) form a complex that can separate the strands of DNA while also inserting primers [65]. Amenamevir (AMV; Figure 4A), approved for clinical use in Japan [66], and pritelivir (PTV; Figure 4B; still in clinical trials) are two of the most promising HPIs developed [67]. Both are active in their native state and require no modifications in order to inhibit the virus. Both drugs act similarly, likely by preventing the helicase–primase complex from forming by preventing the precise protein–protein interactions required between the UL5- and UL52-encoded proteins [67].

While it is not entirely understood at a molecular level exactly how the HPIs prevent the helicase–primase complex from forming, drug resistance appears through mutations to either the helicase, the primase, or both [68]. Most HPI resistance mutations already exist in the HSV population at a frequency of about 10^{-6} [69,70], and those mutants are not necessarily induced or selected by exposure to the inhibitors [68]. Nonetheless, these HPI-resistant mutants maintain wild-type levels of virulence in vivo [70].

9. Binding and Entry Inhibition

Other antiviral drugs act on the host cell to inhibit the virus [71]. The advantage to this approach is that resistance to the drug is less likely to appear, especially because these drugs are not subject to TK activation and ACV resistance mutations in that locus; while random mutations occur in both viruses and hosts, the mutation rate in viruses is much higher than it is in host cells [71–74]. On the other hand, targeting a host cell function may lead to higher toxicity, potentially limiting therapeutic use to only viral strains that are resistant to safer therapies.

n-Docosanol (Figure 5) is a long-chain, 22-carbon, primary alcohol offered over the counter. It likely inhibits a broad range of enveloped viruses that uncoat at the plasma membrane of target cells [75,76]. The drug appears to prevent binding and entry of HSVs by interfering directly with the cell surface phospholipids, which are required by the viruses for entry, and stabilizing them [76]. This activity tends to work well against ACV-resistant HSVs [75] and can even act synergistically with other anti-HSV drugs [77]. *n*-Docosanol is applied topically during prodrome to lessen the effect of a recurrent HSV outbreak; the drug even lessens the severity and duration of overt lesions. *n*-Docosanol is used only against labial, not genital, herpes outbreaks [78–80]. The parent compound itself is metabolized within cells primarily into phosphatidylethanolamine and phosphatidylcholine, typical cellular phospholipids, and it appears that these new derivatives of the drug exhibit the observed anti-HSV activity [76].

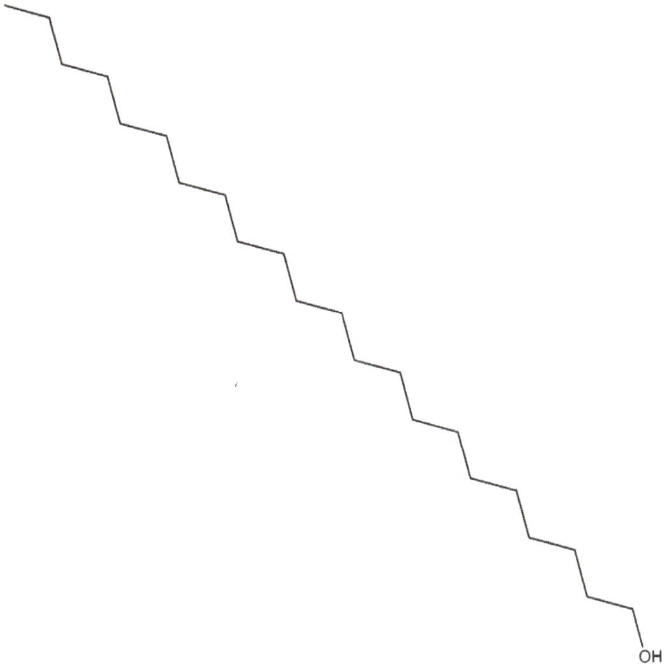

Figure 5. n-Docosanol.

10. Licensed Drugs for Other Infectious Agents Can Also Inhibit Herpesviruses

Another drug that inhibits the virus by affecting the host cell is nelfinavir (NFV) (Figure 6), which also does not require activation by TK. Nelfinavir is a protease inhibitor used for HIV treatment that has curiously also been shown to inhibit HSV [5]. In the presence of NFV, the HSV capsids do not undergo secondary envelopment and therefore never reach maturity [5]. Even so, the mechanisms for this inhibitory effect are not well understood, although there is speculation that NFV interferes with intracellular membrane sorting and trafficking [48]. Since NFV has not been used clinically against HSVs, little is known about its overall safety and efficacy for such treatment schemes.

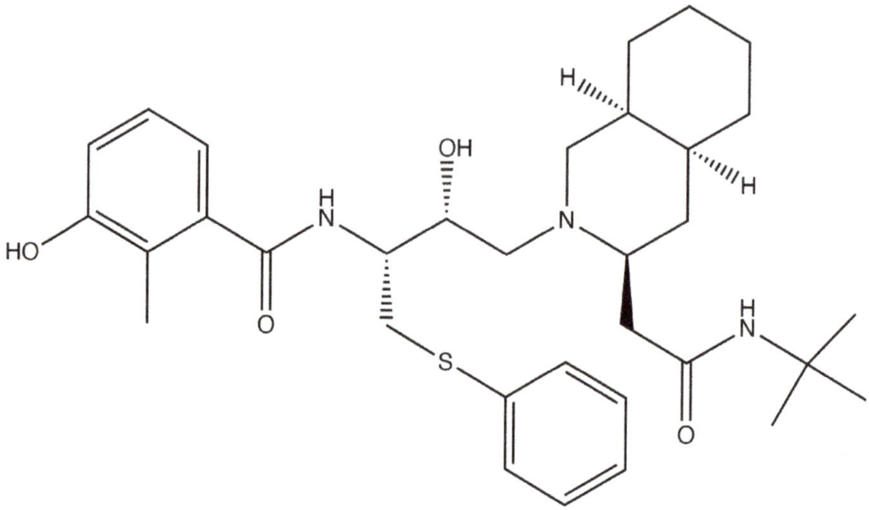

Figure 6. Nelfinavir.

Emtricitabine (Figure 1M), a nucleoside analog typically used in pre-exposure prophylaxis (PrEP) schemes against HIV-1 in conjunction with the nucleotide analog tenofovir (Figure 2G; shown as its prodrug tenofovir disoproxil in Figure 2H) [81], has also found utility against HSV-2 [82,83]. Emtricitabine appears to be phosphorylated solely by cellular kinases [84]. Studies were originally designed to assess daily oral emtricitabine plus tenofovir (FTC/TDF) as a means to protect HIV-negative partners from acquiring that virus from HIV-positive partners [85]. As a side effect, it was shown that the same nucleoside/nucleotide analog regimen used to combat HIV-1 seroconversion could also reduce the risk of acquiring HSV-2 to 2.1 incidents per 100 person-years [86]; however, one study found that emtricitabine alone did not wholly lessen the chance of contracting HSV-2 [82]. Depending on the amount and means of drug delivery among other existing variables, FTC/TDF has been found to be effective at reducing the presence and severity of genital ulcers, a common HSV symptom [82].

11. Summary

While the arsenal of pharmacologic weapons we have to treat HSV infections is substantial, there is always room for improvement. To wit, IDU and TFT were supplanted by ACV and PCV, which have been further improved with VaCV and FamCV. The discovery of HPIs has revealed new HSV loci against which we can intervene, but it is likely that even these antiherpetics will be improved over the course of time. Moreover, time and effort in basic virology and pharmacology will inevitably lead to finding new molecular targets for intervention.

Regardless, none of these treatments are prophylactic, nor are they curative; these criteria may be overcome with an effective vaccine. Each antiviral agent mentioned above does not necessarily target or prevent primary infection. They also almost always require active replication, which means they cannot be used to rid the body of latent virus. Furthermore, as long as gene expression of latent virus is limited, the array of antiviral targets will similarly be constrained; more in-depth research must continue to be explored in the future to definitively aim at these much more complex problems.

Author Contributions: Conceptualization, L.A.S., R.U., Z.W.G. and B.J.M.; Writing—Original Draft Preparation, L.A.S., R.U., Z.W.G. and B.J.M.; Writing—Review and Editing, B.J.M.; Supervision, B.J.M.; Project Administration, B.J.M. All authors have read and agreed to the published version of the manuscript.

Funding: This research received no external funding.

Conflicts of Interest: The authors declare no conflict of interest.

References

1. Kaufman, H.; Martola, E.L.; Dohlman, C. Use of 5-iodo-2′-deoxyuridine (IDU) in treatment of herpes simplex keratitis. *Arch. Ophthalmol.* **1962**, *68*, 235–239. [CrossRef]
2. Kaufman, H.E. Clinical cure of herpes simplex keratitis by 5-iodo-2-deoxyuridine. *Proc. Soc. Exp. Biol. Med.* **1962**, *109*, 251–252. [CrossRef] [PubMed]
3. Roizman, B.; Knipe, D.M.; Whitley, R.J. Herpes Simplex Viruses. In *Fields Virology*, 6th ed.; Knipe, D.M., Howley, P.M., Cohen, J.I., Griffin, D.E., Lamb, R.A., Martin, M.A., Racaniello, V.R., Roizman, B., Eds.; Wolters Kluwer/Lippincott Williams & Wilkins: Philadelphia, PA, USA, 2013; pp. 1823–1897.
4. Looker, K.J.; Garnett, G.P. A systematic review of the epidemiology and interaction of herpes simplex virus types 1 and 2. *Sex. Transm. Infect.* **2005**, *81*, 103–107. [CrossRef]
5. Kalu, N.N.; Desai, P.J.; Shirley, C.M.; Gibson, W.; Dennis, P.A.; Ambinder, R.F. Nelfinavir inhibits maturation and export of herpes simplex virus 1. *J. Virol.* **2014**, *88*, 5455–5461. [CrossRef]
6. Jia, X.; Schols, D.; Meier, C. Lipophilic Triphosphate Prodrugs of Various Nucleoside Analogues. *J. Med. Chem.* **2020**, *63*, 6991–7007. [CrossRef]
7. Berdis, A.J. DNA polymerases as therapeutic targets. *Biochemistry* **2008**, *47*, 8253–8260. [CrossRef] [PubMed]
8. Elion, G.B. Mechanism of action and selectivity of acyclovir. *Am. J. Med.* **1982**, *73*, 7–13. [CrossRef]
9. Furman, P.A.; St Clair, M.H.; Spector, T. Acyclovir triphosphate is a suicide inactivator of the herpes simplex virus DNA polymerase. *J. Biol. Chem.* **1984**, *259*, 9575–9579. [CrossRef]
10. Yajima, M.; Yamada, H.; Takemoto, M.; Daikoku, T.; Yoshida, Y.; Long, T.; Okuda, T.; Shiraki, K. Profile of anti-herpetic action of ASP2151 (amenamevir) as a helicase-primase inhibitor. *Antivir. Res.* **2017**, *139*, 95–101. [CrossRef]
11. Xiong, X.; Smith, J.L.; Chen, M.S. Effect of incorporation of cidofovir into DNA by human cytomegalovirus DNA polymerase on DNA elongation. *Antimicrob. Agents Chemother.* **1997**, *41*, 594–599. [CrossRef] [PubMed]
12. Cunha, A.C.; Ferreira, V.F.; Vaz, M.G.F.; Cassaro, R.A.A.; Resende, J.; Sacramento, C.Q.; Costa, J.; Abrantes, J.L.; Souza, T.M.L.; Jordao, A.K. Chemistry and anti-herpes simplex virus type 1 evaluation of 4-substituted-1H-1,2,3-triazole-nitroxyl-linked hybrids. *Mol. Divers.* **2020**. [CrossRef]
13. McGuirt, P.V.; Furman, P.A. Acyclovir inhibition of viral DNA chain elongation in herpes simplex virus-infected cells. *Am. J. Med.* **1982**, *73*, 67–71. [CrossRef]
14. Topalis, D.; Gillemot, S.; Snoeck, R.; Andrei, G. Distribution and effects of amino acid changes in drug-resistant alpha and beta herpesviruses DNA polymerase. *Nucleic Acids Res.* **2016**, *44*, 9530–9554. [PubMed]
15. Crumpacker, C.S.; Schnipper, L.E.; Chartrand, P.; Knopf, K.W. Genetic mechanisms of resistance to acyclovir in herpes simplex virus. *Am. J. Med.* **1982**, *73*, 361–368. [CrossRef]
16. Van Dyke, R.B.; Connor, J.D.; Wyborny, C.; Hintz, M.; Keeney, R.E. Pharmacokinetics of orally administered acyclovir in patients with herpes progenitalis. *Am. J. Med.* **1982**, *73*, 172–175. [CrossRef]
17. Gurgel Assis, M.S.; Fernandes Pedrosa, T.C.; de Moraes, F.S.; Caldeira, T.G.; Pereira, G.R.; de Souza, J.; Ruela, A.L.M. Novel Insights to Enhance Therapeutics with Acyclovir in the Management of Herpes Simplex Encephalitis. *J. Pharm. Sci.* **2021**, *110*, 1557–1571. [CrossRef] [PubMed]
18. Birkmann, A.; Zimmermann, H. HSV antivirals-current and future treatment options. *Curr. Opin. Virol.* **2016**, *18*, 9–13. [CrossRef] [PubMed]
19. Lai, L.; Xu, Z.; Zhou, J.; Lee, K.D.; Amidon, G.L. Molecular basis of prodrug activation by human valacyclovirase, an alpha-amino acid ester hydrolase. *J. Biol. Chem.* **2008**, *283*, 9318–9327. [CrossRef] [PubMed]
20. Marsillach, J.; Suzuki, S.M.; Richter, R.J.; McDonald, M.G.; Rademacher, P.M.; MacCoss, M.J.; Hsieh, E.J.; Rettie, A.E.; Furlong, C.E. Human valacyclovir hydrolase/biphenyl hydrolase-like protein is a highly efficient homocysteine thiolactonase. *PLoS ONE* **2014**, *9*, e110054. [CrossRef] [PubMed]
21. Earnshaw, D.L.; Bacon, T.H.; Darlison, S.J.; Edmonds, K.; Perkins, R.M.; Vere Hodge, R.A. Mode of antiviral action of penciclovir in MRC-5 cells infected with herpes simplex virus type 1 (HSV-1), HSV-2, and varicella-zoster virus. *Antimicrob. Agents Chemother.* **1992**, *36*, 2747–2757. [CrossRef]
22. Boyd, M.R.; Bacon, T.H.; Sutton, D. Antiherpesvirus activity of 9-(4-hydroxy-3-hydroxymethylbut-1-yl) guanine (BRL 39123) in animals. *Antimicrob. Agents Chemother.* **1988**, *32*, 358–363. [CrossRef] [PubMed]
23. Gill, K.S.; Wood, M.J. The clinical pharmacokinetics of famciclovir. *Clin. Pharm.* **1996**, *31*, 1–8. [CrossRef]

24. Vere Hodge, R.A.; Sutton, D.; Boyd, M.R.; Harnden, M.R.; Jarvest, R.L. Selection of an oral prodrug (BRL 42810; famciclovir) for the antiherpesvirus agent BRL 39123 [9-(4-hydroxy-3-hydroxymethylbut-l-yl)guanine; penciclovir]. *Antimicrob. Agents Chemother.* **1989**, *33*, 1765–1773. [CrossRef]
25. Filer, C.W.; Allen, G.D.; Brown, T.A.; Fowles, S.E.; Hollis, F.J.; Mort, E.E.; Prince, W.T.; Ramji, J.V. Metabolic and pharmacokinetic studies following oral administration of 14C-famciclovir to healthy subjects. *Xenobiotica* **1994**, *24*, 357–368. [CrossRef]
26. Clarke, S.E.; Harrell, A.W.; Chenery, R.J. Role of aldehyde oxidase in the in vitro conversion of famciclovir to penciclovir in human liver. *Drug Metab. Dispos.* **1995**, *23*, 251–254.
27. Agrahari, V.; Mandal, A.; Agrahari, V.; Trinh, H.M.; Joseph, M.; Ray, A.; Hadji, H.; Mitra, R.; Pal, D.; Mitra, A.K. A comprehensive insight on ocular pharmacokinetics. *Drug Deliv. Transl. Res.* **2016**, *6*, 735–754. [CrossRef]
28. Silvestri, D.L.; Corey, L.; Holmes, K.K. Ineffectiveness of topical idoxuridine in dimethyl sulfoxide for therapy for genital herpes. *JAMA* **1982**, *248*, 953–959. [CrossRef] [PubMed]
29. Yamashita, F.; Komoto, I.; Oka, H.; Kuwata, K.; Takeuchi, M.; Nakagawa, F.; Yoshisue, K.; Chiba, M. Exposure-dependent incorporation of trifluridine into DNA of tumors and white blood cells in tumor-bearing mouse. *Cancer Chemother. Pharm.* **2015**, *76*, 325–333. [CrossRef]
30. Sharma, S.; Mehndiratta, S.; Kumar, S.; Singh, J.; Bedi, P.M.; Nepali, K. Purine Analogues as Kinase Inhibitors: A Review. *Recent Pat. Anticancer Drug Discov.* **2015**, *10*, 308–341. [CrossRef] [PubMed]
31. Whitley, R.J.; Tucker, B.C.; Kinkel, A.W.; Barton, N.H.; Pass, R.F.; Whelchel, J.D.; Cobbs, C.G.; Diethelm, A.G.; Buchanan, R.A. Pharmacology, tolerance, and antiviral activity of vidarabine monophosphate in humans. *Antimicrob. Agents Chemother.* **1980**, *18*, 709–715. [CrossRef]
32. Aebersold, P.M. Relative mutagenicity of nucleoside virostatic drugs in Chinese hamster ovary cells. *Adv. Ophthalmol.* **1979**, *38*, 214–221.
33. Seley-Radtke, K.L.; Yates, M.K. The evolution of nucleoside analogue antivirals: A review for chemists and non-chemists. Part 1: Early structural modifications to the nucleoside scaffold. *Antivir. Res.* **2018**, *154*, 66–86. [CrossRef] [PubMed]
34. Kaufman, H.E. Antimetabolite drug therapy in herpes simplex. *Ophthalmology* **1980**, *87*, 135–139. [CrossRef]
35. De Clercq, E. Discovery and development of BVDU (brivudin) as a therapeutic for the treatment of herpes zoster. *Biochem. Pharmacol.* **2004**, *68*, 2301–2315. [CrossRef]
36. Wassilew, S.W.; Wutzler, P.; Brivddin Herpes Zoster Study Group. Oral brivudin in comparison with acyclovir for herpes zoster: A survey study on postherpetic neuralgia. *Antivir. Res.* **2003**, *59*, 57–60. [CrossRef]
37. Andrei, G.; Balzarini, J.; Fiten, P.; De Clercq, E.; Opdenakker, G.; Snoeck, R. Characterization of herpes simplex virus type 1 thymidine kinase mutants selected under a single round of high-dose brivudin. *J. Virol.* **2005**, *79*, 5863–5869. [CrossRef] [PubMed]
38. Noble, S.; Faulds, D. Ganciclovir. An update of its use in the prevention of cytomegalovirus infection and disease in transplant recipients. *Drugs* **1998**, *56*, 115–146. [CrossRef]
39. Gilbert, C.; Bestman-Smith, J.; Boivin, G. Resistance of herpesviruses to antiviral drugs: Clinical impacts and molecular mechanisms. *Drug Resist. Updates* **2002**, *5*, 88–114. [CrossRef]
40. Cheng, Y.C.; Grill, S.P.; Dutschman, G.E.; Nakayama, K.; Bastow, K.F. Metabolism of 9-(1,3-dihydroxy-2-propoxymethyl)guanine, a new anti-herpes virus compound, in herpes simplex virus-infected cells. *J. Biol. Chem.* **1983**, *258*, 12460–12464. [CrossRef]
41. Cheng, Y.C.; Huang, E.S.; Lin, J.C.; Mar, E.C.; Pagano, J.S.; Dutschman, G.E.; Grill, S.P. Unique spectrum of activity of 9-[(1,3-dihydroxy-2-propoxy)methyl]-guanine against herpesviruses in vitro and its mode of action against herpes simplex virus type 1. *Proc. Natl. Acad. Sci. USA* **1983**, *80*, 2767–2770. [CrossRef]
42. Jung, D.; Dorr, A. Single-dose pharmacokinetics of valganciclovir in HIV- and CMV-seropositive subjects. *J. Clin. Pharmacol.* **1999**, *39*, 800–804. [CrossRef]
43. Brown, F.; Banken, L.; Saywell, K.; Arum, I. Pharmacokinetics of valganciclovir and ganciclovir following multiple oral dosages of valganciclovir in HIV-and CMV-seropositive volunteers. *Clin. Pharm.* **1999**, *37*, 167–176. [CrossRef]
44. Morfin, F.; Thouvenot, D. Herpes simplex virus resistance to antiviral drugs. *J. Clin. Virol.* **2003**, *26*, 29–37. [CrossRef]
45. Bronson, J.J.; Ho, H.T.; De Boeck, H.; Woods, K.; Ghazzouli, I.; Martin, J.C.; Hitchcock, M.J. Biochemical pharmacology of acyclic nucleotide analogues. *Ann. N. Y. Acad Sci.* **1990**, *616*, 398–407. [CrossRef]
46. Andrei, G.; Snoeck, R.; De Clercq, E.; Esnouf, R.; Fiten, P.; Opdenakker, G. Resistance of herpes simplex virus type 1 against different phosphonylmethoxyalkyl derivatives of purines and pyrimidines due to specific mutations in the viral DNA polymerase gene. *J. Gen. Virol.* **2000**, *81*, 639–648. [CrossRef] [PubMed]
47. Razonable, R.R. Drug-resistant cytomegalovirus: Clinical implications of specific mutations. *Curr. Opin. Organ. Transpl.* **2018**, *23*, 388–394. [CrossRef]
48. Meier, P.; Dautheville-Guibal, S.; Ronco, P.M.; Rossert, J. Cidofovir-induced end-stage renal failure. *Nephrol. Dial. Transpl.* **2002**, *17*, 148–149. [CrossRef] [PubMed]
49. Ahmed, A. Antiviral treatment of cytomegalovirus infection. *Infect. Disord. Drug Targets* **2011**, *11*, 475–503. [CrossRef]
50. Marty, F.M.; Winston, D.J.; Chemaly, R.F.; Mullane, K.M.; Shore, T.B.; Papanicolaou, G.A.; Chittick, G.; Brundage, T.M.; Wilson, C.; Morrison, M.E.; et al. A Randomized, Double-Blind, Placebo-Controlled Phase 3 Trial of Oral Brincidofovir for Cytomegalovirus Prophylaxis in Allogeneic Hematopoietic Cell Transplantation. *Biol. Blood Marrow Transpl.* **2019**, *25*, 369–381. [CrossRef]
51. Griffiths, P.; Lumley, S. Cytomegalovirus. *Curr. Opin. Infect. Dis.* **2014**, *27*, 554–559. [CrossRef] [PubMed]

52. Balzarini, J.; Naesens, L.; De Clercq, E. New antivirals-mechanism of action and resistance development. *Curr. Opin. Microbiol.* **1998**, *1*, 535–546. [CrossRef]
53. Aduma, P.; Connelly, M.C.; Srinivas, R.V.; Fridland, A. Metabolic diversity and antiviral activities of acyclic nucleoside phosphonates. *Mol. Pharmacol.* **1995**, *47*, 816–822.
54. Foster, S.A.; Cerny, J.; Cheng, Y.C. Herpes simplex virus-specified DNA polymerase is the target for the antiviral action of 9-(2-phosphonylmethoxyethyl)adenine. *J. Biol. Chem.* **1991**, *266*, 238–244. [CrossRef]
55. Huang, C.; Yang, X.H.; Yang, Y.L.; Huang, A.L.; Shi, X.F. Clinical-features analysis on 926 patients with virological breakthrough in chronic hepatitis B receiving nucleos(t)ide analogues. *Eur. J. Intern. Med.* **2018**, *53*, e9–e10. [CrossRef] [PubMed]
56. Cundy, K.C.; Barditch-Crovo, P.; Walker, R.E.; Collier, A.C.; Ebeling, D.; Toole, J.; Jaffe, H.S. Clinical pharmacokinetics of adefovir in human immunodeficiency virus type 1-infected patients. *Antimicrob. Agents Chemother.* **1995**, *39*, 2401–2405. [CrossRef]
57. Law, S.T.; Li, K.K.; Ho, Y.Y. Acquired Fanconi syndrome associated with prolonged adefovir dipivoxil therapy in a chronic hepatitis B patient. *Am. J. Ther.* **2013**, *20*, e713–e716. [CrossRef] [PubMed]
58. Vashishtha, A.K.; Kuchta, R.D. Effects of Acyclovir, Foscarnet, and Ribonucleotides on Herpes Simplex Virus-1 DNA Polymerase: Mechanistic Insights and a Novel Mechanism for Preventing Stable Incorporation of Ribonucleotides into DNA. *Biochemistry* **2016**, *55*, 1168–1177. [CrossRef]
59. Crumpacker, C.S. Mechanism of action of foscarnet against viral polymerases. *Am. J. Med.* **1992**, *92*, S3–S7. [CrossRef]
60. Leowattana, W. Antiviral Drugs and Acute Kidney Injury (AKI). *Infect. Disord. Drug Targets* **2019**, *19*, 375–382. [CrossRef]
61. Mareri, A.; Lasorella, S.; Iapadre, G.; Maresca, M.; Tambucci, R.; Nigro, G. Anti-viral therapy for congenital cytomegalovirus infection: Pharmacokinetics, efficacy and side effects. *J. Matern. Fetal Neonatal Med.* **2016**, *29*, 1657–1664. [CrossRef] [PubMed]
62. Jacobson, M.A.; Gambertoglio, J.G.; Aweeka, F.T.; Causey, D.M.; Portale, A.A. Foscarnet-induced hypocalcemia and effects of foscarnet on calcium metabolism. *J. Clin. Endocrinol. Metab.* **1991**, *72*, 1130–1135. [CrossRef]
63. Jayaweera, D.T. Minimising the dosage-limiting toxicities of foscarnet induction therapy. *Drug Saf.* **1997**, *16*, 258–266. [CrossRef]
64. Stenberg, K.; Skog, S.; Tribukait, B. Concentration-dependent effects of foscarnet on the cell cycle. *Antimicrob. Agents Chemother.* **1985**, *28*, 802–806. [CrossRef]
65. Matthews, J.T.; Terry, B.J.; Field, A.K. The structure and function of the HSV DNA replication proteins: Defining novel antiviral targets. *Antivir. Res.* **1993**, *20*, 89–114. [CrossRef]
66. Shoji, N.; Tanese, K.; Sasaki, A.; Horiuchi, T.; Utsuno, Y.; Fukuda, K.; Hoshino, Y.; Noda, S.; Minami, H.; Asakura, W.; et al. Pharmaceuticals and Medical Device Agency approval summary: Amenamevir for the treatment of herpes zoster. *J. Dermatol.* **2020**, *47*, 683–688. [CrossRef]
67. Shiraki, K. Antiviral Drugs Against Alphaherpesvirus. *Adv. Exp. Med. Biol.* **2018**, *1045*, 103–122.
68. Field, H.J.; Biswas, S. Antiviral drug resistance and helicase-primase inhibitors of herpes simplex virus. *Drug Resist. Updates* **2011**, *14*, 45–51. [CrossRef]
69. Biswas, S.; Jennens, L.; Field, H.J. Single amino acid substitutions in the HSV-1 helicase protein that confer resistance to the helicase-primase inhibitor BAY 57-1293 are associated with increased or decreased virus growth characteristics in tissue culture. *Arch. Virol.* **2007**, *152*, 1489–1500. [CrossRef] [PubMed]
70. Liuzzi, M.; Kibler, P.; Bousquet, C.; Harji, F.; Bolger, G.; Garneau, M.; Lapeyre, N.; McCollum, R.S.; Faucher, A.M.; Simoneau, B.; et al. Isolation and characterization of herpes simplex virus type 1 resistant to aminothiazolylphenyl-based inhibitors of the viral helicase-primase. *Antivir. Res.* **2004**, *64*, 161–170. [CrossRef] [PubMed]
71. Lin, K.; Gallay, P. Curing a viral infection by targeting the host: The example of cyclophilin inhibitors. *Antivir. Res.* **2013**, *99*, 68–77. [CrossRef] [PubMed]
72. Drake, J.W.; Hwang, C.B. On the mutation rate of herpes simplex virus type 1. *Genetics* **2005**, *170*, 969–970. [CrossRef] [PubMed]
73. Renner, D.W.; Szpara, M.L. Impacts of Genome-Wide Analyses on Our Understanding of Human Herpesvirus Diversity and Evolution. *J. Virol.* **2018**, *92*, e00908-17. [CrossRef]
74. Sanjuán, R.; Nebot, M.R.; Chirico, N.; Mansky, L.M.; Belshaw, R. Viral mutation rates. *J. Virol.* **2010**, *84*, 9733–9748. [CrossRef]
75. Katz, D.H.; Marcelletti, J.F.; Khalil, M.H.; Pope, L.E.; Katz, L.R. Antiviral activity of 1-docosanol, an inhibitor of lipid-enveloped viruses including herpes simplex. *Proc. Natl. Acad. Sci. USA* **1991**, *88*, 10825–10829. [CrossRef]
76. Pope, L.E.; Marcelletti, J.F.; Katz, L.R.; Lin, J.Y.; Katz, D.H.; Parish, M.L.; Spear, P.G. The anti-herpes simplex virus activity of n-docosanol includes inhibition of the viral entry process. *Antivir. Res.* **1998**, *40*, 85–94. [CrossRef]
77. Marcelletti, J.F. Synergistic inhibition of herpesvirus replication by docosanol and antiviral nucleoside analogs. *Antivir. Res.* **2002**, *56*, 153–166. [CrossRef]
78. Woo, S.B.; Challacombe, S.J. Management of recurrent oral herpes simplex infections. *Oral Surg. Oral Med. Oral Pathol. Oral Radiol. Endodontol.* **2007**, *103* (Suppl. S12), e1–e18. [CrossRef] [PubMed]
79. Usatine, R.P.; Tinitigan, R. Nongenital herpes simplex virus. *Am. Fam. Phys.* **2010**, *82*, 1075–1082.
80. Leung, D.T.; Sacks, S.L. Docosanol: A topical antiviral for herpes labialis. *Expert Opin. Pharm.* **2004**, *5*, 2567–2571. [CrossRef]
81. Deeks, E.D. Bictegravir/Emtricitabine/Tenofovir Alafenamide: A Review in HIV-1 Infection. *Drugs* **2018**, *78*, 1817–1828. [CrossRef]
82. Marcus, J.L.; Glidden, D.V.; McMahan, V.; Lama, J.R.; Mayer, K.H.; Liu, A.Y.; Montoya-Herrera, O.; Casapia, M.; Hoagland, B.; Grant, R.M. Daily oral emtricitabine/tenofovir preexposure prophylaxis and herpes simplex virus type 2 among men who have sex with men. *PLoS ONE* **2014**, *9*, e91513. [CrossRef]

83. Celum, C.; Morrow, R.A.; Donnell, D.; Hong, T.; Hendrix, C.W.; Thomas, K.K.; Fife, K.H.; Nakku-Joloba, E.; Mujugira, A.; Baeten, J.M. Daily oral tenofovir and emtricitabine-tenofovir preexposure prophylaxis reduces herpes simplex virus type 2 acquisition among heterosexual HIV-1-uninfected men and women: A subgroup analysis of a randomized trial. *Ann. Intern. Med.* **2014**, *161*, 11–19. [CrossRef] [PubMed]
84. Figueroa, D.B.; Madeen, E.P.; Tillotson, J.; Richardson, P.; Cottle, L.; McCauley, M.; Landovitz, R.J.; Andrade, A.; Hendrix, C.W.; Mayer, K.H.; et al. Genetic Variation of the Kinases That Phosphorylate Tenofovir and Emtricitabine in Peripheral Blood Mononuclear Cells. *AIDS Res. Hum. Retrovir.* **2018**, *34*, 421–429. [CrossRef] [PubMed]
85. Baeten, J.M.; Donnell, D.; Mugo, N.R.; Ndase, P.; Thomas, K.K.; Campbell, J.D.; Wangisi, J.; Tappero, J.W.; Bukusi, E.A.; Cohen, C.R.; et al. Single-agent tenofovir versus combination emtricitabine plus tenofovir for pre-exposure prophylaxis for HIV-1 acquisition: An update of data from a randomised, double-blind, phase 3 trial. *Lancet Infect. Dis.* **2014**, *14*, 1055–1064. [CrossRef]
86. Chaix, M.L.; Charreau, I.; Pintado, C.; Delaugerre, C.; Mahjoub, N.; Cotte, L.; Capitant, C.; Raffi, F.; Cua, E.; Pialoux, G.; et al. Effect of On-Demand Oral Pre-exposure Prophylaxis With Tenofovir/Emtricitabine on Herpes Simplex Virus-1/2 Incidence Among Men Who Have Sex With Men: A Substudy of the ANRS IPERGAY Trial. *Open Forum Infect. Dis.* **2018**, *5*, ofy295. [CrossRef] [PubMed]

viruses

Review

Amenamevir, a Helicase-Primase Inhibitor, for the Optimal Treatment of Herpes Zoster

Kimiyasu Shiraki [1,*], Shinichiro Yasumoto [2], Nozomu Toyama [3] and Hiroaki Fukuda [4]

1 Faculty of Nursing, Senri Kinran University, 5-25-1 Fujishirodai, Suita, Osaka 565-0873, Japan
2 Yasumoto Dermatology Clinic, Tsukushino, Fukuoka 818-0083, Japan; shinyhc55103@extra.ocn.ne.jp
3 Toyama Dermatologic Clinic, Aburatsu, Nichinan City, Miyazaki 887-0001, Japan; nontoyama@miyazaki.med.or.jp
4 Maruho Co., Ltd., Nakatsu, Osaka 531-0071, Japan; fukuda_cis@mii.maruho.co.jp
* Correspondence: k-shiraki@cs.kinran.ac.jp; Tel.: +81-6-6872-7139

Abstract: Acyclovir, valacyclovir, and famciclovir are used for the treatment of herpes simplex virus (HSV) and varicella-zoster virus (VZV) infections. Helicase-primase inhibitors (HPIs) inhibit replication fork progression that separates double DNA strands into two single strands during DNA synthesis. The HPIs amenamevir and pritelivir have novel mechanisms of anti-herpetic action, and their once-daily administration has clinical efficacy for genital herpes. Among HPIs, amenamevir has anti-VZV activity. The concentrations of HSV-1 and VZV required for the 50% plaque reduction of amenamevir were 0.036 and 0.047 μM, respectively. We characterized the features of amenamevir regarding its mechanism, resistance, and synergism with acyclovir. Its antiviral activity was not influenced by the viral replication cycle, in contrast to acyclovir. A clinical trial of amenamevir for herpes zoster demonstrated its non-inferiority to valacyclovir. To date, amenamevir has been successfully used in over 1,240,000 patients with herpes zoster in Japan. Post-marketing surveillance of amenamevir in Japan reported side effects with significant potential risk identified by the Japanese Risk Management Plan, including thrombocytopenia, gingival bleeding, and palpitations, although none of these were serious. The clinical efficacy and safety profiles of amenamevir were established in patients with herpes zoster. Therefore, amenamevir as an HPI opens a new era of anti-herpes therapy.

Keywords: amenamevir; helicase-primase inhibitor; herpes simplex virus; varicella-zoster virus; herpes zoster; antivirals

Citation: Shiraki, K.; Yasumoto, S.; Toyama, N.; Fukuda, H. Amenamevir, a Helicase-Primase Inhibitor, for the Optimal Treatment of Herpes Zoster. *Viruses* **2021**, *13*, 1547. https://doi.org/10.3390/v13081547

Academic Editor: Barry J. Margulies

Received: 30 June 2021
Accepted: 3 August 2021
Published: 5 August 2021

1. Introduction

Varicella-zoster virus (VZV) infection, which causes varicella and herpes zoster, is treated with antivirals. Elion developed acyclovir for systemic administration to treat herpes simplex virus (HSV) and VZV infections [1–3]. Penciclovir, valacyclovir, and famciclovir are currently used for preventing and treating HSV and VZV infections [4].

The antiherpetic drugs valacyclovir (acyclovir) and famciclovir (penciclovir) have been developed for the treatment and prevention of apparent HSV and VZV infections. New antiherpetic drugs with different mechanisms of action have been developed as novel helicase-primase (HP) inhibitors (HPIs) of HSV and VZV. Double-stranded DNA is separated into two single strands (replication fork) before DNA synthesis, and complementary strands are synthesized from each DNA strand to produce two new double-stranded DNA molecules during DNA replication, as shown in Figure 1. The HP complex unwinds viral DNA at the replication fork, separating double-stranded DNA into two single strands, and synthesizing RNA primers followed by Okazaki fragments in the lagging strand for DNA synthesis. Then, DNA polymerase initiates complementary DNA synthesis in the two separated DNA strands. The HP complex consists of three proteins: HSV UL5/VZVORF55 (helicase), HSV UL52/VZVORF6 (primase), and HSV UL8/VZVORF52 (cofactor).

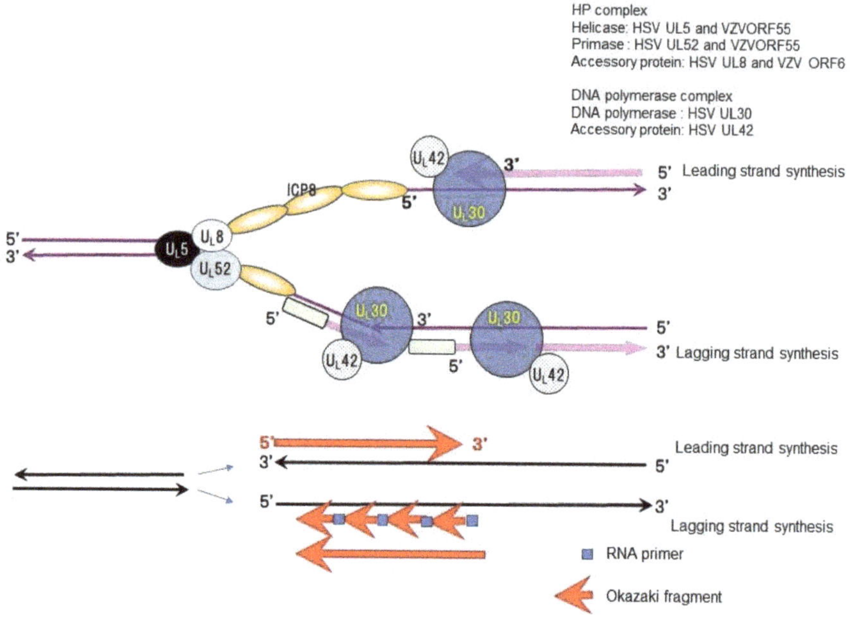

Figure 1. The viral helicase primase (HP) complex in viral DNA synthesis (modified from [5]). The figure shows the role of the HP complex (UL5, UL8, and UL52 of HSV and ORF55, ORF6, and ORF52 of VZV), the DNA polymerase complex (UL42 and UL30 of HSV and ORF28 of VZV: DNA polymerase), and the ICP8 single-stranded DNA binding protein of HSV (ORF29 of VZV). HSV UL5 and VZVORF55 (helicase) relax double-stranded DNA and separate double strands into two single strands, forming a replication fork. HSV UL52 and VZVORF55 (primase) synthesize RNA primers (followed by Okazaki fragments) for lagging strand DNA synthesis. DNA polymerase contains intrinsic ribonuclease H (RNase H) activity that specifically degrades RNA/DNA heteroduplexes formed from RNA primer-Okazaki fragments and the template DNA complex. DNA polymerase and its accessory protein (UL42) bind to each single strand and synthesize complementary DNA to each strand of the replication fork. The single-stranded DNA binding protein with helix destabilizing activity, ICP8 (UL29 of HSV and VZV), binds to a single-stranded template DNA with helix destabilizing activity. The arrows indicate the direction of movement of the DNA replication proteins.

A 2-amino thiazole compound, T157602, was reported as an HSV-2 HPI [6] and thereafter two HPIs, BILS 22 BS and Bay 57-1293 (pritelivir), were shown to have anti-HSV activity in vitro and therapeutic activity in murine HSV models [7–9]. Next, three classes of herpesvirus HPIs were developed: thiazole urea (pritelivir [9]), 2-amino-thiazolylphenyl derivatives (BILS 179 BS [8]), and oxadiazolylphenyl type (ASP2151, amenamevir) [10]. Amenamevir has anti-HSV and anti-VZV activity, while, in contrast, pritelivir and BILS 22 BS have anti-HSV activity but lack anti-VZV activity. Clinical studies of HPIs on genital herpes using amenamevir and pritelivir have been conducted [11–13].

We characterized the profile of the anti-HSV and anti-VZV activities of amenamevir [14–18]. The antiviral activity of amenamevir was not influenced by viral DNA synthesis, although that of acyclovir was attenuated [17,18]. Amenamevir was licensed for the treatment of herpes zoster on the basis of a clinical trial on herpes zoster treatment in September 2017 [19]. In this review, we focus on the anti-HSV and anti-VZV activities of amenamevir and discuss the differences in its antiviral activity compared with acyclovir.

2. Role of HP in DNA Synthesis

Double-stranded DNA needs to be separated into two single strands (replication fork) for DNA synthesis, and these two separated complementary strands proceed to form two new double-stranded DNA molecules during DNA replication (Figure 1). HP is an essential enzyme complex for DNA synthesis conserved from *Escherichia coli* to *Homo sapiens*. HSV, VZV, and host cells produce specific HP as an essential and indispensable gene product related to their DNA replication.

The HP complex possesses multiple enzymatic activity, including DNA-dependent ATPase, helicase, and primase activities, all of which are required for the functions of HP in viral DNA replication. The helicase relaxes the duplex DNA ahead of the replication fork and separates the double strand into two single strands. The primase sets RNA primers for DNA synthesis on the single-stranded DNA and the DNA polymerase extends the DNA (Okazaki fragment) as a new complementary DNA following the RNA primer in the lagging strand. Okazaki fragments are ligated and DNA synthesis in the lagging strand is completed.

The HP enzyme complex of herpesviruses consists of three proteins—UL5 (helicase, VZVORF55), UL52 (primase, VZVORF6), and UL8 (cofactor, VZVORF52)—which are well conserved among the Herpesviridae. Helicase unwinds duplex DNA ahead of the fork and separates the double strand into two single strands. Primase lays down RNA primers that the DNA polymerase complex (UL30/UL42) extends. The HP complex possesses multi-enzymatic activities mediated by DNA-dependent ATPase, helicase, and primase.

3. HP Inhibitors of HSV

HPIs bind to the helicase-primase complex and inhibit single-stranded, DNA- dependent ATPase, helicase, and primase activities [10,14,20,21]. T157602 was first reported as an HPI of the HSV UL5-UL8-UL52 complex with the use of a high-throughput biochemical DNA helicase assay [6]. T157602 inhibited helicase activity, primase activity, and the replication of HSV types 1 and 2 without cytotoxicity. Seven independently isolated T157602-resistant mutant viruses (four HSV type 2 and three HSV type 1) carried a single base pair mutation in UL5 that resulted in a single amino acid change in the UL5 protein. When the mutated UL5 gene from T157602-resistant HSV was transferred to a sensitive HSV, it acquired T157602 resistance.

Three HPIs, pritelivir, BILS 179 BS, and amenamevir, have anti-HSV activity, whereas amenamevir alone has anti-VZV activity [8–10,22]. Amenamevir was more effective than valacyclovir for treating HSV skin lesions in HSV mutant-infected mice, and HPI-resistant HSV mutants were susceptible to acyclovir with attenuated growth in vitro and reduced pathogenicity compared with the parent virus [14]. Mutations in the helicase or primase of the HP complex against amenamevir impaired viral replication and pathogenicity. Amenamevir showed better efficacy than valacyclovir at treating HSV zosteriform skin lesions in immunocompromised mice [23].

4. Comparison of Anti-Herpes Virus Activity in Three HPIs

Figure 2 shows the structures of four HPIs. These HPIs are virus-specific with low cytotoxicity in vitro. Pritelivir and amenamevir are orally available, effective against HSV infection, and are well tolerated in mice and humans. The target molecules of HPIs are different from acyclovir, penciclovir, foscarnet, and vidarabine; therefore, their mechanism of action and antiviral and pharmacokinetic profiles are unique to HPIs. HPIs have a lower EC_{50} for HSV compared with acyclovir. Furthermore, the anti-VZV activity of amenamevir is markedly different from the other anti-herpetic HPIs. The EC_{50} of HPIs for HSV-1 and HSV-2 were low (0.014–0.060 μM and 0.023–0.046 μM, respectively) and amenamevir (0.038–0.10 μM) was more potent against all VZV strains tested compared with acyclovir (1.3–5.9 μM) [10]. Only amenamevir has anti-VZV activity with a similar IC_{50} value to HSV; however, pritelivir and BILS 22 BS had 100–200 times higher IC_{50} values than amenamevir. Amenamevir has a unique antiviral spectrum for HSV and VZV. Furthermore, it had efficacy against HSV-1, HSV-2, and acyclovir-resistant/TK-deficient virus infection and exhibited synergistic activity against HSV-1 and HSV-2 with acyclovir and valacyclovir in vitro and in vivo, respectively [3,16,24].

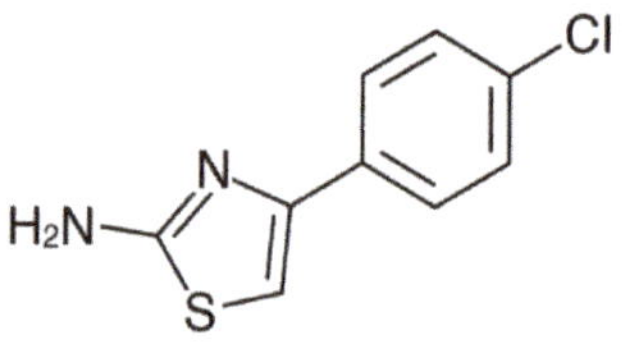

2-amino thiazole compound (T157602)

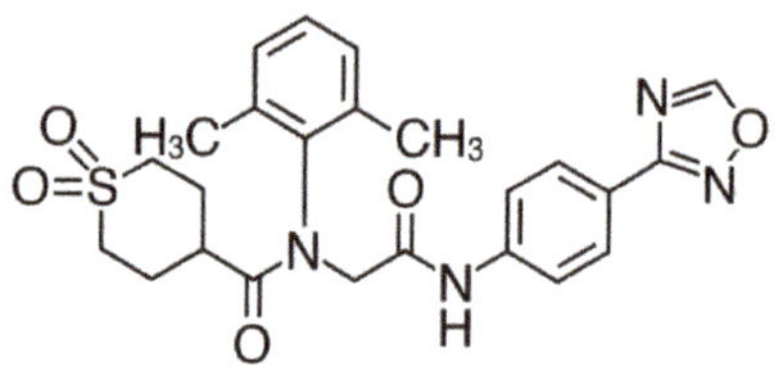

amenamevir (ASP2151)

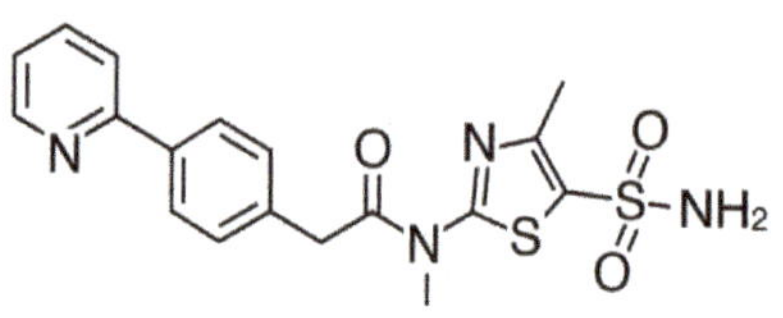

pritelivir (AIC316, Bay 57-1293)

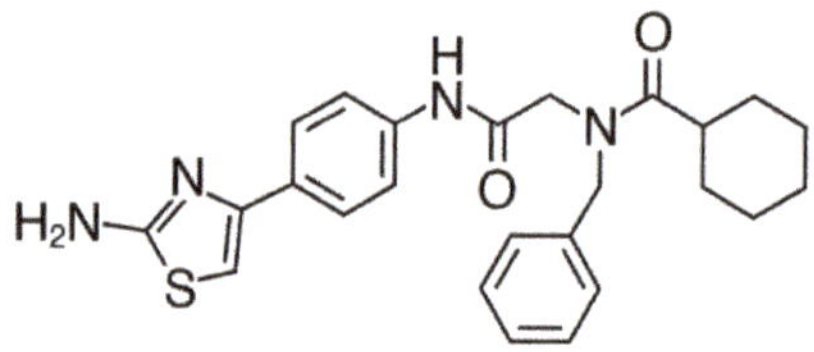

BILS 22 BS

Figure 2. Structures of helicase-primase inhibitors.

Amenamevir had a better antiviral activity profile during the DNA synthesis phase compared with acyclovir when used as an anti-HSV and anti-VZV drug, and compared with acyclovir, the anti-VZV and anti-HSV activities of amenamevir were not affected by viral DNA synthesis in the infected cells [17,18]. Acyclovir is effective against infected cells after infection and before viral DNA synthesis, but it is not effective against infected cells with abundant viral DNA synthesis. Conversely, amenamevir is equally effective against infected cells immediately after infection or in the late phase of infection, when viral DNA synthesis is abundant. This suggests that amenamevir would have high efficacy in treating severe VZV and HSV infections with a high viral load.

5. Amenamevir Resistance

Amenamevir-resistant viruses have been isolated, and sequencing analyses revealed several single-base-pair substitutions resulting in amino acid changes in the helicase and primase of amenamevir-resistant HSV mutants [10]. Amino acid alterations in the helicase subunit were clustered near helicase motif IV in the UL5 helicase gene of HSV-1 and HSV-2, whereas the primase subunit substitution was found only in amenamevir-resistant HSV-1 mutants. The combined mutation of R367H and S364G in the UL52 primase gene affords greater resistance to amenamevir than the S364G mutation alone. The accumulation of mutations increases the resistance to amenamevir, as shown in Table 1. Amenamevir-resistant HSV mutants had reduced growth capability in vitro and pathogenicity compared with the parent virus in HSV-infected mice [14].

Because the HP is essential for virus growth, an HP-deficient virus cannot replicate, in contrast to a TK-deficient virus. Any mutation in the thymidine kinase gene resulting in TK deficiency or reduced activity becomes an acyclovir-resistant mutant. Amenamevir-resistant viruses can replicate in the presence of amenamevir by avoiding interactions with HP. Acyclovir-resistant mutants of HSV and VZV with TK deficiency are similarly as susceptible as wild-type strains to amenamevir (Table 2) [16]. Thus, acyclovir-resistant HSV and VZV are susceptible to amenamevir, and this is consistent with the fact that the targets of acyclovir and amenamevir are thymidine kinase and helicase-primase, respectively, with no cross resistance. Accordingly, amenamevir-resistant HSV was as susceptible to acyclovir and penciclovir as the wild-type strain.

Table 1. Amino acid substitutions in the helicase and primase of ASP2151-resistant HSV-1 and HSV-2 mutants, and susceptibility to ASP2151 [14].

Virus	Strains/ Mutants [a]	Helicase Gene (UL5)	Primase Gene (UL52)	EC_{50} (μmol/L) [b]	Fold Increase
HSV-1	KOS	- [c]	-	0.037	-
	K2151^{r}m	G352V, M355I	S364G, R367X [d]	131.8	3562
	K2151^{r}m#B9	G352V, M355I	S364G, R367H	105.4	2849
	K2151^{r}m#D9	G352V, M355I	S364G	19.6	530
	K2151^{r}m#G11	G352V, M355I	S364G	28.2	762
	K2151^{r}m#H10	G352V, M355I	S364G, R367H	118.0	3189
HSV-2	Lyon	-	-	0.12	-
	L2151^{r}m#C1	K355N, K451R	-	>150	>1250

[a] K2151rm#B9, K2151rm#D9, K2151rm#G11, and K2151rm#H10 were derived from K2151rm and L2151rm8#C1 was derived from L2151rm by single plaque isolation. [b] The 50% effective concentration (EC50) was calculated via nonlinear regression analysis using a sigmoid-Emax model from one (HSV-2) or three (HSV-1) independent experiments performed in triplicate. [c] Identical to the parental sequence, or no substitutions were observed. [d] 'X' indicates Arg (R) or His (H) due to the detection of a mixed-base signal at the 367th Arg codon. The authors obtained permission from *Biochemical Pharmacology* to reuse this table [14].

Table 2. EC_{50} values of ASP2151 and ACV against ACV-resistant or ACV-susceptible HSV-1, HSV-2, and VZV strains (plaque reduction assay) [15].

Virus	Strains	EC50 (95% Confidence Interval) (μM) [a]		Susceptibility (Amenamevir/ Acyclovir) [d]
		Amenamevir (ASP2151)	Acyclovir	
HSV-1	KOS	0.010 (0.0082–0.012)	0.400 (0.32–0.50)	+/+
	A4-3	0.067 (0.049–0.091)	1.15 (98.8–133)	+/−
HSV-2	Genital isolate	0.012 (0.006–0.023)	1.34 (0.51–3.56)	+/+
	Whitlow 2	0.012 (0.006–0.022)	65.9 (31.9–136)	+/−
VZV	Kawaguchi [b]	0.064 (0.043–0.094)	1.61 (0.99–2.63)	+/+
	TK-deficient mutant	0.068 (0.052–0.088)	12.8 (9.5–17.3)	+/−
	A2 [c]	0.11 (0.078–0.16)	11.5 (6.5–20.3)	+/−
	A3 [c]	0.11 (0.049–0.26)	19.2 (11.1–33.1)	+/−
	A7 [c]	0.065 (0.045–0.093)	41.4 (21.6–79.2)	+/−
	A8 [c]	0.10 (0.062–0.162)	82.2 (72.7–92.9)	+/−

[a] Means of four independent experiments. [b] Parental strain of TK-deficient mutants, A2, A3, A7, and A8. [c] DNA polymerase mutant. [d] Susceptibility of virus strains to each compound: +, susceptible; -, resistant. The authors obtained permission from *Antiviral Research* to reuse this table [15].

The mean frequencies of amenamevir- and acyclovir-resistant HSV variants were 1.19×10^{-6} and 1.65×10^{-3}, respectively, from four or two strains of wild HSV-1 and HSV-1 virus stocks, respectively, and the frequency of pre-existing amenamevir-resistant HSV variants was 1389 times lower than that of acyclovir-resistant variants [14]. The frequency of acyclovir-resistant mutants in the virus stock was approximately 1 in 1000 plaque forming units. Amenamevir-mutants should preserve the function of HP to replicate carrying the restricted amino acid change in UL5 or UL52 and the frequency of amenamevir-resistant virus was approximately 1 in 10^6 plaque-forming units [10,14]. Thus, amenamevir resistance is lower than acyclovir resistance, which suggests that the effectiveness of amenamevir is partly related to the lack of amenamevir-resistant strains.

Amenamevir-resistant mutants had attenuated growth and pathogenicity compared with the wild-type strain [14]. Furthermore, amenamevir had antiviral activity against VZV [10,14–16].

6. Nucleotides and DNA Synthesis

Figure 3 illustrates nucleotide metabolism and the viral enzymes involved in viral DNA synthesis. Purines and deoxyribonucleotide triphosphates (dXTP) are synthesized from amino acids to inosine-monophosphate (IMP) and then to the ribosyl form of adenosine-MP (rAMP), guanosine-MP, cytosine-MP, and uridine-MP. Ribonucleotide-MP are in the form of ribose (rNMP: RNA type), and their triphosphate forms (rNTPs) are substrates for RNA. The ribose forms of ribonucleotide diphosphate (rNDP) are then converted to the deoxyribose forms of dNDPs by ribonucleotide reductase (RR) and further to dNTP to become the substrates for DNA. Uridine diphosphate (dUDP) is converted to the monophosphate forms dUMP and dUMP, substrates for thymidylate synthase (TS), which are converted into thymidine-MP (dTMP) and then successively to dTTP for DNA synthesis.

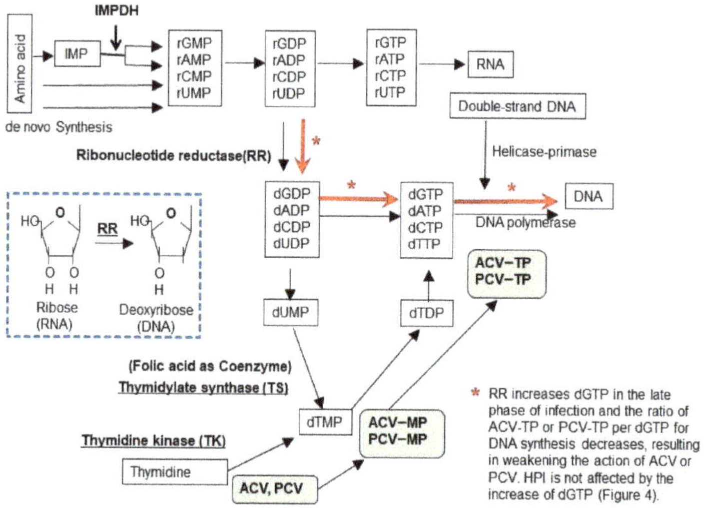

Figure 3. Biosynthesis of nucleotides. Purines and pyrimidines are synthesized de novo from amino acids as the ribose form of nucleotides and inosine monophosphate (IMP) that are modified by IMP dehydrogenase to adenosine-monophosphate (rAMP) and guanosine-monophosphate (rGMP). Next, nucleotide monophosphate (rNMP) is phosphorylated to a triphosphate form (rNTP), which is the substrate for RNA. The ribose form of nucleotide diphosphate (rNDP) is converted to the 2′-deoxyribose form (dNDP) by cellular or viral ribonucleotide reductase (RR), as shown in the lower box. When viral RR is induced by HSV and VZV infection, dNDPs are synthesized in the early phase of infection and are used for viral DNA synthesis, even in cells that do not actively synthesize cellular DNA. Thymidine is an important substrate of DNA and is supplied in two ways—by the conversion of uridine monophosphate (UMP) to thymidine monophosphate (TMP) via thymidylate synthase (TS) (de novo pathway) and from the systemic circulation by thymidine kinase (TK) (salvage pathway). Acyclovir (ACV) and penciclovir (PCV) are phosphorylated by viral TK and are further phosphorylated to the triphosphate form by cellular enzymes, as shown in the green-shaded boxes. ACV-TP and PCV-TP are incorporated into viral DNA by viral DNA polymerase, which results in chain termination. Foscarnet (PFA) and amenamevir (ASP2151) directly inhibit viral DNA synthesis by inhibiting DNA polymerase and HP, respectively. Nucleotides are used for RNA synthesis in the early phase of viral replication. ACV and PCV are efficiently phosphorylated by viral TK and inhibit viral DNA synthesis because the supply of dGTP is limited in infected cells. This efficient inhibition of viral replication by ACV continues for 5 h after infection. In the late phase of viral replication, ribonucleotides are converted to deoxyribonucleotides by viral RR for viral DNA synthesis as indicated by red arrows. Accordingly, large amounts of dGTP are supplied for DNA synthesis (approximately 60,000 and 90,000 dGTPs per DNA molecule of VZV and HSV, respectively) and this attenuates the inhibition of viral DNA synthesis by reducing the ratio of ACV-TP:dGTP. PFA and ASP2151 directly inhibit viral DNA synthesis and are not influenced by the supply of dGTP, which results in the efficient inhibition of viral growth in contrast to ACV.

Basal cells in the skin synthesize DNA for cell proliferation and differentiation to keratinocytes; however, most skin cells do not synthesize DNA, and instead they synthesize RNA and proteins to maintain cellular functions. Because skin cells contain low amounts of deoxyribonucleotides for DNA synthesis, when HSV or VZV infection induces thymidine kinase, acyclovir or penciclovir is phosphorylated and further converted to acyclovir or penciclovir triphosphate, which results in the efficient inhibition of viral DNA synthesis by chain termination. When viral RR and TS are induced, rNTP, a substrate for RNA, is converted to dNTP, which increases dGTP. dGTP is increased in HSV-infected cells at 4 h after infection. Therefore, HSV and VZV traffic between infected cells to facilitate viral DNA synthesis by converting RNA synthesis to viral DNA synthesis via the induction of enzymes in the newly infected cells [18]. One molecule of the VZV and HSV genome contains 60,000 and 90,000 guanosines, respectively, and abundant dGTP competes with acyclovir- or penciclovir-TP for DNA polymerase, which results in the inefficient inhibition of viral DNA synthesis, when viral DNA synthesis is abundant, as shown in Figure 4.

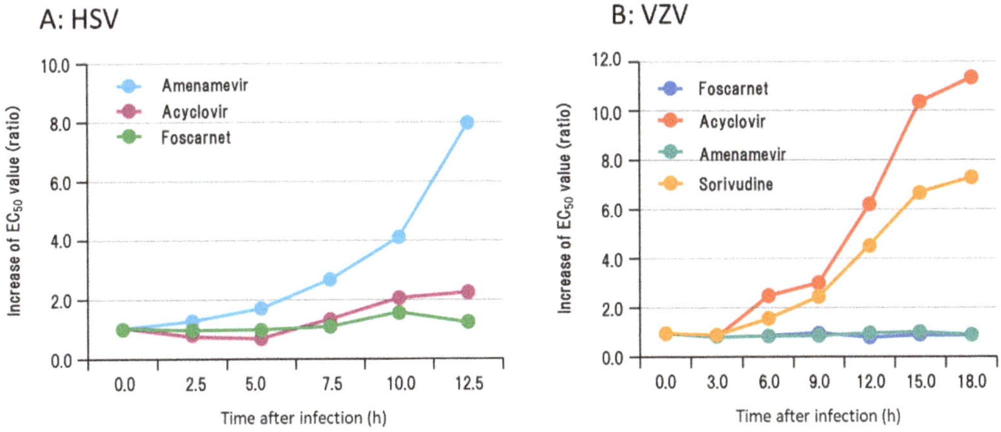

Figure 4. Time course of changes in susceptibility of HSV- and VZV-infected cells to acyclovir, amenamevir, foscarnet, and sorivudine [17,18]. The susceptibility of (**A**) HSV- and (**B**) VZV-infected cells to acyclovir, amenamevir, foscarnet, and sorivudine was assessed serially after infection to examine when and how the susceptibility of infected cells to antiviral drugs might change during the replication cycle of HSV and VZV. EC_{50} values of infected cells to anti-herpetic drugs were determined at the indicated times after infection, and the increase in EC_{50} values is expressed as the ratio of those at 0 h. The authors obtained permission from *Antiviral Research* to reuse these figures [17,18].

7. Antiviral Activity of Amenamevir Is Not Influenced by the Replication Cycle

Cells infected with viruses are treated with antiviral drugs immediately after infection, and the drug concentration at 50% plaque formation of the inoculated virus is expressed as the EC_{50}. After infection, cells will be at various stages of viral DNA synthesis (immediately after infection and prior to viral DNA synthesis, viral DNA synthesis initiated, and production of viruses during viral DNA synthesis). Therefore, it might be possible to determine the actual concentrations of antiviral drugs required to inhibit virus growth in vivo by examining the susceptibility of infected cells to antiviral drugs at various stages after virus infection. We investigated the susceptibility of infected cells to acyclovir and amenamevir after infection with HSV and VZV.

The time course of the antiviral activity of amenamevir and acyclovir after HSV and VZV showed contrasting profiles related to the concentration required for the 50% plaque reduction of infected cells (Figure 4). The EC_{50} values of acyclovir were increased 5.0–7.5 h after HSV infection and reached approximately 10 and 8 times the EC_{50} of 0 h at 12.5 h in contrast to ASP2151 and foscarnet [17,18]. The EC_{50} values of amenamevir and foscarnet were not affected 0 to 12.5 h after HSV infection. The EC_{50} values of acyclovir and sorivudine increased 6 h after VZV infection and reached approximately 10 times the EC_{50} of 0 h at 18 h [18].

Conversely the EC_{50} values of amenamevir and foscarnet were not affected 0 to 18 h after VZV infection. The increase in the EC_{50} values of infected cells to acyclovir began at the time of HSV and VZV DNA synthesis and the effects of viral DNA synthesis and its related cellular events clearly influenced the antiviral activity of acyclovir. The antiviral activity of amenamevir was not affected by the replication cycle of VZV and HSV, whereas the late phase of infected cells was 10 times less susceptible to acyclovir than immediately after infection [17,18].

The susceptibility of infected cells to acyclovir after viral DNA synthesis was decreased because of the increased amount of dGTP present for viral DNA synthesis in the late phase of viral replication (Figures 4 and 5). Acyclovir triphosphate competes with dGTP for viral DNA polymerase in infected cells, and when the dGTP supply becomes abundant, anti-HSV activity is attenuated by competing with acyclovir triphosphate, which results in an increase in the EC_{50} values of acyclovir. Viral RR converts the ribose form of guanosine diphosphate (rGTP) to the deoxyribose form of deoxyguanosine diphosphate (dGDP), which is converted to dGTP, a substrate for viral DNA polymerase. Hydroxyurea is an inhibitor of RR that inhibits the supply of dGTP. Acyclovir and hydroxyurea treatment did not reduce the acyclovir susceptibility of HSV-infected cells 12.5 h after viral DNA synthesis or of cells without hydroxyurea dGTP supplied by viral RR, which competes with acyclovir triphosphate, which decreases the anti-HSV and anti-VZV activity of acyclovir in the late phase of cells infected with HSV and VZV [17,18,25]. Conversely, HPIs target the HP and not DNA polymerase, and the nucleoside analog is not a substrate of the HP. The anti-HSV activity of amenamevir was not influenced by the time course of infection, the status of infected cells, or the replication cycle of the virus, which is a major advantage of the HPIs over the current anti-herpetic drugs, acyclovir, valacyclovir, and famciclovir.

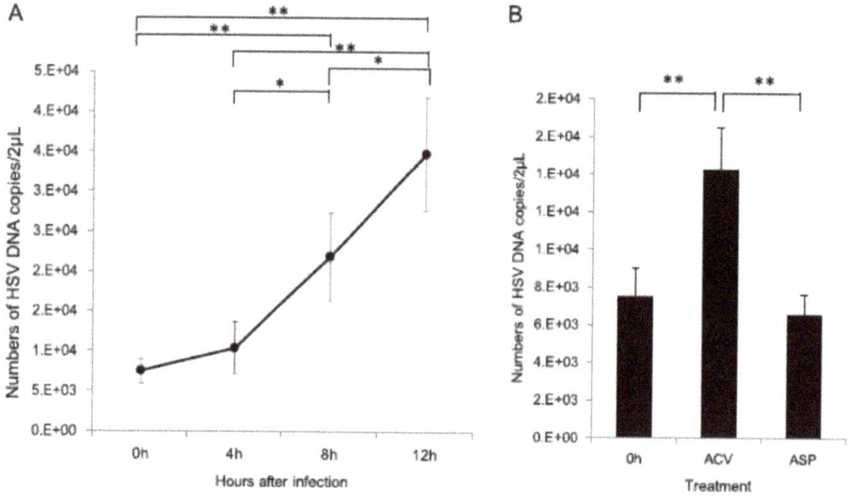

Figure 5. *Cont.*

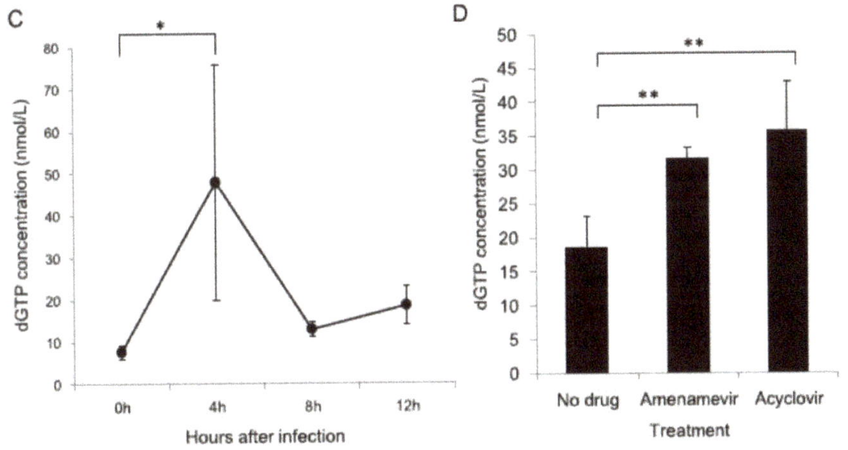

Figure 5. Time-dependent growth of HSV and concentration of dGTP after infection [18]. HSV DNA copy number and dGTP concentration were assessed serially in untreated HSV-infected cells or cells treated with acyclovir and amenamevir. (**A**) Time-dependent increase in HSV DNA copy number after infection. An increase in the copy number was observed later than 4 h after infection. (**B**) Comparison of HSV DNA copy number in cells immediately after infection at 0 h and in cells 12 h after infection treated with 10 times the EC_{50} of amenamevir and acyclovir. The HSV DNA copy number was significantly higher in cells treated with acyclovir than in cells infected at 0 h and cells infected at 12 h and treated with amenamevir. (**C**) Time-dependent changes in the concentration of dGTP after infection. The concentration of dGTP was significantly increased at 4 h after infection and decreased thereafter. (**D**) The concentration of dGTP in infected cells at 12 h without drug treatment was significantly lower than that in infected cells treated with amenamevir and acyclovir. * and ** indicated $p < 0.05$ and $p < 0.01$, respectively. The authors obtained permission from *Antiviral Research* to reuse these figures [18].

8. Synergism of Amenamevir with Other Antiherpetic Drugs

We analyzed the antiviral interactions of amenamevir with acyclovir and penciclovir when used to treat HSV and VZV infection by isobologram in a plaque reduction assay using the response surface model. The combination of amenamevir with acyclovir had statistically significant synergistic antiviral activity against the tested strains of HSV-1, HSV-2, and VZV ($p < 0.0001$, $p = 0.0009$, $p = 0.0005$, respectively) [15]. The antiviral activity of amenamevir combined with acyclovir and penciclovir against wild-type HSV-1, HSV-2, and VZV demonstrated statistically significant synergistic activity at all concentrations ($p < 0.05$) (Figure 6). Amenamevir with vidarabine showed additive effects against wild-type HSV-2 and synergistic effects against VZV. Low concentrations of amenamevir had stronger synergism with acyclovir or penciclovir compared with higher concentrations of amenamevir in the isobologram analysis for HSV-1, HSV-2, and VZV.

The increased efficacy of amenamevir at lower concentrations with acyclovir and penciclovir for HSV and VZV indicated that amenamevir might reduce the number of viral DNA replication forks and allow acyclovir to inhibit the reduced sites of viral DNA synthesis. This is an important pharmacological issue for combination therapy with amenamevir and acyclovir. A single dose of amenamevir maintains an antiviral blood level throughout the day, which reduces the number of replication forks and DNA synthesis sites. Thus, an effective concentration of amenamevir is effective in cells immediately after infection and cells in which viral DNA synthesis is abundant. However, acyclovir is effective for cells in the early stage of infection, but not for cells with abundant viral DNA synthesis. Amenamevir and acyclovir are effective for cells in the early stages of infection. Although acyclovir is not effective in cells with abundant viral DNA synthesis, amenamevir inhibits viral DNA synthesis by reducing the number of forks and reducing the number of replication forks susceptible to acyclovir, even in cells with abundant viral

DNA synthesis. Amenamevir and acyclovir not only have synergism in cells in the early stage of infection, as shown by the plaque reduction method, but also have efficacy on cells with advanced infection and abundant viral DNA synthesis.

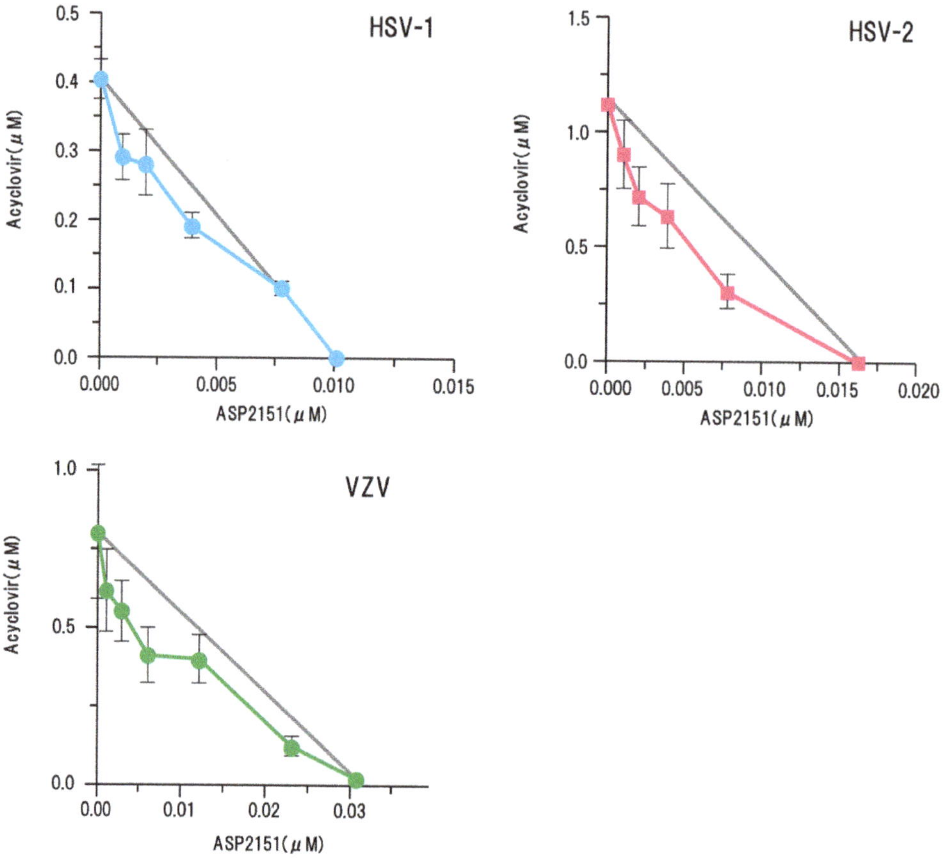

Figure 6. Synergism of amenamevir (ASP2151) with acyclovir against HSV-1, HSV-2, and VZV [15]. Synergism of amenamevir with acyclovir was analyzed by isobologram, and the solid straight line (gray) indicates the theoretical additive antiviral activity in combination with amenamevir and acyclovir. Each point (EC_{50}) is the mean ± standard error from four independent experiments. Significant synergism was observed for the combination of amenamevir and acyclovir ($p = 0.0005$), and low concentrations of amenamevir showed stronger synergism with acyclovir than the higher concentrations of amenamevir. The authors obtained permission from *Antiviral Research* to reuse these figures [15].

Synergism of amenamevir and valacyclovir related to antiviral activity was examined in a mouse HSV zosteriform model, and the inhibition of progression of zosteriform lesions by combination therapy was more potent than that of either drug as a monotherapy [15]. The efficacy of amenamevir was not affected by the host's immune status in terms of effective oral doses in immunocompromised mice [23]. Amenamevir was effective at treating severe skin infections, even when the start of treatment was delayed, whereas valacyclovir was ineffective.

These results indicate that combination therapies of amenamevir with acyclovir have synergistic anti-herpes effects against HSV and VZV infections in vitro and in vivo. Therefore, the combination of amenamevir with acyclovir may be a useful approach to treat herpes infections and might be a more effective therapeutic option than monotherapy for the treatment of herpes encephalitis or immunosuppressed patients.

In severe VZV and HSV infections, where viral replication is abundant, the susceptibility to acyclovir is low because of DNA synthesis and the effect is unlikely, as shown in Figure 5. However, amenamevir is not affected by viral DNA synthesis, even if viral DNA synthesis is abundant. Moreover, because replication fork formation is restricted by the action of amenamevir, acyclovir at low concentrations inhibits DNA synthesis in the presence of amenamevir, as shown in Figure 6. Therefore, combination therapy that takes advantage of the characteristics of acyclovir and amenamevir is recommended for severe VZV and HSV infections.

9. Pharmacokinetic Advantage of Amenamevir

Acyclovir and penciclovir are excreted in the urine as renal excretory drugs, and their oral administration two or three times a day is necessary to maintain a drug concentration in the blood that preserves their antiviral activity over a whole day. Administration of 1000 mg of valacyclovir reached 5.65 $\pm$ 2.37 μg/mL of acyclovir in the serum, with an elimination half-life of 3.03 $\pm$ 0.13 h. The concentration decreased to 2 μg/mL or less within 4 h (Weller et al., 1993). The EC_{50} of VZV-infected cells was 0.745 μg/mL at 0 h after infection, >2 μg/mL at 6 h, and after 6 h, acyclovir did not exhibit sufficient anti-VZV activity against VZV-infected cells (Figure 4) [18].

Approximately 75% of amenamevir is excreted in the feces and 20% in the urine. Amenamevir is not a renal excretion type drug and therefore its blood concentration can be maintained for a long time. A single dose of 300 mg of amenamevir preserved a mean plasma concentration over 9 times higher than the EC_{50} after 24 h [26]. Plasma amenamevir concentrations required to completely suppress HSV-1 growth were seven times higher than the EC_{50} in a mouse skin infection model [27]. A once-daily dose can maintain an antiviral concentration for 24 h, and this pharmacokinetic profile is longer than that of renal excretion type drugs, such as acyclovir and penciclovir, especially for recurrent genital herpes. Suppressive therapy with valacyclovir, famciclovir, or acyclovir successfully suppresses recurrent episodes but they do not maintain an effective antiviral concentration, which allows asymptomatic viral shedding and transmission. HPIs can maintain an antiviral concentration for a whole day, thereby completely suppressing viral replication, including the complete inhibition and viral shedding of genital herpes. HPIs are expected to demonstrate their true value as an antiviral for the suppressive treatment of recurrent genital herpes.

10. The Fate of HSV- and VZV-Infected Cells

Immune responses to VZV and HSV consist of innate immunity and adaptive immunity. Furthermore, cell-mediated immunity specific to VZV and HSV causes eruptions and vesicles in the skin. Erythema multiforme occurred at the site of apparently normal skin recovered from HSV skin lesions 1–3 weeks after infection and HSV DNA was detected in the cells of erythema multiforme lesions [28]. Although VZV is strongly cytolytic in cell cultures, the process by which infected cells become apparently normal cells with viral DNA was reproduced in cell culture by antigenic modulation with an anti-gH neutralizing antibody [29]. The skin lesions caused by HSV and VZV reverted to apparently normal skin over time without causing erosions/ulcers or skin defects related to extensive cell necrosis. Infected cells that have completed viral DNA synthesis are resistant to acyclovir (Figure 4) and continue to survive and express viral antigens. These cells become the target of the immune response until returning to normal.

11. Innate and Adaptive Cell-Mediated Immunity Related to the Clinical Image of Viral Infection

Typical inflammation caused by adaptive immune responses characterized by cell-mediated immunity is termed delayed type hypersensitivity (DTH) or type IV hypersensitivity—tuberculin tests, contact dermatitis, or urushiol-induced dermatitis are examples. DTH occurs as redness and swelling at 5–6 h and peaks at 48–72 h after contact with an antigen, and even in the absence of the initial antigen, which then resolve 1 week later.

Photodistribution revealed the role of innate immune responses to HSV and VZV (Figure 7) [30]. Sunburn (ultraviolet light) allows virus growth before inducing a phase of adaptive immunity by impairing innate immunity related to the function of Langerhans cells in the skin. This results in more severe skin lesions in the sunburned skin compared with non-sunburned skin in the adaptive immunity phase [31].

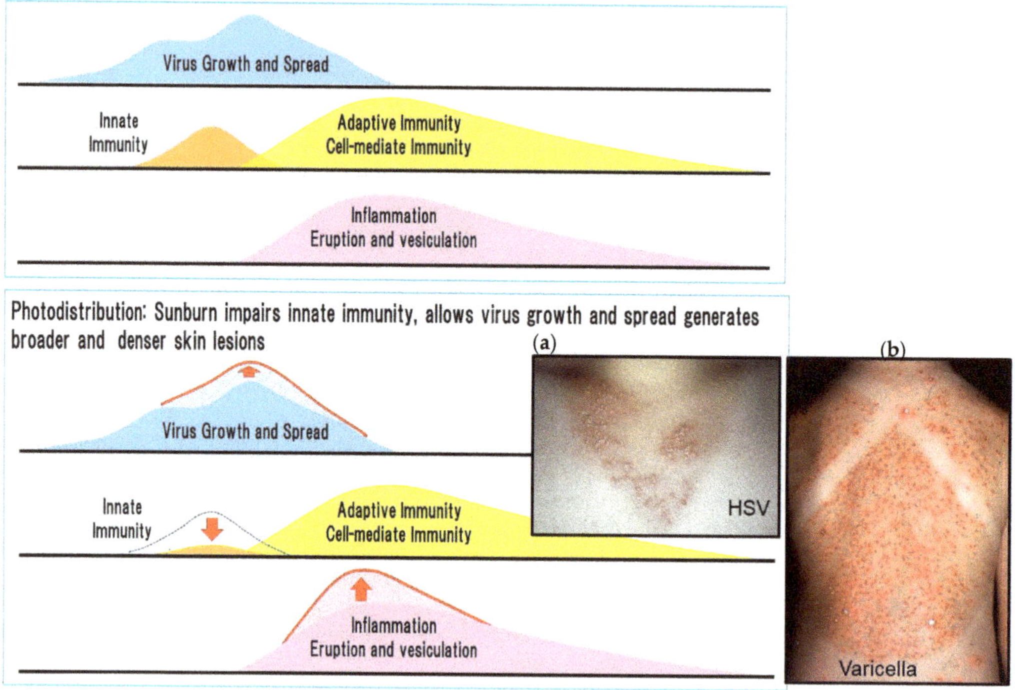

Figure 7. Innate and adaptive immunity and photodistribution [30]. The figure shows the relationship between virus proliferation, innate and adaptive immunity, and rash in HSV and VZV infection. Sunburn modifies virus proliferation, innate and adaptive immunity, and rash as shown by the red arrow in the figure on the right, and causes characteristic photodistribution as shown in the photographs. Exacerbated and dense distribution of skin lesions of HSV and VZV infection related to the inhibition of innate immunity by sunlight exposure (ultraviolet rays). (**a**) A woman in her 20s developed vesicles that were consistently distributed throughout an anterior cervical area exposed to the sun 2 days previously. Denser uniform vesicles and erythema are present in the sun-exposed areas compared with the unexposed areas. The sparse distribution of skin lesions in the area unexposed to sunlight is related to the lack of inhibition of innate immune responses by sun exposure. HSV-1 was present in blister fluid (photodistribution by HSV). (**b**) An 8-year-old girl was diagnosed with varicella with fever and vesicles 3 days after bathing in the sea. Dense uniform vesicles were clustered in the sunburned area, whereas the distribution of eruptions was sparse in the unexposed area where the shoulder straps were located because varicella lesions were inhibited by innate immunity (photodistribution by VZV). In these two cases, innate immunity in the skin was not impaired in areas without sunburn and VZV infection resulted in mild varicella. Thus, innate immunity is important for alleviating dense lesions by inhibiting the growth, spread, and distribution of the virus before inducing adaptive cell-mediated immunity. The photographs were provided by Dr. Yasumoto.

Skin lesions are generally only present in areas where viral spread is not suppressed by innate immunity. However, ultraviolet rays impair innate immune responses, especially those mediated by Langerhans cells, which allows the initial viral infection to spread, which results in broader, denser, and more severe skin lesions generated by an adaptive cell-mediated immune response termed photodistribution. The extent of viral lesions is determined by the size of the virus replicated area before adaptive cell-mediated immune responses are induced. This demonstrates that innate immunity has an important role in the distribution and density of viral skin lesions by suppressing viral spread.

This is consistent with the idea that early treatment before the appearance of lesions alleviates skin lesions in varicella and recurrent genital herpes. Treatment with acyclovir in the latter half of the incubation period of chickenpox resulted in subclinical or mild varicella [32]. Furthermore, for recurrent genital herpes, treatment at the prodromal stage before the appearance of skin lesions blocks their appearance in one-third of patients [33,34]. If antiviral agents are administered before the adaptive cell-mediated immune response is initiated, they can prevent virus localization, distribution, and replication, which results in mild or subclinical skin lesions and alleviated disease. This concept of prophylactic or preemptive therapy was achieved in cytomegalovirus (CMV) pneumonia in immunocompromised patients by starting ganciclovir treatment before apparent CMV replication appeared [35,36].

Anti-inflammatory steroids reduced inflammation of urushiol-induced dermatitis caused by adaptive cell-mediated immunity (DTH), but did not shorten the duration of inflammation. Similarly, antiviral drugs prevented the appearance of new skin lesions and halted the progression to vesiculation, but did not shorten the time to the elimination of inflammation, even when prednisolone was administered [19,37,38]. Inflammation appeared 3 days after contact with a viral antigen and inflammation induced by herpes zoster was exacerbated 3 to 5 days after the onset of inflammation by the continuous presence of infected cells and continued for 3 weeks (Figure 7). The infected cells continued to receive antigen stimulation and inflammation peaks 3 to 5 days after the appearance of the rash. Antiviral drugs halted the appearance of new lesions and the enlargement of skin lesions but did not suppress inflammation once it was induced. The inflammatory process continued for 3 weeks before being resolved, even under the intervention of amenamevir treatment initiated on day 2 of herpes zoster infection (Figure 7).

12. Timing of Antiviral Therapy

The effectiveness of antiviral drugs can be maximized by limiting the spread, distribution, and size of viral infections before the onset of adaptive cell-mediated immunity as observed in photodistribution. Therefore, antiviral therapy should be started in the prodromal period when innate immunity is available or as soon as VZV and HSV infections are diagnosed (Figure 8).

Anti-VZV drug treatment for varicella is started within 24 h after the onset of symptoms and continues for 7 days. However, eruptions do not always progress to vesiculation, ending in an abortive form of infection. Varicella is highly contagious and exposure to it causes approximately 80% of infections within a family. After exposure to varicella, family members were prophylactically treated with acyclovir during the first and second halves of the incubation period of about 14 days, and infection was assessed by an increase in antibody titers [32]. In the first half group of 11 patients, varicella developed in 91% of cases and 9% was subclinical, whereas in the second half group of 11 patients, a very mild disease occurred in 27% of cases and subclinical disease developed in 73%. Prophylactic administration converted overt varicella to an asymptomatic infection in the second half of the incubation period. Acyclovir inhibited viral replication in the skin when administered immediately before the onset of varicella (corresponding to the prodromal period), which resulted in subclinical or mild disease. Although prophylactic acyclovir treatment was convenient and useful, the introduction of universal varicella vaccination has superseded it [39,40].

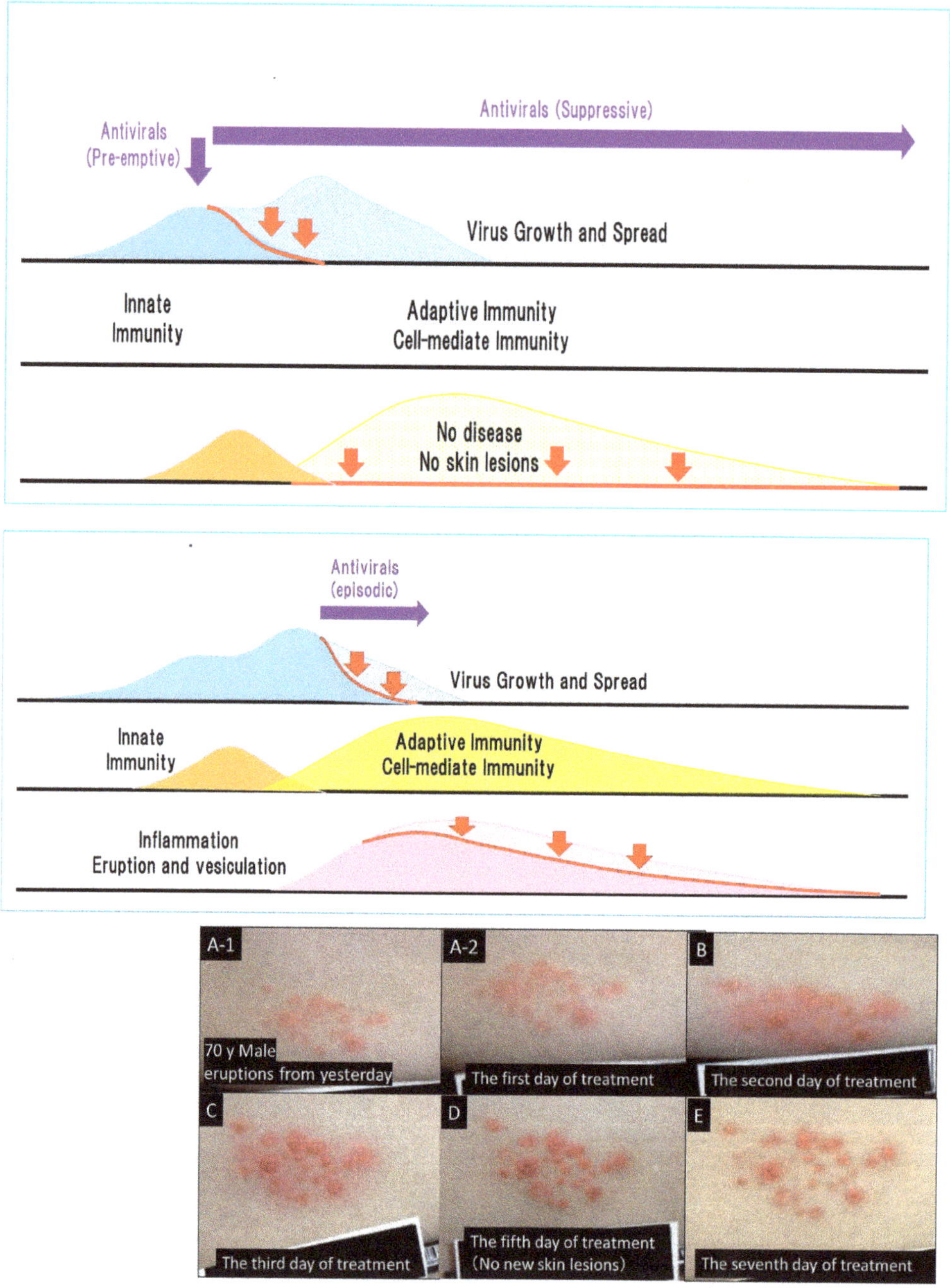

Figure 8. Antiviral treatment at the prodrome and after the onset of herpes zoster. Antiviral therapy inhibits virus growth and spread, as shown by the red arrows. Antiviral treatments started before the prodrome, which are susceptible to photodistribution, include suppressive therapy for HSV, preemptive therapy, and the latter half of the incubation period of varicella. These treatments prevent the onset of overt diseases, which prevents skin lesions. Once the overt disease has occurred, skin

lesions continue for 1 week for HSV, 1–2 weeks for varicella, and 3 weeks for herpes zoster. Apparent deterioration of inflammation and improvement of herpes zoster lesions related to cell-mediated immune responses after the initiation of antiviral treatment. Photograph: A 70-year-old male patient noticed a rash on the left-hand side of his waist and treatment with amenamevir was started the day after its appearance [19,22]. Amenamevir inhibited the enlargement of the lesions and new lesion formation and cured the lesions up to the erythema without proceeding to vesicles (abortive infection). (**A-1**,**A-2**) show a panoramic view and a close view of the skin lesions, respectively, on the first day of amenamevir therapy, which was the day after the eruptions were observed. (**B–E**) show the 2nd, 3rd, 5th, and 7th days, respectively, of amenamevir treatment. Inflammation in the central part of the eruption increased as assessed by redness and swelling from days 1–5, but the redness and inflammation in the peripheral part of the erythema (red halo) gradually disappeared after day 3. (**B**) shows the skin lesions on the second day after treatment where redness and swelling had increased and spread around the lesions, which indicates that the inflammatory response was augmented by the maturation and enhancement of the cell-mediated immune response to VZV when compared with day 1. (**C**,**D**) show the contrasting course of reduced peripheral inflammation in the red halo areas and increased inflammation in the central part of lesions, with the peak of inflammation at day 5. Urushiol-induced dermatitis peaked on day 3 after antigen contact, and any viral lesions present at the start of treatment appeared as a rash on day 3. There was no new eruption in this patient on day 4, which indicates that antiviral treatment blocked the formation of new lesions and prevented the spread of the eruption and the formation of new lesions. Inflammation represented by redness and swelling was exacerbated despite antiviral treatment. The therapeutic effect of the antiviral drug is not related to the reduction in inflammation, which makes it difficult to determine the therapeutic efficacy of antiviral drugs. The inflammation became more severe between days 3 and 5, even after antiviral treatment. The photograph was provided by Dr. Toyama.

Herpes zoster is uncommon with an annual incidence of approximately 1 in 100 people aged > 60 years old [41,42]. Seventy to eighty percent of patients with herpes zoster experience prodromal symptoms, such as burning, shooting, stabbing, or throbbing pain in the dermatome(s), which represent allodynia [43,44]. Sclerotomal pain usually precedes dermatomal pain by a few days in the prodrome [45]. Although the preemptive use of antiherpetic drugs at the prodromal symptom stage might be the optimal timepoint to alleviate the severity of herpes zoster, it is not easy to differentially diagnose the prodrome of herpes zoster from other causative symptoms.

Recurrent genital herpes causes the appearance of unpleasant vesicles, erosions, and ulcers that last for approximately 1 week. Prodromal treatment with anti-HSV drugs prevents uncomfortable genital lesions in up to one third of patients and helps to maintain a comfortable daily life [33,34]. The oral administration of acyclovir, valacyclovir, and famciclovir starting within 24 h of the onset of recurrent herpes and continuing for a period of 5 days is effective at reducing the duration of symptoms by a median of 1–2 days.

CMV pneumonia was treated with ganciclovir in transplant recipients and immunocompromised patients in the 1980s, and current guidelines have been established to prevent the development of refractory CMV pneumonia by the administration of prophylactic or preemptive treatment with ganciclovir or letermovir [35,36,46]. The optimal timing for the treatment of herpes virus diseases is prodromal and preemptive therapies with antiherpetic drugs block the onset of diseases such as varicella, herpes zoster, genital herpes, and CMV pneumonia. Although it is difficult to diagnose the prodromal stage in VZV infections, it is easier for HSV and CMV infections. The optimal timepoint for the antiviral treatment of VZV infection is at least within 24 h for varicella and within 72 h for herpes zoster, as soon as possible after the onset or diagnosis.

13. Clinical Trials of Herpes Zoster Treatment with Amenamevir

Current suppressive therapies for genital herpes using acyclovir, valacyclovir, and famciclovir are effective, but these drugs do not provide efficacious antiviral concentrations over the whole day because they are renal excretory drugs [26], and this allows viral shedding and viral replication.

On the basis of the promising preclinical profiles related to the antiviral activity and pharmacokinetics of HPIs, pritelivir and amenamevir were evaluated in two phase 2 clinical studies of patients with genital herpes [11–13]. HPIs have an excellent pharmacokinetic profile, and when administered daily, they maintain anti-HSV activity for the whole day, which results in the inhibition of HSV replication, reactivation, and shedding, and lesion formation in patients with genital herpes, as well as the transmission of HSV from asymptomatic and symptomatic cases of genital herpes. Although one of the indications for HPI treatment is the suppressive treatment of genital herpes, sufficient clinical efficacy has not been achieved, and they have not replaced current suppressive therapies.

The efficacy and safety of amenamevir 400 mg once daily were evaluated in a phase 3 randomized, double-blind, valacyclovir-controlled phase 3 study when compared with valacyclovir 1000 mg three times daily in 751 Japanese patients with herpes zoster within 72 h after the onset of rash [19]. The proportion of cases with reduced new lesion formation by day 4 (primary efficacy endpoint) was 81.1% (197/243) for amenamevir and 75.1% (184/245) for valacyclovir and the non-inferiority of amenamevir to valacyclovir was confirmed using a closed testing procedure. Furthermore, 10.0% (25/249) and 12.0% (30/249) of patients receiving amenamevir or valacyclovir, respectively, experienced drug-related adverse events. Days to cessation of new lesion formation, complete crusting, healing, pain resolution, and virus disappearance (secondary endpoints) were not statistically different between the amenamevir and valacyclovir groups.

Although amenamevir has excellent pharmacokinetics and anti-VZV properties compared with acyclovir, it did not show clinically superior efficacy over valacyclovir in immunocompetent subjects with herpes zoster [19]. Sorivudine 40 mg once daily had better efficacy against herpes zoster than acyclovir 800 mg five times daily in patients infected with human immunodeficiency virus [47,48]. The target period of the administration of anti-VZV agents to inhibit viral replication in the skin of immunocompetent subjects with herpes zoster might be limited to a few days, but longer in immunocompromised patients, which might demonstrate the beneficial action of amenamevir over acyclovir in immunocompromised subjects. Amenamevir (Amenalief®) has been approved as an anti-herpes zoster drug and has been successfully used to treat approximately 1,240,000 herpes zoster patients in Japan.

14. Post Marketing Surveillance

At the time of approval in Japan, "renal disorder," "cardiovascular event," and "platelets decreased" were set as important potential risks in the Japanese risk management plan (RMP) to be monitored during routine pharmacovigilance (PV) activities. As of June 2020, "erythema multiform" was added as an important identified risk, and "toxic epidermal necrolysis" and "Stevens–Johnson syndrome" were added as important potential risks into the Japanese RMP.

As an additional PV activity to further evaluate and demonstrate the efficacy and safety of amenamevir in herpes zoster patients in a clinical setting, data were collected by a Special Drug Use Surveillance program (an observational study, protocol No. AME11) [49]. This study specifically collects information on the efficacy and safety of amenamevir in routine clinical practice in patients who use the drug for herpes zoster. In addition, pain status was followed to examine post-herpetic neuralgia. This study plans to enroll 3000 patients; as of 2 January 2019, 1446 patients have been enrolled. The safety analysis set includes 1346 patients, of which 11 experienced adverse drug reactions, with an incidence of 0.82% (11/1,346 patients). Among the 11 reported cases of adverse drug reactions, two patients had abdominal pain and two had diarrhea and fever. Regarding safety issues related to the important potential risks identified in the Japanese RMP, one case of thrombocytopenia and one case of gingival bleeding were reported as events associated with "platelets decreased", and one case of palpitation was reported as an event associated with "cardiovascular event". None of these were serious.

In Japan, everyone has health insurance, which covers most patients with shingles who are treated at medical institutions. The estimated number of patients with herpes zoster treated with Amenalief® from its launch in September 2017 to February 2021 is approximately 1,240,000 based on sales data and the estimated dose per patient in Japan.

From estimations using the number of prescriptions in 2020, the total number of new herpes zoster patients in Japan is approximately 940,000 per year, of which 240,000 (25.5%) are treated with amenamevir.

15. Cumulative Number of Adverse Drug Reactions in Post-Marketing

Table 3 shows the number of adverse drug reactions related to oral anti-herpetic drugs (valaciclovir, acyclovir, famciclovir, and amenamevir) in the database (Japanese Adverse Drug Event Report database) maintained by the Pharmaceuticals and Medical Devices Agency (PMDA), the Japanese regulatory authority. Overall, 500–700 adverse drug reactions related to oral anti-herpetic drugs are reported every year, and most events are categorized as "nervous system disorders" and "renal and urinary disorders." The incidence of adverse drug reactions is not calculated, because they are spontaneous reports from healthcare providers or consumers to a pharmaceutical company and/or regulatory authority such as the PMDA. Because the Ministry of Health, Labor and Welfare of Japan requires the widespread reporting of cases with suspected side effects/adverse events, each report states that there is a causal relationship between the drug and the symptoms and abnormal findings. Furthermore, the same case may be reported by multiple reporters. All reported cases are listed, but the relationship with the drug has not been evaluated and should be interpreted with caution. Accordingly, it is not possible to simply evaluate or compare the safety of drugs based on the number of cases in the case reports or the number of cases in the list of reported adverse drug reactions. However, the information obtained here includes data that cannot be obtained by the post-marketing surveillance of amenamevir, although our interpretation should be carefully evaluated with the understanding of the limitations of the above information. These events are a medical problem for current nucleoside analogs such as valaciclovir, acyclovir, and famciclovir in clinical practice. The type and the number of events related to amenamevir are shown in parenthesis (Table 3).

Table 3. Cumulative number of adverse drug reactions related to oral anti-herpetic drugs (as of 16 May 2021).

System Organ Class	2015	2016	2017	2018	2019	2020
Nervous system disorders	221	257	272 (15)	255 (21)	271 (14)	254 (5)
Renal and urinary disorders	235	212	144 (1)	195 (5)	211 (6)	134 (6)
Psychiatric disorders	31	31	29 (1)	10 (1)	22 (1)	15 (0)
Infections and infestations	11	9	21 (5)	38 (9)	40 (1)	16 (2)
Skin and subcutaneous tissue disorders	14	6	27 (7)	25 (15)	34 (10)	22 (10)
General disorders and administration site conditions	17	15	19 (4)	36 (19)	24 (7)	16 (3)
Metabolism and nutrition disorders	7	12	13 (2)	33 (11)	16 (2)	23 (4)
Others	69	78	105 (11)	108 (25)	98 (11)	82 (12)
Total	605	620	630 (44)	700 (106)	716 (52)	562 (42)

Number (including amenamevir). Adverse drug reaction reports to the PMDA are reported by pharmaceutical companies or medical institutions, and the PMDA has not individually evaluated their relevance to the pharmaceutical products. In addition, because the number of reported adverse drug reactions varies depending on the number of patients administered each product and the availability of information from pharmaceutical companies, it is not possible to evaluate or compare the safety of pharmaceutical products based on the number of reported adverse drug reactions. (Japanese Adverse Drug Event Report database: https://www.info.pmda.go.jp/fsearchnew/jsp/menu_fukusayou_base.jsp, accessed on 30 July 2021).

16. Amenamevir against Herpes Zoster Caused by Acyclovir-Resistant VZV

A 64-year-old male patient with adult T-cell lymphoma with stem cell transplantation suffered herpes zoster and was treated with acyclovir. VZV was isolated from 12 vesicles and the susceptibility of the 12 isolated viruses from each vesicle was examined to acyclovir and amenamevir 14 days after acyclovir treatment was investigated. Half of the 12 isolated viruses were a mixture of acyclovir-susceptible and acyclovir-resistant viruses with reduced susceptibility to acyclovir compared with the wild-type strain, which indicates that the isolated viruses were in the transition phase of susceptible VZV to resistant VZV harboring mutations (p.Phe139Serfs*25, p.Try144Phefs*20) in the thymidine kinase gene. Amenamevir treatment quickly terminated the appearance of new vesicles that subsequently scabbed over 10 days later [50]. Furthermore, amenamevir showed efficacy against acyclovir-resistant VZV infection in one case, as expected from the finding that amenamevir has efficacy against acyclovir resistance in vitro (Table 2) [15,16].

17. Conclusions and Overall Perspectives

HPIs have been developed as new anti-herpes drugs, but currently only amenamevir among the HPIs is used for the treatment of herpes zoster. Amenamevir has a low EC_{50} to HSV and VZV and its efficacy in HSV-infected animals and synergism with acyclovir and penciclovir was indicated for the combinational treatment of severe infection with HSV or VZV [14–18]. The target enzymes of amenamevir and acyclovir are different—amenamevir is effective against acyclovir-resistant viruses and has been used successfully to treat acyclovir-resistant VZV in a patient with herpes zoster caused by acyclovir-resistant VZV [50]. Amenamevir (Amenalief®) has been approved as an anti-herpes zoster drug and has been successfully used to treat approximately 1,240,000 herpes zoster patients in Japan. To date, the numbers of adverse reactions in amenamevir-treated patients seem to be lower than for other anti-herpetic drugs (Table 3).

The relationship between viral replication in HSV and VZV infections and innate and adaptive immunity is explained by the pathophysiology of photodistribution, which affects the distribution of skin lesions, as stated in Section 11. The optimal treatment timepoint is at the prodrome during photodistribution, which prevents the formation of skin lesions. This is supported by clinical observations that antiviral treatment in the latter half of the latent period of chickenpox and prodromal treatment in recurrent herpes can prevent the appearance of skin lesions [32–34]. However, it is difficult to start treatment for chickenpox and herpes zoster from the prodrome; therefore, it is best to start treatment immediately after the onset and diagnosis. Vesiculation of herpetic lesions can be prevented by the early treatment of HSV skin lesions and chickenpox as an abortive form. Treatment after the onset of herpes zoster can stop the appearance of new skin lesions and prevent its spread after 4 days, but it has no effect on the exacerbation of inflammation induced by adaptive immunity, and the inflammation is augmented even after the start of antiviral treatment. Approximately 3 weeks of inflammation cannot be shortened by the use of anti-inflammatory drugs. As described above, the efficacy of antiviral drugs and inflammation caused by adaptive immune responses should be evaluated separately because viral replication and generating adaptive immunity are independent pathophysiologic events. Therefore, antiviral agents can stop viral spread but cannot alleviate adaptive immunity, which exacerbates inflammation after the start of antiviral therapy. Before starting antiviral treatment, it is recommended to explain the following to the patient: inflammation related to lesions already present will worsen for the next 3 days, which is unavoidable because it is an immune response, but antiviral drugs will alleviate herpes zoster by stopping viral replication and limiting the extent of the lesion and preventing the spread of the infection.

The long-lasting antiviral concentration of HPIs can inhibit HSV replication throughout the whole day, which prevents the reactivation of HSV from ganglia, subsequent viral shedding, and its sexual transmission. The excellent pharmacokinetic profile of HPIs for the suppressive therapy of genital herpes indicates that they might provide greater benefit than current therapy with valacyclovir and famciclovir, although this has not been reported to date. Thus, HPIs might have favorable characteristics as antiherpetic drugs for suppressive therapy.

The clinical efficacy and safety profiles of amenamevir have been established in patients with herpes zoster, which indicates that amenamevir as an HPI might be an anti-herpes therapy. This review introduced the newly developed HPI, amenamevir, and suggests that HPIs might be next-generation drugs for HSV and VZV infections.

Author Contributions: Conceptualization, K.S.; resources, N.T., S.Y., H.F.; writing—original draft preparation, K.S., N.T., S.Y., H.F.; writing—review and editing, all authors. All authors have read and agreed to the published version of the manuscript.

Funding: This research received no external funding.

Institutional Review Board Statement: Not applicable.

Informed Consent Statement: Not applicable.

Data Availability Statement: Not applicable.

Acknowledgments: The authors thank Yasuhiro Kawasaki for help with the tables, illustrations, and designs for the figure panels.

Conflicts of Interest: K.S. reports the receipt of consulting fees from Maruho Co., Ltd., lecture fees form Maruho Co., Ltd., MSD, and Novartis, and research funding from Maruho Co., Ltd., MSD, and Japan Blood Products Organization; all payments to the institution. The other authors declare no conflict of interest.

References

1. Elion, G.B.; Furman, P.A.; Fyfe, J.A.; de Miranda, P.; Beauchamp, L.; Schaeffer, H.J. Selectivity of action of an antiherpetic agent, 9-(2-hydroxyethoxymethyl) guanine. *Proc. Natl. Acad. Sci. USA* **1977**, *74*, 5716–5720. [CrossRef]
2. Elion, G.B. Nobel lecture in physiology or medicine–1988. The purine path to chemotherapy. *In Vitro Cell Dev. Biol.* **1989**, *25*, 321–330. [CrossRef] [PubMed]
3. Shiraki, K. Antiviral drugs against alphaherpesvirus. *Adv. Exp. Med. Biol.* **2018**, *1045*, 103–122. [PubMed]
4. Boyd, M.R.; Bacon, T.H.; Sutton, D. Antiherpesvirus activity of 9-(4-hydroxy-3-hydroxymethylbut-1-yl) guanine (BRL 39123) in animals. *Antimicrob. Agents Chemother.* **1988**, *32*, 358–363. [CrossRef] [PubMed]
5. Boehmer, P.E.; Lehman, I.R. Herpes simplex virus DNA replication. *Annu. Rev. Biochem.* **1997**, *66*, 347–384. [CrossRef] [PubMed]
6. Spector, F.C.; Liang, L.; Giordano, H.; Sivaraja, M.; Peterson, M.G. Inhibition of herpes simplex virus replication by a 2-amino thiazole via interactions with the helicase component of the UL5-UL8-UL52 complex. *J. Virol.* **1998**, *72*, 6979–6987. [CrossRef] [PubMed]
7. Crumpacker, C.S.; Schaffer, P.A. New anti-HSV therapeutics target the helicase-primase complex. *Nat. Med.* **2002**, *8*, 327–328. [CrossRef] [PubMed]
8. Crute, J.J.; Grygon, C.A.; Hargrave, K.D.; Simoneau, B.; Faucher, A.M.; Bolger, G.; Kibler, P.; Liuzzi, M.; Cordingley, M.G. Herpes simplex virus helicase-primase inhibitors are active in animal models of human disease. *Nat. Med.* **2002**, *8*, 386–391. [CrossRef]
9. Kleymann, G.; Fischer, R.; Betz, U.A.; Hendrix, M.; Bender, W.; Schneider, U.; Handke, G.; Eckenberg, P.; Hewlett, G.; Pevzner, V.; et al. New helicase-primase inhibitors as drug candidates for the treatment of herpes simplex disease. *Nat. Med.* **2002**, *8*, 392–398. [CrossRef]
10. Chono, K.; Katsumata, K.; Kontani, T.; Kobayashi, M.; Sudo, K.; Yokota, T.; Konno, K.; Shimizu, Y.; Suzuki, H. ASP2151, a novel helicase-primase inhibitor, possesses antiviral activity against varicella-zoster virus and herpes simplex virus types 1 and 2. *J. Antimicrob. Chemother.* **2010**, *65*, 1733–1741. [CrossRef]
11. Tyring, S.; Wald, A.; Zadeikis, N.; Dhadda, S.; Takenouchi, K.; Rorig, R. ASP2151 for the treatment of genital herpes: A randomized, double-blind, placebo- and valacyclovir-controlled, dose-finding study. *J. Infect. Dis.* **2012**, *205*, 1100–1110. [CrossRef]
12. Wald, A.; Corey, L.; Timmler, B.; Magaret, A.; Warren, T.; Tyring, S.; Johnston, C.; Kriesel, J.; Fife, K.; Galitz, L.; et al. Helicase-primase inhibitor pritelivir for HSV-2 infection. *N. Engl. J. Med.* **2014**, *370*, 201–210. [CrossRef]
13. Wald, A.; Timmler, B.; Magaret, A.; Warren, T.; Tyring, S.; Johnston, C.; Fife, K.; Selke, S.; Huang, M.L.; Stobernack, H.P.; et al. Effect of pritelivir compared with valacyclovir on genital HSV-2 shedding in patients with frequent recurrences: A randomized clinical trial. *JAMA* **2016**, *316*, 2495–2503. [CrossRef]
14. Chono, K.; Katsumata, K.; Kontani, T.; Shiraki, K.; Suzuki, H. Characterization of virus strains resistant to the herpes virus helicase-primase inhibitor ASP2151 (Amenamevir). *Biochem. Pharmacol.* **2012**, *84*, 459–467. [CrossRef]
15. Chono, K.; Katsumata, K.; Suzuki, H.; Shiraki, K. Synergistic activity of amenamevir (ASP2151) with nucleoside analogs against herpes simplex virus types 1 and 2 and varicella-zoster virus. *Antiviral Res.* **2013**, *97*, 154–160. [CrossRef]
16. Himaki, T.; Masui, Y.; Chono, K.; Daikoku, T.; Takemoto, M.; Haixia, B.; Okuda, T.; Suzuki, H.; Shiraki, K. Efficacy of ASP2151, a helicase-primase inhibitor, against thymidine kinase-deficient herpes simplex virus type 2 infection in vitro and in vivo. *Antiviral Res.* **2012**, *93*, 301–304. [CrossRef] [PubMed]
17. Yajima, M.; Yamada, H.; Takemoto, M.; Daikoku, T.; Yoshida, Y.; Long, T.; Okuda, T.; Shiraki, K. Profile of anti-herpetic action of ASP2151 (amenamevir) as a helicase-primase inhibitor. *Antiviral Res.* **2017**, *139*, 95–101. [CrossRef]

18. Shiraki, K.; Tan, L.; Daikoku, T.; Takemoto, M.; Sato, N.; Yoshida, Y. Viral ribonucleotide reductase attenuates the anti-herpes activity of acyclovir in contrast to amenamevir. *Antiviral Res.* **2020**, *180*, 104829. [CrossRef] [PubMed]
19. Kawashima, M.; Nemoto, O.; Honda, M.; Watanabe, D.; Nakayama, J.; Imafuku, S.; Kato, T.; Katsuramaki, T.; study investigators. Amenamevir, a novel helicase-primase inhibitor, for treatment of herpes zoster: A randomized, double-blind, valaciclovir-controlled phase 3 study. *J. Dermatol.* **2017**, *44*, 1219–1227. [CrossRef]
20. Biswas, S.; Sukla, S.; Field, H.J. Helicase-primase inhibitors for herpes simplex virus: Looking to the future of non-nucleoside inhibitors for treating herpes virus infections. *Future Med. Chem.* **2014**, *6*, 45–55. [CrossRef] [PubMed]
21. James, S.H.; Larson, K.B.; Acosta, E.P.; Prichard, M.N. Helicase-primase as a target of new therapies for herpes simplex virus infections. *Clin. Pharmacol. Ther.* **2015**, *97*, 66–78. [CrossRef]
22. Shiraki, K. Helicase-primase inhibitor amenamevir for herpesvirus infection: Towards practical application for treating herpes zoster. *Drugs Today* **2017**, *53*, 573–584. [CrossRef]
23. Katsumata, K.; Chono, K.; Suzuki, H. Antiviral efficacy of the helicase-primase inhibitor amenamevir in murine models of severe herpesvirus infection. *Biochem. Pharmacol.* **2018**, *158*, 201–206. [CrossRef]
24. Katsumata, K.; Chono, K.; Sudo, K.; Shimizu, Y.; Kontani, T.; Suzuki, H. Effect of ASP2151, a herpesvirus helicase-primase inhibitor, in a guinea pig model of genital herpes. *Molecules* **2011**, *16*, 7210–7223. [CrossRef]
25. Shiraki, K.; Ochiai, H.; Namazue, J.; Okuno, T.; Ogino, S.; Hayashi, K.; Yamanishi, K.; Takahashi, M. Comparison of antiviral assay methods using cell-free and cell-associated varicella-zoster virus. *Antiviral Res.* **1992**, *18*, 209–214. [CrossRef]
26. Kusawake, T.; Keirns, J.J.; Kowalski, D.; den Adel, M.; Groenendaal-van de Meent, D.; Takada, A.; Ohtsu, Y.; Katashima, M. Pharmacokinetics and safety of amenamevir in healthy subjects: Analysis of four randomized phase 1 studies. *Adv. Ther.* **2017**, *34*, 2625–2637. [CrossRef]
27. Katsumata, K.; Chono, K.; Kato, K.; Yoshiaki, O.; Shoji, T.; Toru, K.; Hiroshi, S. Pharmacokinetics and pharmacodynamics of ASP2151, a helicase-primase inhibitor, in a murine model of herpes simplex virus infection. *Antimicrob. Agents Chemother.* **2013**, *57*, 1339–1346. [CrossRef]
28. Miura, S.; Smith, C.C.; Burnett, J.W.; Aurelian, L. Detection of viral DNA within skin of healed recurrent herpes simplex infection and erythema multiforme lesions. *J. Invest. Dermatol.* **1992**, *98*, 68–72. [CrossRef] [PubMed]
29. Shiraki, K.; Daikoku, T.; Takemoto, M.; Yoshida, Y.; Suzuki, K.; Akahori, Y.; Okuno, T.; Kurosawa, Y.; Asano, Y. Neutralizing anti-gH antibody of varicella-zoster virus modulates distribution of gH and induces gene regulation, mimicking latency. *J. Virol.* **2011**, *85*, 8172–8180. [CrossRef] [PubMed]
30. Gilchrest, B.; Baden, H.P. Photodistribution of viral exanthems. *Pediatrics* **1974**, *54*, 136–138.
31. Aberer, W.; Schuler, G.; Stingl, G.; Hönigsmann, H.; Wolff, K. Ultraviolet light depletes surface markers of Langerhans cells. *J. Invest. Dermatol.* **1981**, *76*, 202–210. [CrossRef] [PubMed]
32. Suga, S.; Yoshikawa, T.; Ozaki, T.; Asano, Y. Effect of oral acyclovir against primary and secondary viraemia in incubation period of varicella. *Arch. Dis. Child.* **1993**, *69*, discussion 642–643. [CrossRef]
33. Patel, R.; Green, J.; Clarke, E.; Seneviratne, K.; Abbt, N.; Evans, C.; Bickford, J.; Nicholson, M.; O'Farrell, N.; Barton, S.; et al. 2014 UK national guideline for the management of anogenital herpes. *Int. J. STD AIDS* **2015**, *26*, 763–776. [CrossRef] [PubMed]
34. Patel, R.; Kennedy, O.J.; Clarke, E.; Geretti, A.; Nilsen, A.; Lautenschlager, S.; Green, J.; Donders, G.; van der Meijden, W.; Gomberg, M.; et al. 2017 European guidelines for the management of genital herpes. *Int. J. STD AIDS* **2017**, *28*, 1366–1379. [CrossRef]
35. Razonable, R.R.; Humar, A. Cytomegalovirus in solid organ transplant recipients-Guidelines of the American Society of Transplantation Infectious Diseases Community of Practice. *Clin. Transplant.* **2019**, *33*, e13512. [CrossRef]
36. Ljungman, P.; de la Camara, R.; Robin, C.; Crocchiolo, R.; Einsele, H.; Hill, J.A.; Hubacek, P.; Navarro, D.; Cordonnier, C.; Ward, K.N. 2017 European Conference on Infections in Leukaemia group. Guidelines for the management of cytomegalovirus infection in patients with haematological malignancies and after stem cell transplantation from the 2017 European Conference on Infections in Leukaemia (ECIL 7). *Lancet Infect. Dis.* **2019**, *19*, e260–e272. [PubMed]
37. Balfour, H.H., Jr.; Bean, B.; Laskin, O.L.; Ambinder, R.F.; Meyers, J.D.; Wade, J.C.; Zaia, J.A.; Aeppli, D.; Kirk, L.E.; Segreti, A.C.; et al. Acyclovir halts progression of herpes zoster in immunocompromised patients. *N. Engl. J. Med.* **1983**, *308*, 1448–1453. [CrossRef]
38. Wood, M.J.; Ogan, P.H.; McKendrick, M.W.; Care, C.D.; McGill, J.I.; Webb, E.M. Efficacy of oral acyclovir treatment of acute herpes zoster. *Am. J. Med.* **1988**, *85*, 79–83.
39. Toyama, N.; Shiraki, K. Universal varicella vaccination reduced the incidence of herpes zoster in vaccine recipients 1 to 4 years of age. *J. Dermatol. Sci.* **2018**, *92*, 284–286. [CrossRef]
40. Toyama, N.; Shiraki, K. Universal varicella vaccination increased the incidence of herpes zoster in the child-rearing generation as its short-term effect. *J. Dermatol. Sci.* **2018**, *92*, 89–96. [CrossRef] [PubMed]
41. Shiraki, K.; Toyama, N.; Daikoku, T.; Yajima, M. Herpes zoster and recurrent herpes zoster. *Open Forum Infect. Dis.* **2017**, *4*, ofx007. [CrossRef]
42. Toyama, N.; Shiraki, K. Epidemiology of herpes zoster and its relationship to varicella in Japan: A 10-year survey of 48,388 herpes zoster cases in Miyazaki prefecture. *J. Med. Virol.* **2009**, *81*, 2053–2058. [CrossRef] [PubMed]

43. Hama, Y.; Shiraki, K.; Yoshida, Y.; Maruyama, A.; Yasuda, M.; Tsuda, M.; Honda, M.; Takahashi, M.; Higuchi, H.; Takasaki, I.; et al. Antibody to varicella-zoster virus immediate-early protein 62 augments allodynia in zoster via brain-derived neurotrophic factor. *J. Virol.* **2010**, *84*, 1616–1624. [CrossRef] [PubMed]
44. Dworkin, R.H.; Johnson, R.W.; Breuer, J.; Gnann, J.W.; Levin, M.J.; Backonja, M.; Betts, R.F.; Gershon, A.A.; Haanpaa, M.L.; McKendrick, M.W.; et al. Recommendations for the management of herpes zoster. *Clin. Infect. Dis.* **2007**, *44*, 1–26. [CrossRef] [PubMed]
45. Lewis, G.W. Zoster sine herpete. *Br. Med. J.* **1958**, *2*, 418–421. [CrossRef] [PubMed]
46. Chemaly, R.F.; Ullmann, A.J.; Stoelben, S.; Richard, M.P.; Bornhäuser, M.; Groth, C.; Einsele, H.; Silverman, M.; Mullane, K.M.; Brown, J.; et al. Letermovir for cytomegalovirus prophylaxis in hematopoietic-cell transplantation. *N. Engl. J. Med.* **2014**, *370*, 1781–1789. [CrossRef] [PubMed]
47. Gnann, J.W., Jr.; Crumpacker, C.S.; Lalezari, J.P.; Smith, J.A.; Tyring, S.K.; Baum, K.F.; Borucki, M.J.; Joseph, W.P.; Mertz, G.J.; Steigbigel, R.T.; et al. Sorivudine versus acyclovir for treatment of dermatomal herpes zoster in human immunodeficiency virus-infected patients: Results from a randomized, controlled clinical trial. Collaborative Antiviral Study Group/AIDS Clinical Trials Group, Herpes Zoster Study Group. *Antimicrob. Agents Chemother.* **1998**, *42*, 1139–1145.
48. Bodsworth, N.J.; Boag, F.; Burdge, D.; Généreux, M.; Borleffs, J.C.; Evans, B.A.; Modai, J.; Colebunders, R.; Thomas, M.; DeHertogh, D.; et al. Evaluation of sorivudine (BV-araU) versus acyclovir in the treatment of acute localized herpes zoster in human immunodeficiency virus-infected adults. The Multinational Sorivudine Study Group. *J. Infect. Dis.* **1997**, *176*, 103–111. [CrossRef]
49. Imafuku, S.; Korematsu, K.; Mori, N.; Kani, T.; Matsui, K. Investigation of the safety and efficacy of Amenamevir (Amenalief® tablet 200 mg) in patients with herpes zoster (interim report from a Special drug use-result survey). *J. Jpn. Organ. Clin. Dermatol.* **2020**, *37*, 641–649.
50. Onaka, T.; Shiraki, K.; Yonezawa, A. Improvement of acyclovir-resistant herpes zoster infection by amenamevir. *J. Dermatol.* **2021**, in press. [CrossRef] [PubMed]

viruses

MDPI

Review

Recent Advances in Developing Treatments of Kaposi's Sarcoma Herpesvirus-Related Diseases

Eleonora Naimo [1,2], Jasmin Zischke [1,2] and Thomas F. Schulz [1,2,3,*]

1 Institute of Virology, Hannover Medical School, 30625 Hannover, Germany; naimo.eleonora@mh-hannover.de (E.N.); zischke.jasmin@mh-hannover.de (J.Z.)
2 German Centre for Infection Research, Hannover-Braunschweig Site, 38023 Braunschweig, Germany
3 Cluster of Excellence 2155 RESIST, Institute of Virology, Hannover Medical School, 30625 Hannover, Germany
* Correspondence: Schulz.Thomas@mh-hannover.de

Abstract: Kaposi-sarcoma-associated herpesvirus (KSHV) or human herpesvirus 8 (HHV-8) is the causative agent of several malignancies, including Kaposi's sarcoma (KS), primary effusion lymphoma (PEL), and multicentric Castleman's disease (MCD). Active KSHV replication has also been associated with a pathological condition called KSHV inflammatory cytokine syndrome (KICS), and KSHV may play a role in rare cases of post-transplant polyclonal lymphoproliferative disorders. Several commonly used herpesviral DNA polymerase inhibitors are active against KSHV in tissue culture. Unfortunately, they are not always efficacious against KSHV-induced diseases. To improve the outcome for the patients, new therapeutics need to be developed, including treatment strategies that target either viral proteins or cellular pathways involved in tumor growth and/or supporting the viral life cycle. In this review, we summarize the most commonly established treatments against KSHV-related diseases and review recent developments and promising new compounds that are currently under investigation or on the way to clinical use.

Keywords: KSHV; HHV-8; Kaposi's sarcoma; multicentric Castleman's disease; primary effusion lymphoma; DNA polymerase; LANA; TK (ORF21); PK (ORF36); ORF59; vFLIP; RTA; LANA; CRISPR-Cas9

Citation: Naimo, E.; Zischke, J.; Schulz, T.F. Recent Advances in Developing Treatments of Kaposi's Sarcoma Herpesvirus-Related Diseases. *Viruses* **2021**, *13*, 1797. https://doi.org/10.3390/v13091797

Academic Editor: Barry J. Margulies

Received: 30 July 2021
Accepted: 1 September 2021
Published: 9 September 2021

1. Introduction

Kaposi's sarcoma-associated herpesvirus (KSHV) is a double-stranded DNA virus, discovered in 1994 by Patrick Moore and Yuan Chang and classified as a human gamma2-herpesvirus [1]. KSHV is associated with three neoplastic diseases: Kaposi's sarcoma (KS) [1], multicentric Castleman's disease (MCD) [2] and primary effusion lymphoma (PEL) [3]; As reviewed elsewhere, it meets the epidemiological and basic research requirements for recognition as an oncogenic agent and has thus been classified as a class I human carcinogen by the International Agency for Research against Cancer (IARC) [4,5]. Additionally, KSHV has also been associated with a pathological condition called KSHV inflammatory cytokine syndrome (KICS) [6] and rare cases of post-transplant polyclonal lymphoproliferative disorders [7,8] as well as with cases of plasmablastic lymphoma emerging from MCD [9].

The histopathological features of KS include atypical vascularization and neoangiogenesis with extensive infiltrates of inflammatory cells and the proliferation of atypical endothelial spindle cells [10]. Based on epidemiological criteria, KS has been classified into four different forms that are histologically similar [11]. Moritz Kaposi described KS for the first time in 1872 as a rare tumor endemic in the Mediterranean area that mostly affected middle-aged and older men. This "classic" KS is characterized by indolent skin lesions and viscera are only rarely involved [12].

In East and Central Africa, a more aggressive form of KS (the "endemic African" KS) in HIV-negative patients involves internal organs and lymph nodes in children and adults [13,14]. The "iatrogenic" KS affects up to 25% (in KSHV endemic regions) of transplant recipients under immunosuppressive therapy who were previously infected with KSHV [15,16]. This form of KS often recedes after the interruption of the immunosuppressive therapy [17,18].

In the 1980s, following the emergence of HIV/AIDS, the AIDS-associated or epidemic KS became a common manifestation among HIV-infected people [19]. AIDS-KS is the most aggressive form of KS. It can involve the lungs and the gastrointestinal tract [20]. After the introduction of the antiretroviral combination therapy (ART) against HIV, the incidence of this variant of KS was significantly reduced [19,21–24].

Primary effusion lymphoma (PEL) or body cavity-based lymphoma (BCBL) is a B cell non-Hodgkin lymphoma characterized by lymphomatous effusions in the pleural, pericardial and peritoneal body cavities [25]. PEL often arises in HIV-infected individuals and it is estimated to account for 2–5% of HIV-associated lymphomas [26]. PEL can also occur in transplant recipients [27]. KSHV DNA detection in the tumor cells is a diagnostic criterion for PEL [28,29].

Multicentric Castleman's disease is characterized by systemic inflammation, increased levels of cytokines IL-6, IL-10 and vIL6 and by clinical symptoms like lymphadenopathy, fever, diarrhea and weight loss. The patients with MCD are more prone to non-Hodgkin lymphomas and organ failure [30–33].

KSHV replication in KSHV-HIV positive patients may induce a systemic inflammation characterized by high levels of IL-6 and IL-10 and high KSHV viral load in the blood. This non-malignant clinical manifestation is called KSHV associated inflammatory cytokine syndrome (KICS). As the clinical symptoms and laboratory abnormalities overlap with those seen in MCD, the diagnosis of KICS is predicated on the absence of the lymphadenopathy seen in MCD. KICS can also arise in KS or PEL patients and is often associated with a more severe disease course [6,34].

Current antiviral treatments against KSHV mainly rely on herpesviral DNA polymerase inhibitors. Although some of them efficiently inhibit KSHV replication in tissue culture, their efficacy against KSHV-associated disease is limited. Surgery, radiotherapy, and chemotherapy combined with antiviral agents and immunomodulatory molecules are used to obtain the best outcome for these patients. In trying to develop novel approaches to an effective pharmacological treatment of KSHV-associated diseases, either the combination of antiviral drugs directed against different viral targets, or the targeting of cellular proteins that are required for viral persistence, replication ('dependency factors') or the growth of tumor cells are being explored.

2. KSHV DNA Polymerase Inhibitors

Since the discovery of KSHV, nucleoside inhibitors of the viral DNA polymerase such as ganciclovir, cidofovir, foscarnet, brivudine, and adefovir have provided the most potent inhibitors of KSHV replication in tissue culture [35–40]. In patients, some studies reported ganciclovir, valganciclovir, valacyclovir, famciclovir, cidofovir or foscarnet to reduce the shedding of KSHV in oral samples or KSHV viral load in peripheral blood, while others failed to notice pronounced effects of these drugs in treated patients [41–43]. With few exceptions [44], herpesviral DNA polymerase inhibitors (foscarnet, cidofovir, ganciclovir, valganciclovir) were found to be largely ineffective when used to treat established KS lesions [45–48]. In addition to these drugs, which are already approved for clinical use against other herpesviruses, several new promising nucleoside inhibitors have been identified in preclinical studies but are not yet approved or available for clinical treatments (for more details, see: [37,40,49–51].

The disappointing efficacy of herpesviral DNA polymerase inhibitors against KS is likely related to the fact that they are nucleoside analogs that, except for foscarnet, need to be phosphorylated to become active drugs. The first phosphorylation step is mediated by KSHV-encoded kinases, while generation of the nucleoside di- and triphosphates is due to the action of cellular kinases [40]. There are two KSHV kinases capable of activating nucleoside prodrugs by phosphorylation: a Ser/Thr kinase (vPK) encoded by open reading frame (ORF) 36 and a thymidine kinase (TK) encoded by ORF21. Both viral kinases are only expressed during the lytic phase of the viral cycle, and may thus only be able to exert their function in the relatively small number of infected cells in KS tumors that undergo lytic replication (see below).

Genes for herpesviral TKs occur in alpha- and gammaherpesviruses, but not in betaherpesviruses. In alpha- and gammaherpesviruses, the TK homologs are conserved: UL23 of herpes simplex virus 1 and 2 (HSV-1/2), ORF36 of varicella-zoster virus (VZV), BXLF1 of Epstein-Barr virus (EBV), and ORF21 of KSHV (52). Herpesviral TKs differ in their capacity to phosphorylate nucleoside analogs. Pyrimidine nucleosides such as brivudine and azidothymidine (zidovudine, the anti-HIV nucleoside reverse transcriptase inhibitor) are efficiently phosphorylated by KSHV TK [40,52]. Instead, PK/ORF36 efficiently phosphorylates purine analogs like valganciclovir [53].

As in the case of KS, the use of these viral DNA polymerase inhibitors against PEL and MCD has also in most cases only produced unsatisfactory clinical results [41,54–58]. The only notable exception is the combination of high dose ganciclovir and zidovudine in patients with MCD, which has shown promising clinical response rates [59]. This drug regimen is based on the activation of the prodrug zidovudine to a toxic moiety by KSHV TK, in combination with the antiviral effects of ganciclovir [59].

The limited efficacy of the DNA polymerase inhibitors pushed the scientific community to identify other suitable targets with different molecular mechanisms to treat KSHV-associated disease.

3. Antivirals Targeting Other Steps in the Viral Life Cycle

KSHV, like the other members of the Herpesviridae family, has a biphasic life cycle characterized by distinct patterns of viral gene expression [60]. KSHV establishes a permanent infection that lasts for the entire life of the infected host. During the KSHV latent phase, the viral DNA is maintained as a circular episome in the infected cells, replicated in dividing cells together with the cellular DNA [61,62], and a few latency-associated genes are transcribed: these encode the latency-associated nuclear antigen (LANA, encoded by ORF73), the viral homolog of cyclin D (vCyc-D/ORF72), the viral homolog of the fas-associated death domain-like interleukin-1-β-converting enzyme (FLICE-) inhibitory protein (vFLIP/ORF71), Kaposin (A, B and C encoded by K12) and 25 mature microRNAs [63–66]. In order to produce new viral progeny, KSHV has to periodically reactivate from latency and to switch into the productive ('lytic') phase of its life cycle. During the immediate-early and early stages of productive KSHV infection, only a subset of lytic viral genes is expressed. Following the replication of the viral DNA, viral genes encoding viral structural proteins are switched on ('late' phase of the productive replication cycle) in order to allow the production of new viral progeny [67].

In KS and PEL, the majority of KSHV infected cells adopt the latent program; therefore, a considerable effort has been made to target latent viral proteins or cellular pathways in which they interfere.

LANA (latency-associated nuclear antigen) is expressed in all the latently KSHV-infected cells [35,68]. In PEL cells, decreasing LANA expression with shRNA [69], by treatment with glycyrrhizic acid [70] or HSP90 inhibitors [71] induces cell death. The gene-editing technique, CRISPR-Cas9, has also been used successfully in two studies to target KSHV LANA and to target KSHV latency [72,73]. These findings suggest that LANA may be a promising viral target to disrupt KSHV latency. Its C-terminal DNA-binding domain (DBD) binds the latent KSHV replication origin in the terminal repeat (TRs) region of the viral genome; this interaction ensures the viral genome replication and segregation during cell mitosis [62,74–77]. The structure of the LANA DBD alone and in complex with the viral latent replication origin has been solved [76,78], allowing Kirsch and colleagues to discover and optimize new small compounds able to inhibit the binding of LANA to viral DNA in the low micromolar range [79–81]. In addition, Mubritinib (TAK165) was identified as a potent inhibitor of LANA-DNA binding and strongly reduced living KSHV PEL cells in vitro and in vivo [82].

Another potential target of the latent KSHV cycle is the viral FLICE-inhibitory protein (vFLIP). vFLIP is a potent activator of the NF-kB pathway and counteracts Fas-induced apoptosis [83,84]. Silencing vFLIP using siRNA [85] or using NF-kB inhibitors such as Bay 11-7082 [83,86–88] induces PEL cell apoptosis, suggesting that vFLIP may also represent an attractive therapeutic target. In order to activate the NF-kB pathway, vFLIP directly interacts with IKKγ/NEMO, a key player in the canonical NF-kB pathway [85,89]. The structure of a fragment of the coiled-coil domains of IKKγ/NEMO in complex with vFLIP has been solved [90], which provided the basis for a structure-guided development of vFLIP inhibitors. A conformationally constrained, stapled IKKγ peptide derived from the IKKγ–vFLIP interaction site interferes with the binding of IKKγ to vFLIP and enhances apoptosis in PEL cell lines [91]. Also, a tertiary protein structure mimic of the vFLIP-interaction site in the IKKγ/NEMO helix was able to induce cell death in PEL cell lines and to delay tumor growth in a PEL xenograft mouse model [88]. These findings indicate that it may be feasible to develop small molecule inhibitors targeting the vFLIP-IKKγ/NEMO interaction and showing a therapeutic effect against some KSHV-associated diseases.

New approaches to target the productive ('lytic') phase of the KSHV life cycle have also been developed but remain at a preclinical stage. Among the viral immediate early proteins to be expressed early after lytic reactivation are RTA, K-bZIP, and pORF45, crucial regulatory proteins and/or transcription factors [92,93]. RTA (encoded by ORF50) is necessary and sufficient to trigger the KSHV lytic phase, thus it is called "the master of KSHV lytic-switch" [94]. Long and colleagues recently described the efficiency of Gallic acid (GA) to inhibit RTA transcriptional activity by preventing its binding to target promoters. GA induces apoptosis in a PEL cell line in a dose-dependent manner [95].

Another novel viral target is the KSHV protein encoded by ORF59. pORF59 is a homologue of the DNA polymerase-associated processivity factor, which occurs in pro- as well as eukaryotes and in all herpesviruses. By acting in concert with the KSHV DNA polymerase encoded by ORF9, it facilitates the elongation of newly synthesized viral DNA. The compound NSC373989 was shown to target the pORF9/pORF59 complex and to inhibit viral DNA synthesis in vitro as well as KSHV lytic reactivation in PEL cells [96]. An inhibitor of pORF59 could provide an alternative approach to inhibiting viral DNA replication during the lytic phase of the replication and could potentially be used in combination with established competitive DNA polymerase inhibitors.

The structural similarity between the RNAse H-like nucleotidyltransferase domain contained in the HIV integrase and the two single-strand DNA (ssDNA) binding proteins essential for herpesviral DNA replication allowed the identification of XZ45, an HIV integrase inhibitor, as a compound that also inhibits the replication of KSHV and other herpesviruses [97]. Raltegravir and Dolutegravir, two HIV integrase inhibitors approved for clinical use against HIV, were successfully tested in vitro for their inhibition of the KSHV large terminase subunit encoded by pORF29. The C-terminal domain of KSHV pORF29 also shows a high degree of similarity with RNAse H-like nucleotidyltransferases and its inhibition impairs KSHV lytic reactivation in tissue culture [98].

In the case of herpes simplex virus (HSV), Varicella-Zoster virus (VZV), and human cytomegalovirus (HCMV), structure-based drug design has been employed to target capsid proteins, capsid assembly, and DNA encapsidation and this approach has already shown promising results [99–102]. One compound, letermovir, targets the HCMV terminase and the incorporation of viral DNA into newly formed viral capsids and has been approved for clinical use in stem cell transplant recipients [103]. However, it is not active against KSHV or other human herpesviruses. For KSHV, inhibitors of the pORF17 scaffold/protease polyprotein, which transiently fills the newly assembled capsid and is then released by autoproteolytic cleavage to allow packaging of capsids with viral DNA [104], have been developed and some have shown potency in tissue culture [105–107]. Nelfinavir, an HIV protease inhibitor, has been shown by Gantt and colleagues to inhibit KSHV, HSV and

HCMV replication. Whether the KSHV pORF17 scaffold/protease is the key target of nelfinavir however still remains unclear [108,109].

Attempts were also made to target viral glycoproteins expressed on the surface of KSHV infected cells such as K8.1 and gH, by using immunotoxins that bind to these viral proteins. These immunotoxins could induce cell death in KSHV-infected cells in tissue culture, and a combination with ganciclovir increased their effect [110,111].

An opposite approach to inhibiting the viral lytic replication cycle involves its activation, with the aiming of taking advantage of the cell death occurring in lytically reactivated cells. Different treatments aimed to induce the viral lytic cycle in latently KSHV-infected cells have been attempted. Treatment with histone deacetylase (HADAC) inhibitors like sodium butyrate (NaB/SB), 12-*O*-tetradecanoylphorbol-13-acetate (TPA), and trichostatin (TSA), with the DNA methyltransferase inhibitor 5-Azacytidine (5-AZaC) or with some African autochthonous plant extracts can induce the lytic reactivation in vitro [112–115]. The proteasome inhibitor bortezomib induces KSHV and EBV lytic reactivation and it was successfully used in a clinical trial in combination with ganciclovir to treat MCD [57]. Liang and colleagues used the CRISPR-Cas9 system to inhibit the expression of KSHV miRNAs in latently KSHV positive PEL cells. This alters the expression of the mature miRNAs and induces upregulation of the viral lytic genes [116]. Recently, the suberoyl bis-hydroxamic acid (SAHA) was selected for its ability to induce KSHV lytic reactivation and apoptosis in a dose-dependent manner in PEL cells, indicating its possible therapeutic use [117].

Another possible strategy to counteract KSHV infection could be inhibition of virus entry into the target cell. This has so far proved difficult, because KSHV entry is mediated through diverse receptors, depending on the cell type that is to be infected. Binding of KSHV to the cell surface is achieved by heparan sulfate-proteoglycans (HSPGs) and DC-SIGN and entry is mediated through Ephrin receptors (EPHA2, 4, 5 and 7), integrins ($\alpha3\beta1$, $\alpha V\beta3$, $\alpha V\beta5$, and $\alpha5\beta1$) and xCT (reviewed in [118]).

4. Cellular Targets to Inhibit KSHV Replication

Instead of targeting the virus replication directly by inhibiting a viral protein, there are several ways of inhibiting the virus by targeting cellular processes that are essential for the virus to survive. As viruses hijack the host cells and exploit the cell machinery, there are several cellular proteins that play an important role in the viral life cycle and that can be targeted pharmacologically. A potential drawback of this approach is that these cellular processes are also important for cellular functions and that the inhibition of these targets may be accompanied by side effects.

4.1. Kinase Inhibitors

In KSHV infected cells, cellular tyrosine kinases play an essential role during the KSHV life cycle. Therefore, targeting cellular receptor tyrosine kinases such as c-kit, PDGFR, VEGFR, and Eph2A for antiviral treatment was investigated in several clinical studies. Treatment of KS patients with imatinib, a c-abl tyrosine kinase inhibitor in clinical use for the treatment of chronic myelogenous leukemia, resulted in clinical and histological regression of KS lesions in some patients [119,120]. Furthermore, sorafenib, which inhibits the VEGF receptor and is used to treat several malignancies like hepatocellular carcinoma or kidney carcinoma, was shown in a case report to achieve a complete remission of KS lesions in one patient [121]. Unfortunately, sorafenib showed only moderate effects when used to treat KS in a phase 1b clinical trial [122].

Of the more than 20 currently available inhibitors of cellular tyrosine kinases, five compounds (dasatinib, ponatinib, bosutinib, gefitinib, and nilotinib) were shown to also inhibit KSHV thymidine kinase (TK/pORF21), which, in contrast to its name, acts as an efficient protein tyrosine kinase [52,123]. Dasatinib and ponatinib also strongly inhibited KSHV early viral gene expression and the production of new viral progeny in B, endothelial and epithelial cells, most likely as a result of the inhibition of cellular tyrosine kinases, and dasatinib inhibited the growth of KSHV-driven endothelial tumors in a mouse xenograft model [52]. UNC3810A, a small molecule inhibitor of the receptor tyrosine kinase Tyro3, a member of the Tyro3/Axl/Mer (TAM) family of tyrosine kinases that promote the proliferation and survival of several cancers, was shown to be a potent inhibitor of PEL cell growth in a mouse xenograft model [124].

In KSHV infected cells, mTOR, a cellular kinase that belongs to the phosphatidylinositol 3-kinase related family of protein kinases, plays a key role in the life cycle of KSHV by promoting the activation of mTOR downstream of the viral G-protein coupled receptor (GPCR) homologue vGPCR. Blocking mTOR activity by rapamycin (sirolimus) inhibited cell growth in cell culture and tumor growth in a KSHV related mouse model, whereas overstimulation of the mTOR pathway resulted in the opposite, showing that this pathway is important for KSHV [125,126]. Several mTOR inhibitors reduce the growth of PEL cell lines in tissue culture and/or in mouse xenograft models, in particular when combined with an AKT inhibitor [127–129]. An ATP-competitive inhibitor of mTOR, MLN0128 (sapanisertib), induces apoptosis in PEL cells and reduces the growth of PEL in a xenograft model at nanomolar IC50 concentrations and is still effective against doxorubicin- or rapamycin-resistant PEL cell clones [129].

Similarly, the ERK/MAPK pathway was shown to be crucial in KSHV induced pathogenesis [130]. Several experimental compounds, e.g., sangivamycin and capsaicin, as well as trametinib, a MEK1/2 inhibitor approved for clinical use, can inhibit ERK activation and KSHV reactivation, and/or are able to induce apoptosis in PEL cell lines, suggesting that they could perhaps be used for the treatment of PEL [52,131,132]. BI-D1870, a RSK1/2 inhibitor, suppresses KSHV lytic gene expression and virus production. The RSK1/2 serine/threonine kinase is activated by its interaction with KSHV pORF45 and a small peptide blocking this interaction has been shown to inhibit viral lytic gene expression and viral progeny formation [133]. Furthermore, crizotinib, an inhibitor of ALK and c-Met, suppresses the growth of PEL cells in a mouse xenograft model [134].

4.2. HSP90 and HSP70 Inhibitors

HSP90 is a molecular chaperone required for the correct folding of cellular proteins. HSP90 inhibitors have found use as anti-cancer drugs to treat several malignancies, including lung or prostate cancer. Several groups have shown that HSP90 is also involved in essential steps in the KSHV life cycle: vFLIP, a viral latent protein, is found in a complex containing IKKγ/NEMO and HSP90 [135]. HSP90 serves as a co-factor for MAPK activation and latent viral gene expression of KSHV, and the KSHV K1 protein was shown to bind $HSP90_\beta$ [89,136,137].

Several HSP90 inhibitors have been used in cell culture studies and mouse models of KSHV malignancies. In particular treating KSHV positive cells with different HSP90 inhibitors (PU-H71, AUY922, BIIB021, NVP-BEP800, or 17-DMAG) leads to the proteasomal degradation of LANA and Eph2A and inhibited cell growth as well as induced apoptosis in PEL cells [71,138]. Furthermore, PU-H71, BIIB021, and AUY922 also repressed tumor progression in xenograft mouse models [138–140]. These are encouraging data, but HSP90 inhibitors have not yet been tested in clinical trials against KSHV malignancies.

Several HSP70 chaperone family members are involved in the formation of KSHV nuclear replication and transcription compartments (RTCs) during the early stages of the KSHV lytic cycle, and a small molecule HSP70 inhibitor, VER-155008, blocked KSHV RTC formation [141]. Formation of KSHV RTCs also involves neddylation, and the neddylation inhibitor MLN 4924 induces apoptosis in PEL cells [142].

4.3. Other Cellular Targets

Another promising drug candidate for treating patients with KSHV malignancies is bortezomib, a proteasome inhibitor, which has been shown to promote the KSHV and EBV lytic cycle. Bortezomib activates JNK and induces autophagy and apoptosis in PEL cell lines [143,144] and in a xenograft mouse model [145]. Further clinical studies confirmed this drug as a potential treatment against AIDS-associated KS in a pilot trial study, AMC-063 [146] and in combination with ganciclovir against MCD in a case report [55].

Recently, Chen et al. could show that pemetrexed, an anti-cancer drug already in clinical use, is able to inhibit the lytic replication of KSHV by blocking the dTMP synthesis in infected cells [147].

Other cellular factors that are important for the KSHV replication machinery and which could be targeted pharmacologically include topoisomerase II: (+)-Rutamarin, a topoisomerase II inhibitor that efficiently inhibits KSHV lytic DNA replication in BCBL-1 cells [148].

Hypoxia and hypoxia-mediated signaling are important factors that drive KSHV replication and may play a role in KSHV-associated malignancies. Thus, hypoxia-inducible factors (HIFs), the first mediators of the cellular response to hypoxia, play a crucial role in KSHV induced tumors and have been shown to activate KSHV lytic replication [149]. HIF1α can directly activate RTA, LANA, as well as the ORF34-37 cluster of lytic genes [150,151]. A small molecule inhibitor of HIF1α, PX-478, was shown to achieve a significant inhibition of PEL cell growth in tissue culture, suggesting that HIF1α could be a suitable target for treating this disease [152].

Other cellular metabolic targets include the metabolic sensor SIRT1 that is functionally required for sustaining the proliferation and survival of PEL cells. Inhibition of SIRT with the inhibitor tenovin-6 induced cell cycle arrest and apoptosis in PEL cell culture and significantly extended the survival of mice in a murine PEL model [153].

Heme oxygenase 1 (HO-1) is highly expressed in KSHV-infected HUVECs cells. Targeting HO-1 by siRNA or by the chemical inhibitor SnPP induces cell death in KSHV-infected endothelial cells and inhibits their growth as tumors in nude mice [154].

However, with the exceptions mentioned above, most of these inhibitors directed at cellular targets have so far not been studied in clinical trials. Nevertheless, these findings show the potential of targeting cellular mechanisms for the treatment of KSHV-associated diseases.

5. Monoclonal Antibodies and Immunomodulatory Therapies

Several monoclonal antibodies have been used to treat KSHV-related diseases. One of the targets to have been explored in this manner is the vascular endothelial growth factor (VEGF). Bevacizumab, a humanized monoclonal antibody against VEGF-A, showed an overall response rate of 31% in patients with HIV-associated KS [155,156]. Furthermore, rituximab, a monoclonal antibody against CD20 that is widely used to treat several types of B-cell lymphoma and autoimmune diseases, is effective in clinical trials against multicentric Castleman's disease, either alone or in combination with liposomal doxorubicin [157]. However, treatment with rituximab can also cause the progression of KS in these patients [158,159].

Tocilizumab, a monoclonal antibody directed against the inteleukin-6 receptor that is currently used to treat rheumatoid arthritis and other autoimmune diseases, has also been shown to be beneficial in treating MCD [160–162].

The combination of lenalidomide, an immunomodulatory drug, with arsenic trioxide (ATO), which is normally used to treat acute promyelocytic leukemia, has been reported to produce encouraging results when treating PEL in a xenograft mouse model. In this study, lenalidomide/ATO treatment decreased the proliferation of PEL cells and downregulated the expression of KSHV latent viral proteins. This was associated with less NF-kB expression and downregulation of IL-6 and IL-10 as well as the inhibition of VEGF and the induction of apoptosis [163].

Pomalidomide, another immunomodulatory drug, has been shown to act against KS in HIV-negative and HIV-positive people in a clinical Phase I/II trial. Pomalidomide induced an increase in ICAM-1 and B7-2 expression in PEL cells, thereby leading to T cell activation and NK cell-mediated killing of PEL cells, which makes pomalidomide a promising candidate for the treatment of KSHV related malignancies [164,165].

6. KSHV Tropism and Models to Study the Virus

KSHV shows a relatively strict species tropism for humans. In vivo, viral DNA has been detected in human B cells [166], macrophages [167], keratinocytes, endothelial cells [168,169] and epithelial cells [170]. In vitro, KSHV can infect a broad spectrum of different cells including epithelial cells, endothelial cells, keratinocytes, fibroblasts, B- and T-lymphocytes, monocytes, macrophages and dendritic cells [167,168,171,172]. Besides, KSHV can infect non-human cell lines such as owl monkey kidney cells, baby hamster kidney fibroblasts cells, Chinese hamster ovary cells and mouse fibroblasts [173].

The B-cell lines derived from PEL patients are used to study KSHV pathogenesis in vitro as they are able to maintain the viral genome in a latent state. In contrast, the endothelial spindle cells lose the virus after a few passages in cell culture [174].

KSHV-infected lymphatic endothelial cells (LECs) exploit a unique transcription program with the expression of latent and lytic genes, which differs from the latency program described in stably infected blood endothelial cells (HUVECs) [175,176], both models are used to characterize KSHV molecular mechanisms of action.

Because of its restricted species tropism, studying KSHV infection in vivo is not straightforward. There are mainly three ways of how KSHV infection can be studied in vivo (nicely reviewed in [177]): the first is to infect non-human primates like common marmosets with KSHV [178]. The second approach involves the use of KSHV related viruses, like murine herpesvirus 68 (MHV-68), rhesus rhadinovirus (RRV) [179] or herpesvirus saimiri (HVS) [180].

MHV-68 infects mice and is used as a model to mimic KSHV infection, because it has been shown that 90% of the MHV-68 genes have homologs to KSHV [181]. MHV-68 behaves like a natural persisting pathogen in mice but without showing the disease. Therefore, MHV-68 is often used to study immunological topics like immunevasion and infection control by T cells. Nevertheless, this model is not suitable to study host colonialization and viral reactivation nor can it be used to study KSHV related malignancies [182].

The third approach, which is becoming increasingly more important, is to use humanized mice. In a xenograft mouse model, human PEL derived cell lines are implanted into immunodeficient mice to establish a PEL like phenotype [182,183]. McHugh et al. described an animal model, showing that coinfection with EBV establishes persistent KSHV infection in B cells, resulting in a PEL like phenotype in these mice [184].

7. Conclusions

Immunocompromised patients and people living in KSHV-endemic areas are most likely to be affected by KSHV-induced diseases. Despite more than 25 years of research on KSHV, we still lack effective therapies to counteract KSHV infection, reactivation and pathogenicity (Table S1). However, progress has been made over recent years and both new viral as well as cellular 'druggable' targets have emerged. Some of the insights into KSHV pathogenesis that have been made over the last two decades have also laid the ground for the development of active compounds that may find use in other malignancies. As KSHV-related malignancies are not among the most common cancers and often occur in economically disadvantaged countries, the development of effective drugs against KSHV and KSHV-associated diseases faces the obstacle of a lack of interest on the part of the pharmaceutical industry. Focusing on mechanisms of pathogenicity that are shared between KSHV-related and other, more common, malignancies may open up a way forward to overcome this obstacle.

Supplementary Materials: The following are available online at https://www.mdpi.com/article/10.3390/v13091797/s1, Table S1: Therapies in clinical trials.

Funding: This research received no external funding.

Institutional Review Board Statement: Not Applicable.

Informed Consent Statement: Not Applicable.

Data Availability Statement: Not Applicable.

Acknowledgments: Work in TFS' group is supported by by the Deutsche Forschungsgemeinschaft (DFG, German Research Foundation) under Germany's Excellence Strategy—EXC 2155 "RESIST"—Project ID 39087428 and the Collaborative Research Center 900 'Chronic Infections' (Project C1), as well as the German Center for Infection Research (TTU IICH) and the Lower Saxony Ministry of Science and Culture (project 14-76103-184).

Conflicts of Interest: The authors declare no conflict of interest.

References

1. Chang, Y.; Cesarman, E.; Pessin, M.; Lee, F.; Culpepper, J.; Knowles, D.; Moore, P. Identification of herpesvirus-like DNA sequences in AIDS-associated Kaposi's sarcoma. *Science* **1994**, *266*, 1865–1869. [CrossRef] [PubMed]
2. Soulier, J.; Grollet, L.; Oksenhendler, E.; Cacoub, P.; Cazals-Hatem, D.; Babinet, P.; D'Agay, M.F.; Clauvel, J.P.; Raphael, M.; Degos, L. Kaposi's sarcoma-associated herpesvirus-like DNA sequences in multicentric Castleman's disease. *Blood* **1995**, *86*, 1276–1280. [CrossRef]
3. Cesarman, E.; Chang, Y.; Moore, P.; Said, J.W.; Knowles, D.M. Kaposi's Sarcoma–Associated Herpesvirus-Like DNA Sequences in AIDS-Related Body-Cavity–Based Lymphomas. *N. Engl. J. Med.* **1995**, *332*, 1186–1191. [CrossRef]
4. Bouvard, V.; Baan, R.; Straif, K.; Grosse, Y.; Lauby-Secretan, B.; El Ghissassi, F.; Benbrahim-Tallaa, L.; Guha, N.; Freeman, C.; Galichet, L.; et al. A review of human carcinogens—Part B: Biological agents. *Lancet Oncol.* **2009**, *10*, 321–322. [CrossRef]
5. Longnecker, R.; Neipel, F. Introduction to the human γ-herpesviruses. In *Human Herpesviruses: Biology, Therapy, and Immunoprophylaxis*; Arvin, A., Campadelli-Fiume, G., Mocarski, E., Moore, P.S., Roizman, B., Whitley, R., Eds.; Cambridge Ubiversity Press: Cambridge, UK, 2007.
6. Uldrick, T.S.; Wang, V.; O'Mahony, D.; Aleman, K.; Wyvill, K.M.; Marshall, V.; Steinberg, S.M.; Pittaluga, S.; Maric, I.; Whitby, D.; et al. An Interleukin-6–Related Systemic Inflammatory Syndrome in Patients Co-Infected with Kaposi Sarcoma–Associated Herpesvirus and HIV but without Multicentric Castleman Disease. *Clin. Infect. Dis.* **2010**, *51*, 350–358. [CrossRef]
7. Matsushima, A.Y.; Strauchen, J.A.; Lee, G.; Scigliano, E.; Hale, E.E.; Weisse, M.T.; Burstein, D.; Kamel, O.; Moore, P.S.; Chang, Y. Posttransplantation Plasmacytic Proliferations Related to Kaposi's Sarcoma–Associated Herpesvirus. *Am. J. Surg. Pathol.* **1999**, *23*, 1393. [CrossRef] [PubMed]
8. Kapelushnik, J.; Ariad, S.; Benharroch, D.; Landau, D.; Moser, A.; Delsol, G.; Brousset, P. Post renal transplantation human herpesvirus 8-associated lymphoproliferative disorder and Kaposi's sarcoma. *Br. J. Haematol.* **2001**, *113*, 425–428. [CrossRef]
9. Dupin, N.; Diss, T.L.; Kellam, P.; Tulliez, M.; Du, M.-Q.; Sicard, D.; Weiss, R.A.; Isaacson, P.G.; Boshoff, C. HHV-8 is associated with a plasmablastic variant of Castleman disease that is linked to HHV-8–positive plasmablastic lymphoma. *Blood* **2000**, *95*, 1406–1412. [CrossRef] [PubMed]
10. Orenstein, J.M. Ultrastructure of Kaposi Sarcoma. *Ultrastruct. Pathol.* **2008**, *32*, 211–220. [CrossRef]
11. Antman, K.; Chang, Y. Kaposi's sarcoma. *N. Engl. J. Med.* **2000**, *342*, 1027–1038. [CrossRef]
12. Kaposi, M. Idiopathisches multiples Pigmentsarkom der Haut. *Arch. Dermatol. Syph.* **1872**, *4*, 265–273. [CrossRef]
13. Plancoulaine, S.; Abel, L.; van Beveren, M.; Trégouët, D.A.; Joubert, M.; Tortevoye, P. Human herpesvirus 8 transmission from mother to child and between siblings in an endemic population. *Lancet* **2000**, *356*, 1062–1065. [CrossRef]
14. Dedicoat, M.; Newton, R.; Alkharsah, K.R.; Sheldon, J.; Szabados, I.; Ndlovu, B. Mother-to-Child Transmission of Human Herpesvirus-8 in South Africa. *J. Infect. Dis.* **2004**, *190*, 1068–1075. [CrossRef] [PubMed]
15. Lebbé, C.; Legendre, C.; Francès, C. Kaposi sarcoma in transplantation. *Transplant. Rev.* **2008**, *22*, 252–261. [CrossRef]
16. Cattani, P.; Capuano, M.; Graffeo, R.; Ricci, R.; Cerimele, F.; Cerimele, D.; Nanni, G.; Fadda, G. Kaposi's Sarcoma Associated with Previous Human Herpesvirus 8 Infection in Kidney Transplant Recipients. *J. Clin. Microbiol.* **2001**, *39*, 506–508. [CrossRef]
17. Grulich, E.A.; van Leeuwen, M.; Falster, M.; Vajdic, C. Incidence of cancers in people with HIV/AIDS compared with immunosuppressed transplant recipients: A meta-analysis. *Lancet* **2007**, *370*, 59–67. [CrossRef]
18. Francès, C.; Marcelin, A.G.; Legendre, C.; Chevret, S.; Dussaix, E.; Lejeune, J.T. The impact of Preexisting or Acquired Kaposi Sarcoma Herpesvirus infection in Kidney Trasplant Recipiens on Morbidity and Survival. *Am. J. Transpl.* **2009**, *9*, 2580–2586. [CrossRef]
19. Wabinga, H.R.; Nambooze, S.; Amulen, P.M.; Okello, C.; Mbus, L.; Parkin, D.M. Trends in the incidence of cancer in Kampala, Uganda 1991–2010. *Int. J. Cancer.* **2014**, *135*, 432–439. [CrossRef]
20. Friedman-Kien, A.E. Disseminated Kaposi's sarcoma syndrome in young homosexual men. *J. Am. Acad. Dermatol.* **1981**, *5*, 468–471. [CrossRef]
21. Dupin, N.; De Cervens, V.R.; Gorin, I.; Calvez, V.; Pessis, E.; Grandadam, M.; Rabian, C.; Viard, J.P.; Huraux, J.M.; Escande, J.P. The influence of highly active antiretroviral therapy on AIDS-associated Kaposi's sarcoma. *Br. J. Dermatol.* **1999**, *140*, 875–881. [CrossRef]
22. Cattelan, A.; Calabro', M.; Aversa, S.; Zanchetta, M.; Meneghetti, F.; De Rossi, A.; Chieco-Bianchi, L. Regression of AIDS-related Kaposi's sarcoma following antiretroviral therapy with protease inhibitors: Biological correlates of clinical outcome. *Eur. J. Cancer* **1999**, *35*, 1809–1815. [CrossRef]

23. Van Leeuwen, M.; Vajdic, C.; Middleton, M.G.; McDonald, A.M.; Law, M.; Kaldor, J.M.; Grulich, A.E. Continuing declines in some but not all HIV-associated cancers in Australia after widespread use of antiretroviral therapy. *AIDS* **2009**, *23*, 2183–2190. [CrossRef] [PubMed]
24. Grulich, A.E.; Li, Y.; McDonald, A.M.; Correll, P.K.; Law, M.G.; Kaldor, J.M. Decreasing rates of Kaposi's sarcoma and non-Hodgkin's lymphoma in the era of potent combination anti-retroviral therapy. *AIDS* **2001**, *15*, 629–633. [CrossRef] [PubMed]
25. Knowles, D.M.; Inghirami, G.; Ubriaco, A.; Dalla-Favera, R. Molecular Genetic Analysis of Three AIDS-Associated Neoplasms of Uncertain Lineage Demonstrates Their B-Cell Derivation and the Possible Pathogenetic Role of the Epstein-Barr Virus. *Blood* **1989**, *73*, 792–799. [CrossRef] [PubMed]
26. Pan, Z.G.; Zhang, Q.Y.; Lu, Z.B.; Quinto, T.; Rozenvald, I.B.; Liu, L.-T. Extracavitary KSHV-associated large B-Cell lymphoma: A distinct entity or a subtype of primary effusion lymphoma? Study of 9 cases and review of an additional 43 cases. *Am. J. Surg. Pathol.* **2012**, *36*, 1129–1140. [CrossRef]
27. Boulanger, E.; Afonso, P.; Yahiaoui, Y.; Adle-Biassette, H.; Gabarre, J.; Agbalika, F. Human Herpesvirus-8 (HHV-8)-Associated Primary Effusion Lymphoma in two Renal Transplant Recipients Receiving Rapamycin. *Arab. Archaeol. Epigr.* **2008**, *8*, 707–710. [CrossRef]
28. Nador, R.G.; Cesarman, E.; Chadburn, A.; Dawson, D.B.; Ansari, M.Q.; Sald, J.; Knowles, D.M. Primary effusion lymphoma: A distinct clinicopathologic entity associated with the Kaposi's sarcoma-associated herpes virus. *Blood* **1996**, *88*, 645–656. [CrossRef]
29. Song, J.Y.; Jaffe, E.S. HHV-8–positive but EBV-negative primary effusion lymphoma. *Blood* **2013**, *122*, 3712. [CrossRef]
30. Castleman, B.; Towne, V.W. Case Records of the Massachusetts General Hospital: Case No. 40231. *N. Engl. J. Med.* **1954**, *250*, 1001–1005. [CrossRef]
31. Du, M.-Q.; Liu, H.; Diss, T.C.; Ye, H.; Hamoudi, R.A.; Dupin, N. Kaposi sarcoma-associated herpesvirus infects monotypic (IgM lambda) but polyclonal naive B cells in Castleman disease and associated lymphoproliferative disorders. *Blood* **2001**, *97*, 2130–2136. [CrossRef]
32. Aoki, Y.; Tosato, G.; Fonville, T.W.; Pittaluga, S. Serum viral interleukin-6 in AIDS-related multicentric Castleman disease. *Blood* **2001**, *97*, 2526–2527. [CrossRef]
33. Oksenhendler, E.; Boulanger, E.; Galicier, L.; Du, M.-Q.; Dupin, N.; Diss, T.C.; Hamoudi, R.; Daniel, M.-T.; Agbalika, F.; Boshoff, C.; et al. High incidence of Kaposi sarcoma–associated herpesvirus–related non-Hodgkin lymphoma in patients with HIV infection and multicentric Castleman disease. *Blood* **2002**, *99*, 2331–2336. [CrossRef]
34. Polizzotto, M.N.; Uldrick, T.S.; Hu, D.; Yarchoan, R. Clinical Manifestations of Kaposi Sarcoma Herpesvirus Lytic Activation: Multicentric Castleman Disease (KSHV–MCD) and the KSHV Inflammatory Cytokine Syndrome. *Front. Microbiol.* **2012**, *3*, 73. [CrossRef] [PubMed]
35. Kedes, D.H.; Ganem, D. Sensitivity of Kaposi's sarcoma-associated herpesvirus replication to antiviral drugs. Implications for potential therapy. *J. Clin. Investig.* **1997**, *99*, 2082–2086. [CrossRef] [PubMed]
36. Medveczky, M.M.; Horvath, E.; Lund, T.; Medveczky, P.G. In vitro antiviral drug sensitivity of the Kaposi's sarcoma-associated herpesvirus. *AIDS* **1997**, *11*, 1327–1332. [CrossRef]
37. Neyts, J.; De Clercq, E. Antiviral drug susceptibility of human herpesvirus 8. *Antimicrob. Agents Chemother.* **1997**, *41*, 2754–2756. [CrossRef]
38. Sergerie, Y.; Boivin, G. Evaluation of Susceptibility of Human Herpesvirus 8 to Antiviral Drugs by Quantitative Real-Time PCR. *J. Clin. Microbiol.* **2003**, *41*, 3897–3900. [CrossRef]
39. Coen, N.; Singh, U.; Vuyyuru, V.; Oord, J.J.V.D.; Balzarini, J.; Duraffour, S.; Snoeck, R.; Cheng, Y.C.; Chu, C.K.; Andrei, G. Activity and Mechanism of Action of HDVD, a Novel Pyrimidine Nucleoside Derivative with High Levels of Selectivity and Potency against Gammaherpesviruses. *J. Virol.* **2013**, *87*, 3839–3851. [CrossRef] [PubMed]
40. Coen, N.; Duraffour, S.; Topalis, D.; Snoeck, R.; Andrei, G. Spectrum of Activity and Mechanisms of Resistance of Various Nucleoside Derivatives against Gammaherpesviruses. *Antimicrob. Agents Chemother.* **2014**, *58*, 7312–7323. [CrossRef] [PubMed]
41. Luppi, M.; Trovato, R.; Barozzi, P.; Vallisa, D.; Rossi, G.; Re, A.; Ravazzini, L.; Potenza, L.; Riva, G.; Morselli, M.; et al. Treatment of herpesvirus associated primary effusion lymphoma with intracavity cidofovir. *Leukemia* **2005**, *19*, 473–476. [CrossRef]
42. Casper, C.; Krantz, E.M.; Corey, L.; Kuntz, S.R.; Wang, J.; Selke, S.; Hamilton, S.; Huang, M.L.; Wald, A. Valganciclovir for suppression of human herpesvirus-8 replication: A randomized, Double-blind, Placebo-Controlled, Crossover trial. *J. Infect. Dis.* **2008**, *198*, 23–30. [CrossRef]
43. Cattamanchi, A.; Saracino, M.; Selke, S.; Huang, M.-L.; Magaret, A.; Celum, C.; Corey, L.; Wald, A.; Casper, C. Treatment with valacyclovir, famciclovir, or antiretrovirals reduces human herpesvirus-8 replication in HIV-1 seropositive men. *J. Med. Virol.* **2011**, *83*, 1696–1703. [CrossRef] [PubMed]
44. Mazzi, R.; Parisi, S.G.; Sarmati, L.; Uccella, I.; Nicastri, E.; Carolo, G.; Gatti, F.; Concia, E.; Andreoni, M. Efficacy of cidofovir on human herpesvirus 8 viraemia and Kaposi's sarcoma progression in two patients with AIDS. *AIDS* **2001**, *15*, 2061–2062. [CrossRef]
45. Simonart, T.; Noel, J.C.; De Dobbeleer, G.; Parent, D.; Van Vooren, J.P.; De Clercq, E. Treatment of Classical Kaposi's Sarcoma With Intralesional Injections of Cidofovir: Report of a Case. **1998**. *J. Med. Virol.* **1998**, *55*, 215–218. [CrossRef]
46. Little, R.F.; Merced-Galindez, F.; Staskus, K.; Whitby, D.; Aoki, Y.; Humphrey, R.; Pluda, J.M.; Marshall, V.; Walters, M.; Welles, L.; et al. A Pilot Study of Cidofovir in Patients with Kaposi Sarcoma. *J. Infect. Dis.* **2003**, *187*, 149–153. [CrossRef]

47. Krown, S.E.; Dittmer, D.P.; Cesarman, E. Pilot Study of Oral Valganciclovir Therapy in Patients With Classic Kaposi Sarcoma. *J. Infect. Dis.* **2011**, *203*, 1082–1086. [CrossRef] [PubMed]
48. Plachouri, K.; Oikonomou, C.; Sarantopoulos, A.; Koumoundourou, D.; Georgiou, S.; Spiliopoulos, T. Successful treatment and durable remission of human herpesvirus-8-induced Kaposi sarcoma and multicentric Castleman's disease under valganciclovir in an HIV -negative patient. *Dermatol. Ther.* **2020**, *33*, e13419. [CrossRef] [PubMed]
49. Zhu, W.; Burnette, A.; Dorjsuren, D.; Roberts, P.E.; Huleihel, M.; Shoemaker, R.H.; Marquez, V.E.; Agbaria, R.; Sei, S. Potent Antiviral Activity of North-Methanocarbathymidine against Kaposi's Sarcoma-Associated Herpesvirus. *Antimicrob. Agents Chemother.* **2005**, *49*, 4980–4988. [CrossRef] [PubMed]
50. Coen, N.; Duraffour, S.; Snoeck, R.; Andrei, G. KSHV Targeted Therapy: An Update on Inhibitors of Viral Lytic Replication. *Viruses* **2014**, *6*, 4731–4759. [CrossRef] [PubMed]
51. Prichard, M.N.; Williams, J.D.; Komazin-Meredith, G.; Khan, A.R.; Price, N.B.; Jefferson, G.M.; Harden, E.A.; Hartline, C.B.; Peet, N.P.; Bowlin, T.L. Synthesis and Antiviral Activities of Methylenecyclopropane Analogs with 6-Alkoxy and 6-Alkylthio Substitutions That Exhibit Broad-Spectrum Antiviral Activity against Human Herpesviruses. *Antimicrob. Agents Chemother.* **2013**, *57*, 3518–3527. [CrossRef] [PubMed]
52. Beauclair, G.; Naimo, E.; Dubich, T.; Rückert, J.; Koch, S.; Dhingra, A.; Wirth, D.; Schulz, T.F. Targeting Kaposi's Sarcoma-Associated Herpesvirus ORF21 Tyrosine Kinase and Viral Lytic Reactivation by Tyrosine Kinase Inhibitors Approved for Clinical Use. *J. Virol.* **2020**, *94*, e01791-19. [CrossRef]
53. Gustafson, E.A.; Schinazi, R.F.; Fingeroth, J.D. Human Herpesvirus 8 Open Reading Frame 21 Is a Thymidine and Thymidylate Kinase of Narrow Substrate Specificity That Efficiently Phosphorylates Zidovudine but Not Ganciclovir. *J. Virol.* **2000**, *74*, 684–692. [CrossRef]
54. Pastore, R.D.; Chadburn, A.; Kripas, C.; Schattner, E.J. Novel association of haemophagocytic syndrome with Kaposi's sarcoma-associated herpesvirus-related primary effusion lymphoma. *Br. J. Haematol.* **2000**, *111*, 1112–1115.
55. Sbenghe, M.M.; Besa, E.; Mahipal, A.; Florea, A.D.; Bray, P.; Caro, J. HHV-8–Associated Multicentric Castleman's Disease in HIV-Negative Patient: A Novel Therapy for an Orphan Disease. *Oncologist.* **2012**, *17*, 145–146. [CrossRef] [PubMed]
56. Ozbalak, M.; Tokatli, I.; Özdemirli, M.; Tecimer, T.; Ar, M.C.; Ornek, S.; Koroglu, A.; Laleli, Y.; Ferhanoglu, B. Is valganciclovir really effective in primary effusion lymphoma: Case report of an HIV(−) EBV(−) HHV8(+) patient. *Eur. J. Haematol.* **2013**, *91*, 467–469. [CrossRef]
57. Kantarci, F.E.N.; Eren, R.; Gündoğan, C.; Huq, G.E.; Doğu, M.H.; Suyanı, E.; Gündoğdu, C. A HHV-8 positive, HIV negative multicentric Castleman disease treated with R-CEOP chemotherapy and valganciclovir combination. *J. Infect. Chemother.* **2016**, *22*, 483–485. [CrossRef] [PubMed]
58. Murphy, C.; Hawkes, E.; Chionh, F.; Chong, G.; Fracp, C.M.M.B. Durable remission of both multicentric Castleman's disease and Kaposi's sarcoma with valganciclovir, rituximab and liposomal doxorubicin in an HHV-8-positive, HIV-negative patient. *J. Clin. Pharm. Ther.* **2016**, *42*, 111–114. [CrossRef]
59. Uldrick, T.S.; Polizzotto, M.; Aleman, K.; O'Mahony, D.; Wyvill, K.M.; Wang, V.; Marshall, V.; Pittaluga, S.; Steinberg, S.M.; Tosato, G.; et al. High-dose zidovudine plus valganciclovir for Kaposi sarcoma herpesvirus-associated multicentric Castleman disease: A pilot study of virus-activated cytotoxic therapy. *Blood* **2011**, *117*, 6977–6986. [CrossRef]
60. Dittmer, D.; Damania, B. Kaposi sarcoma associated herpesvirus pathogenesis (KSHV)—an update. *Curr. Opin. Virol.* **2013**, *3*, 238–244. [CrossRef]
61. Zhong, W.; Wang, H.; Herndier, B.; Ganem, D. Restricted expression of Kaposi sarcoma-associated herpesvirus (human herpesvirus 8) genes in Kaposi sarcoma. *Proc. Natl. Acad. Sci. USA* **1996**, *93*, 6641–6646. [CrossRef] [PubMed]
62. Ballestas, M.E.; Chatis, P.A.; Kaye, K.M. Efficient Persistence of Extrachromosomal KSHV DNA Mediated by Latency-Associated Nuclear Antigen. *Science* **1999**, *284*, 641–644. [CrossRef]
63. Dittmer, D.; Lagunoff, M.; Renne, R.; Staskus, K.; Haase, A.; Ganem, D. A Cluster of Latently Expressed Genes in Kaposi's Sarcoma-Associated Herpesvirus. *J. Virol.* **1998**, *72*, 8309–8315. [CrossRef] [PubMed]
64. Lan, K.; Kuppers, D.A.; Verma, S.C.; Sharma, N.; Murakami, M.; Robertson, E.S.; Cheung, C.Y.; Poon, L.L.M.; Ng, I.H.Y.; Luk, W.; et al. Induction of Kaposi's Sarcoma-Associated Herpesvirus Latency-Associated Nuclear Antigen by the Lytic Transactivator RTA: A Novel Mechanism for Establishment of Latency. *J. Virol.* **2005**, *79*, 7819–7826. [CrossRef]
65. Lan, K.; Kuppers, D.A.; Verma, S.C.; Robertson, E.S. Kaposi's Sarcoma-Associated Herpesvirus-Encoded Latency-Associated Nuclear Antigen Inhibits Lytic Replication by Targeting Rta: A Potential Mechanism for Virus-Mediated Control of Latency. *J. Virol.* **2004**, *78*, 6585–6594. [CrossRef]
66. Cai, X.; Lu, S.; Zhang, Z.; Gonzalez, C.M.; Damania, B.; Cullen, B.R. Kaposi's sarcoma-associated herpesvirus expresses an array of viral microRNAs in latently infected cells. *Proc. Natl. Acad. Sci. USA* **2005**, *102*, 5570–5575. [CrossRef]
67. Chakraborty, S.; Veettil, M.V.; Chandran, B. Kaposi's Sarcoma Associated Herpesvirus Entry into Target Cells. *Front. Microbiol.* **2012**, *3*, 6. [CrossRef] [PubMed]
68. Dupin, N.; Fisher, C.; Kellam, P.; Ariad, S.; Tulliez, M.; Franck, N. Distribution of human herpesvirus-8 latently infected cells in Kaposi's sarcoma, multicentric Castleman's disease, and primary effusion lymphoma. *Proc. Natl. Acad. Sci. USA* **1999**, *96*, 4546–4551. [CrossRef] [PubMed]
69. Godfrey, A.; Anderson, J.; Papanastasiou, A.; Takeuchi, Y.; Boshoff, C. Inhibiting primary effusion lymphoma by lentiviral vectors encoding short hairpin RNA. *Blood* **2005**, *105*, 2510–2518. [CrossRef] [PubMed]

70. Curreli, F.; Friedman-Kien, A.E.; Flore, O. Glycyrrhizic acid alters Kaposi sarcoma–associated herpesvirus latency, triggering p53-mediated apoptosis in transformed B lymphocytes. *J. Clin. Invest.* **2005**, *115*, 642–652. [CrossRef]
71. Chen, W.; Sin, S.-H.; Wen, K.W.; Damania, B.; Dittmer, D.P. Hsp90 Inhibitors Are Efficacious against Kaposi Sarcoma by Enhancing the Degradation of the Essential Viral Gene LANA, of the Viral Co-Receptor EphA2 as well as Other Client Proteins. *PLoS Pathog.* **2012**, *8*, e1003048. [CrossRef] [PubMed]
72. Tso, F.Y.; West, J.T.; Wood, C. Reduction of Kaposi's Sarcoma-Associated Herpesvirus Latency Using CRISPR-Cas9 To Edit the Latency-Associated Nuclear Antigen Gene. *J. Virol.* **2019**, *93*, e02183-18. [CrossRef]
73. Haddad, C.O.; Kalt, I.; Shovman, Y.; Xia, L.; Schlesinger, Y.; Sarid, R.; Parnas, O. Targeting the Kaposi's sarcoma-associated herpesvirus genome with the CRISPR-Cas9 platform in latently infected cells. *Virol. J.* **2021**, *18*, 1–12. [CrossRef] [PubMed]
74. Ballestas, M.; Kaye, K.M. Kaposi's Sarcoma-Associated Herpesvirus Latency-Associated Nuclear Antigen 1 Mediates Episome Persistence through cis -Acting Terminal Repeat (TR) Sequence and Specifically Binds TR DNA. *J. Virol.* **2001**, *75*, 3250–3258. [CrossRef]
75. Barbera, J.A.; Ballestas, M.E.; Kaye, K.M. The Kaposi's Sarcoma-Associated Herpesvirus Latency-Associated Nuclear Antigen 1 N Terminus Is Essential for Chromosome Association, DNA Replication, and Episome Persistence. *J. Virol.* **2004**, *78*, 294–301. [CrossRef]
76. Hellert, J.; Weidner-Glunde, M.; Krausze, J.; Lünsdorf, H.; Ritter, C.; Schulz, T.F.; Lührs, T. The 3D structure of Kaposi sarcoma herpesvirus LANA C-terminal domain bound to DNA. *Proc. Natl. Acad. Sci. USA* **2015**, *112*, 6694–6699. [CrossRef] [PubMed]
77. Weidner-Glunde, M.; Mariggiò, G.; Schulz, T.F. Kaposi's Sarcoma-Associated Herpesvirus Latency-Associated Nuclear Antigen: Replicating and Shielding Viral DNA during Viral Persistence. *J. Virol.* **2017**, *91*, e01083-16. [CrossRef]
78. Domsic, J.F.; Chen, H.-S.; Lu, F.; Marmorstein, R.; Lieberman, P.M. Molecular Basis for Oligomeric-DNA Binding and Episome Maintenance by KSHV LANA. *PLoS Pathog.* **2013**, *9*, e1003672. [CrossRef]
79. Kirsch, P.E.; Jakob, V.; Oberhausen, K.; Stein, S.C.; Cucarro, I.S.; Schulz, T.F.; Empting, M. Fragment-Based Discovery of a Qualified Hit Targeting the Latency-Associated Nuclear Antigen of the Oncogenic Kaposi's Sarcoma-Associated Herpesvirus/Human Herpesvirus 8. *J. Med. Chem.* **2019**, *62*, 3924–3939. [CrossRef]
80. Kirsch, P.; Stein, S.C.; Berwanger, A.; Rinkes, J.; Jakob, V.; Schulz, T.F.; Empting, M. Hit-to-lead optimization of a latency-associated nuclear antigen inhibitor against Kaposi's sarcoma-associated herpesvirus infections. *Eur. J. Med. Chem.* **2020**, *202*, 112525. [CrossRef] [PubMed]
81. Kirsch, P.; Jakob, V.; Elgaher, W.A.M.; Walt, C.; Oberhausen, K.; Schulz, T.; Empting, M. Discovery of Novel Latency-Associated Nuclear Antigen Inhibitors as Antiviral Agents Against Kaposi's Sarcoma-Associated Herpesvirus. *ACS Chem. Biol.* **2020**, *15*, 388–395. [CrossRef]
82. Calderon, A.; Soldan, S.S.; De Leo, A.; Deng, Z.; Frase, D.M.; Anderson, E.M.; Zhang, Y.; Vladimirova, O.; Lu, F.; Leung, J.C.; et al. Identification of Mubritinib (TAK 165) as an inhibitor of KSHV driven primary effusion lymphoma via disruption of mitochondrial OXPHOS metabolism. *Oncotarget* **2020**, *11*, 4224–4242. [CrossRef]
83. Keller, S.A.; Schattner, E.J.; Cesarman, E. Inhibition of NF-B Induces Apoptosis of KSHV-Infected Primary Effusion Lymphoma Cells. 2000. Available online: https://ashpublications.org/blood/article-pdf/96/7/2537/1668374/h8190002537.pdf (accessed on 30 August 2021).
84. Chugh, P.; Matta, H.; Schamus, S.; Zachariah, S.; Kumar, A.; Richardson, J.A.; Smith, A.L.; Chaudhary, P.M. Constitutive NF- B activation, normal Fas-induced apoptosis, and increased incidence of lymphoma in human herpes virus 8 K13 transgenic mice. *Proc. Natl. Acad. Sci. USA* **2005**, *102*, 12885–12890. [CrossRef]
85. Guasparri, I.; Keller, S.A.; Cesarman, E. KSHV vFLIP Is Essential for the Survival of Infected Lymphoma Cells. *J. Exp. Med.* **2004**, *199*, 993–1003. [CrossRef]
86. Keller, S.A.; Hernandez-Hopkins, D.; Vider, J.; Ponomarev, V.; Hyjek, E.; Schattner, E.J.; Cesarman, E. NF-κB is essential for the progression of KSHV- and EBV-infected lymphomas in vivo. *Blood* **2006**, *107*, 3295–3302. [CrossRef] [PubMed]
87. Baloon, G.; Chen, K.; Perez, R.; Tam, W.; Cesarman, E. Kaposi Sarcoma Herpesvirus (KSHV) VFLIP Oncoprotein Induces B Cell Transdifferentiation and Tumorigenesis in Mice. *J. Clin. Investig.* **2011**, *121*, 1141–1153. [CrossRef]
88. Sadek, J.; Wuo, M.G.; Rooklin, D.; Hauenstein, A.; Hong, S.H.; Gautam, A. Modulation of virus-induced NF-κB signaling by NEMO coiled coil mimics. *Nat Commun.* **2020**, *11*, 1–14. [CrossRef]
89. Field, N.; Low, W.; Daniels, M.; Howell, S.; Daviet, L.; Boshoff, C.; Collins, M. KSHV vFLIP binds to IKK-γ to activate IKK. *J. Cell Sci.* **2003**, *116*, 3721–3728. [CrossRef]
90. Bagnéris, C.; Ageichik, A.V.; Cronin, N.; Wallace, B.; Collins, M.; Boshoff, C.; Waksman, G.; Barrett, T. Crystal Structure of a VFlip-IKKγ Complex: Insights into Viral Activation of the IKK Signalosome. *Mol. Cell* **2008**, *30*, 620–631. [CrossRef] [PubMed]
91. Briggs, L.C.; Chan, A.W.E.; Davis, C.A.; Whitelock, N.; Hotiana, H.A.; Baratchian, M.; Bagnéris, C.; Selwood, D.L.; Collins, M.K.; Barrett, T.E. IKKγ-Mimetic Peptides Block the Resistance to Apoptosis Associated with Kaposi's Sarcoma-Associated Herpesvirus Infection. *J. Virol.* **2017**, *91*, e01170-17. [CrossRef] [PubMed]
92. Zhu, F.X.; Cusano, T.; Yuan, Y. Identification of the Immediate-Early Transcripts of Kaposi's Sarcoma-Associated Herpesvirus. *J. Virol.* **1999**, *73*, 5556–5567. [CrossRef] [PubMed]
93. Purushothaman, P.; Uppal, T.; Verma, S.C. Molecular Biology of KSHV Lytic Reactivation. *Viruses* **2015**, *7*, 116–153. [CrossRef]
94. Sun, R.; Lin, S.-F.; Gradoville, L.; Yuan, Y.; Zhu, F.; Miller, G. A viral gene that activates lytic cycle expression of Kaposi's sarcoma-associated herpesvirus. *Proc. Natl. Acad. Sci. USA* **1998**, *95*, 10866–10871. [CrossRef]

95. Long, W.; Zhao, G.; Wu, Y.; Liu, Y. Gallic acid inhibits Kaposi's Sarcoma-associated herpesvirus lytic reactivation by suppressing RTA transcriptional activities. *Food Sci. Nutr.* **2020**, *9*, 847–854. [CrossRef] [PubMed]
96. Dorjsuren, D.; Burnette, A.; Gray, G.N.; Chen, X.; Zhu, W.; Roberts, P.E.; Currens, M.J.; Shoemaker, R.H.; Ricciardi, R.P.; Sei, S. Chemical library screen for novel inhibitors of Kaposi's sarcoma-associated herpesvirus processive DNA synthesis. *Antivir. Res.* **2006**, *69*, 9–23. [CrossRef] [PubMed]
97. Yan, Z.; Bryant, K.F.; Gregory, S.M.; Angelova, M.; Dreyfus, D.H.; Zhao, X.Z.; Coen, D.M.; Burke, T.R.; Knipe, D.M. HIV Integrase Inhibitors Block Replication of Alpha-, Beta-, and Gammaherpesviruses. *mBio* **2014**, *5*, e01318-14. [CrossRef] [PubMed]
98. Miller, J.T.; Zhao, H.; Masaoka, T.; Varnado, B.; Castro, E.M.C.; Marshall, V.A.; Kouhestani, K.; Lynn, A.Y.; Aron, K.E.; Xia, A.; et al. Sensitivity of the C-Terminal Nuclease Domain of Kaposi's Sarcoma-Associated Herpesvirus ORF29 to Two Classes of Active-Site Ligands. *Antimicrob. Agents Chemother.* **2018**, *62*, e00233-18. [CrossRef]
99. Newcomb, W.W.; Brown, J.C. Inhibition of Herpes Simplex Virus Replication by WAY-150138: Assembly of Capsids Depleted of the Portal and Terminase Proteins Involved in DNA Encapsidation. *J. Virol.* **2002**, *76*, 10084–10088. [CrossRef]
100. Visalli, R.J.; Fairhurst, J.; Srinivas, S.; Hu, W.; Feld, B.; DiGrandi, M.; Curran, K.; Ross, A.; Bloom, J.D.; van Zeijl, M.; et al. Identification of Small Molecule Compounds That Selectively Inhibit Varicella-Zoster Virus Replication. *J. Virol.* **2003**, *77*, 2349–2358. [CrossRef] [PubMed]
101. Visalli, R.J.; Van Zeijl, M. DNA encapsidation as a target for anti-herpesvirus drug therapy. *Antivir. Res.* **2003**, *59*, 73–87. [CrossRef]
102. Kornfeind, E.M.; Visalli, R.J. Human herpesvirus portal proteins: Structure, function, and antiviral prospects. *Rev. Med. Virol.* **2018**, *28*, e1972. [CrossRef]
103. Goldner, T.; Hewlett, G.; Ettischer, N.; Ruebsamen-Schaeff, H.; Zimmermann, H.; Lischka, P. The Novel Anticytomegalovirus Compound AIC246 (Letermovir) Inhibits Human Cytomegalovirus Replication through a Specific Antiviral Mechanism That Involves the Viral Terminase. *J. Virol.* **2011**, *85*, 10884–10893. [CrossRef]
104. Unal, A.; Pray, T.R.; Lagunoff, M.; Pennington, M.W.; Ganem, D.; Craik, C.S. The protease and the assembly protein of Kaposi's sarcoma-associated herpesvirus (human herpesvirus 8). *J. Virol.* **1997**, *71*, 7030–7038. [CrossRef]
105. Shahian, T.; Lee, G.M.; Lazic, A.; Arnold, L.A.; Velusamy, P.; Roels, C.M.; Guy, R.K.; Craik, C.S. Inhibition of a viral enzyme by a small-molecule dimer disruptor. *Nat. Chem. Biol.* **2009**, *5*, 640–646. [CrossRef] [PubMed]
106. Lee, H.-R.; Brulois, K.; Wong, L.; Jung, J.U. Modulation of Immune System by Kaposi's Sarcoma-Associated Herpesvirus: Lessons from Viral Evasion Strategies. *Front. Microbiol.* **2012**, *3*, 44. [CrossRef] [PubMed]
107. Acker, T.M.; Gable, J.E.; Bohn, M.F.; Jaishankar, P.; Thompson, M.C.; Fraser, J.S.; Renslo, A.R.; Craik, C.S. Allosteric Inhibitors, Crystallography, and Comparative Analysis Reveal Network of Coordinated Movement across Human Herpesvirus Proteases. *J. Am. Chem. Soc.* **2017**, *139*, 11650–11653. [CrossRef] [PubMed]
108. Gantt, S.; Carlsson, J.; Ikoma, M.; Gachelet, E.; Gray, M.; Geballe, A.P.; Corey, L.; Casper, C.; Lagunoff, M.; Vieira, J. The HIV Protease Inhibitor Nelfinavir Inhibits Kaposi's Sarcoma-Associated Herpesvirus Replication In Vitro. *Antimicrob. Agents Chemother.* **2011**, *55*, 2696–2703. [CrossRef]
109. Gantt, S.; Cattamanchi, A.; Krantz, E.; Magaret, A.; Selke, S.; Kuntz, S.R.; Huang, M.-L.; Corey, L.; Wald, A.; Casper, C. Reduced human herpesvirus-8 oropharyngeal shedding associated with protease inhibitor-based antiretroviral therapy. *J. Clin. Virol.* **2014**, *60*, 127–132. [CrossRef] [PubMed]
110. Cai, Y.; Berger, E.A. An Immunotoxin Targeting the GH Glycoprotein of KSHV for Selective Killing of Cells in the Lytic Phase of Infection. *Antivir. Res.* **2011**, *90*, 143–1450. [CrossRef]
111. Chatterjee, D.; Chandran, B.; Berger, E.A. Selective Killing of Kaposi's Sarcoma-Associated Herpesvirus Lytically Infected Cells with a Recombinant Immunotoxin Targeting the Viral GpK8.1A Envelope Glycoprotein. *MAbs* **2012**, *4*, 233–242. [CrossRef] [PubMed]
112. Miller, G.; Heston, L.; Grogan, E.; Gradoville, L.; Rigsby, M.; Sun, R.; Shedd, D.; Kushnaryov, V.M.; Grossberg, S.; Chang, Y. Selective switch between latency and lytic replication of Kaposi's sarcoma herpesvirus and Epstein-Barr virus in dually infected body cavity lymphoma cells. *J. Virol.* **1997**, *71*, 314–324. [CrossRef] [PubMed]
113. Chen, J.; Ueda, K.; Sakakibara, S.; Okuno, T.; Parravicini, C.; Corbellino, M.; Yamanishi, K. Activation of latent Kaposi's sarcoma-associated herpesvirus by demethylation of the promoter of the lytic transactivator. *Proc. Natl. Acad. Sci. USA* **2001**, *98*, 4119–4124. [CrossRef]
114. Whitby, D.; Marshall, V.A.; Bagni, R.K.; Miley, W.J.; McCloud, T.G.; Hines-Boykin, R.; Goedert, J.J.; Conde, B.A.; Nagashima, K.; Mikovits, J.; et al. Reactivation of Kaposi's sarcoma-associated herpesvirus by natural products from Kaposi's sarcoma endemic regions. *Int. J. Cancer* **2006**, *120*, 321–328. [CrossRef] [PubMed]
115. Li, Q.; He, M.; Zhou, F.; Ye, F.; Gao, S.-J. Activation of Kaposi's Sarcoma-Associated Herpesvirus (KSHV) by Inhibitors of Class III Histone Deacetylases: Identification of Sirtuin 1 as a Regulator of the KSHV Life Cycle. *J. Virol.* **2014**, *88*, 6355–6367. [CrossRef] [PubMed]
116. Liang, Z.; Qin, Z.; Riker, A.I.; Xi, Y. CRISPR/Cas9 ablating viral microRNA promotes lytic reactivation of Kaposi's sarcoma-associated herpesvirus. *Biochem. Biophys. Res. Commun.* **2020**, *533*, 1400–1405. [CrossRef]
117. Iida, S.; Mine, S.; Ueda, K.; Suzuki, T.; Hasegawa, H.; Katano, H. Suberoyl Bis-Hydroxamic Acid Reactivates Kaposi's Sarcoma-Associated Herpesvirus through Histone Acetylation and Induces Apoptosis in Lymphoma Cells. *J. Virol.* **2021**, *95*, e01785-20. [CrossRef] [PubMed]

118. Van der Meulen, E.; Anderton, M.; Blumenthal, M.; Schäfer, G. Cellular Receptors Involved in KSHV Infection. *Viruses* **2021**, *13*, 118. [CrossRef]
119. Koon, H.B.; Bubley, G.J.; Pantanowitz, L.; Masiello, D.; Smith, B.; Crosby, K.; Proper, J.; Weeden, W.; Miller, T.E.; Chatis, P.; et al. Imatinib-Induced Regression of AIDS-Related Kaposi's Sarcoma. *J. Clin. Oncol.* **2005**, *23*, 982–989. [CrossRef]
120. Koon, H.B.; Krown, S.E.; Lee, J.Y.; Honda, K.; Rapisuwon, S.; Wang, Z.; Aboulafia, D.; Reid, E.G.; Rudek, M.A.; Dezube, B.J.; et al. Phase II Trial of Imatinib in AIDS-Associated Kaposi's Sarcoma: AIDS Malignancy Consortium Protocol 042. *J. Clin. Oncol.* **2014**, *32*, 402–408. [CrossRef]
121. Ardavanis, A.; Doufexis, D.; Kountourakis, P.; Rigatos, G. A Kaposi's Sarcoma Complete Clinical Response after Sorafenib Administration. *Ann. Oncol.* **2008**, *19*, 1658–1659. [CrossRef] [PubMed]
122. Uldrick, T.S.; Gonçalves, P.H.; Wyvill, K.M.; Peer, C.J.; Bernstein, W.; Aleman, K.; Polizzotto, M.; Venzon, D.; Steinberg, S.M.; Marshall, V.; et al. A Phase Ib Study of Sorafenib (BAY 43-9006) in Patients with Kaposi Sarcoma. *Oncology* **2017**, *22*, 505. [CrossRef]
123. Gill, M.B.; Turner, R.; Stevenson, P.G.; Way, M. KSHV-TK is a tyrosine kinase that disrupts focal adhesions and induces Rho-mediated cell contraction. *EMBO J.* **2014**, *34*, 448–465. [CrossRef]
124. Wong, J.P.; Stuhlmiller, T.J.; Giffin, L.C.; Lin, C.; Bigi, R.; Zhao, J.; Zhang, W.; Cruz, A.G.B.; Park, S.I.; Earp, H.S.; et al. Kinome profiling of non-Hodgkin lymphoma identifies Tyro3 as a therapeutic target in primary effusion lymphoma. *Proc. Natl. Acad. Sci. USA* **2019**, *116*, 16541–16550. [CrossRef] [PubMed]
125. Sodhi, A.; Chaisuparat, R.; Hu, J.; Ramsdell, A.K.; Manning, B.D.; Sausville, E.A.; Sawai, E.T.; Molinolo, A.; Gutkind, J.S.; Montaner, S. The TSC2/mTOR pathway drives endothelial cell transformation induced by the Kaposi's sarcoma-associated herpesvirus G protein-coupled receptor. *Cancer Cell* **2006**, *10*, 133–143. [CrossRef]
126. Nichols, L.A.; Adang, L.A.; Kedes, D.H. Rapamycin Blocks Production of KSHV/HHV8: Insights into the Anti-Tumor Activity of an Immunosuppressant Drug. *PLoS ONE* **2011**, *6*, e14535. [CrossRef] [PubMed]
127. Sin, S.-H.; Roy, D.; Wang, L.; Staudt, M.R.; Fakhari, F.D.; Patel, D.D.; Henry, D.; Harrington, W.J.; Damania, B.A.; Dittmer, D.P. Rapamycin Is Efficacious against Primary Effusion Lymphoma (PEL) Cell Lines in Vivo by Inhibiting Autocrine Signaling. *Blood* **2007**, *109*, 2165–2173. [CrossRef] [PubMed]
128. Bhatt, A.P.; Bhende, P.M.; Sin, S.H.; Roy, D.; Dittmer, D.P.; Damania, B. Dual Inhibition of PI3K and MTOR Inhibits Autocrine and Paracrine Proliferative Loops in PI3K/Akt/MTOR-Addicted Lymphomas. *Blood* **2010**, *115*, 4455–4463. [CrossRef]
129. Caro-Vegas, C.; Bailey, A.; Bigi, R.; Damania, B.; Dittmer, D.P. Targeting MTOR with MLN0128 Overcomes Rapamycin and Chemoresistant Primary Effusion Lymphoma. *MBio* **2019**, *10*, e02871-18. [CrossRef]
130. Pan, H.; Xie, J.; Ye, F.; Gao, S.-J. Modulation of Kaposi's Sarcoma-Associated Herpesvirus Infection and Replication by MEK/ERK, JNK, and p38 Multiple Mitogen-Activated Protein Kinase Pathways during Primary Infection. *J. Virol.* **2006**, *80*, 5371–5382. [CrossRef]
131. Wakao, K.; Watanabe, T.; Takadama, T.; Ui, S.; Shigemi, Z.; Kagawa, H.; Higashi, C.; Ohga, R.; Taira, T.; Fujimuro, M. Sangivamycin induces apoptosis by suppressing Erk signaling in primary effusion lymphoma cells. *Biochem. Biophys. Res. Commun.* **2014**, *444*, 135–140. [CrossRef]
132. Moriguchi, M.; Watanabe, T.; Kadota, A.; Fujimuro, M. Capsaicin Induces Apoptosis in KSHV-Positive Primary Effusion Lymphoma by Suppressing ERK and p38 MAPK Signaling and IL-6 Expression. *Front. Oncol.* **2019**, *9*, 83. [CrossRef]
133. Li, X.; Huang, L.; Xiao, Y.; Yao, X.; Long, X.; Zhu, F.; Kuang, E. Development of an ORF45-Derived Peptide To Inhibit the Sustained RSK Activation and Lytic Replication of Kaposi's Sarcoma-Associated Herpesvirus. *J. Virol.* **2019**, *93*, e02154-18. [CrossRef] [PubMed]
134. Dai, L.; Trillo-Tinoco, J.; Cao, Y.; Bonstaff, K.; Doyle, L.; del Valle, L.; Whitby, D.; Qin, Z. Targeting HGF/c-MET Induces Cell Cycle Arrest, DNA Damage, and Apoptosis for Primary Effusion Lymphoma. *Blood J. Am. Soc. Hematol.* **2015**, *126*, 2821–2831. [CrossRef] [PubMed]
135. Nayar, U.; Lu, P.; Vider, J.; Cerchietti, L.; Chiosis, G.; Wang, L.; Blasberg, R.; Cesarman, E. Hsp90 is a viable therapeutic target in the treatment of KSHV-associated primary effusion lymphoma. *Infect. Agents Cancer* **2010**, *5*, 1–2. [CrossRef]
136. Wen, K.W.; Damania, B. Kaposi sarcoma-associated herpesvirus (KSHV): Molecular biology and oncogenesis. *Cancer Lett.* **2010**, *289*, 140–150. [CrossRef]
137. Qin, Z.; Defee, M.; Isaacs, J.S.; Parsons, C. Extracellular Hsp90 serves as a co-factor for MAPK activation and latent viral gene expression during de novo infection by KSHV. *Virology* **2010**, *403*, 92–102. [CrossRef] [PubMed]
138. Higashi, C.; Saji, C.; Yamada, K.; Kagawa, H.; Ohga, R.; Taira, T.; Fujimuro, M. The Effects of Heat Shock Protein 90 Inhibitors on Apoptosis and Viral Replication in Primary Effusion Lymphoma Cells. *Biol. Pharm. Bull.* **2012**, *35*, 725–730. [CrossRef]
139. Gopalakrishnan, R.; Matta, H.; Chaudhary, P.M. A Purine Scaffold HSP90 Inhibitor BIIB021 Has Selective Activity against KSHV-Associated Primary Effusion Lymphoma and Blocks vFLIP K13-Induced NF-κB. *Clin. Cancer Res.* **2013**, *19*, 5016–5026. [CrossRef]
140. Qi, C.-F.; Kim, Y.-S.; Xiang, S.; Abdullaev, Z.; Torrey, T.A.; Janz, S.; Kovalchuk, A.L.; Sun, J.; Chen, D.; Cho, W.C.; et al. Characterization of ARF-BP1/HUWE1 Interactions with CTCF, MYC, ARF and p53 in MYC-Driven B Cell Neoplasms. *Int. J. Mol. Sci.* **2012**, *13*, 6204–6219. [CrossRef]
141. Baquero-Pérez, B.; Whitehouse, A. Hsp70 Isoforms Are Essential for the Formation of Kaposi's Sarcoma-Associated Herpesvirus Replication and Transcription Compartments. *PLoS Pathog.* **2015**, *11*, e1005274. [CrossRef]

142. Hughes, D.; Wood, J.J.; Jackson, B.; Baquero-Perez, B.; Whitehouse, A. NEDDylation Is Essential for Kaposi's Sarcoma-Associated Herpesvirus Latency and Lytic Reactivation and Represents a Novel Anti-KSHV Target. *PLoS Pathog.* **2015**, *11*, e1004771. [CrossRef]
143. Matta, H.; Chaudhary, P.M. The proteasome inhibitor bortezomib (PS-341) inhibits growth and induces apoptosis in primary effusion lymphoma cells. *Cancer Biol. Ther.* **2005**, *4*, 84–89. [CrossRef]
144. Granato, M.; Romeo, M.A.; Tiano, M.S.; Santarelli, R.; Gonnella, R.; Montani, M.S.G.; Faggioni, A.; Cirone, M. Bortezomib promotes KHSV and EBV lytic cycle by activating JNK and autophagy. *Sci. Rep.* **2017**, *7*, 13052. [CrossRef]
145. Sarosiek, K.; Cavallin, L.E.; Bhatt, S.; Toomey, N.L.; Natkunam, Y.; Blasini, W.; Gentles, A.J.; Ramos, J.C.; Mesri, E.A.; Lossos, I.S. Efficacy of bortezomib in a direct xenograft model of primary effusion lymphoma. *Proc. Natl. Acad. Sci. USA* **2010**, *107*, 13069–13074. [CrossRef]
146. Reid, E.G.; Suazo, A.; Lensing, S.Y.; Dittmer, D.P.; Ambinder, R.F.; Maldarelli, F.; Gorelick, R.J.; Aboulafia, D.M.; Mitsuyasu, R.; Dickson, M.A.; et al. Pilot Trial AMC-063: Safety and Efficacy of Bortezomib in AIDS-associated Kaposi Sarcoma. *Clin. Cancer Res.* **2019**, *26*, 558–565. [CrossRef]
147. Chen, J.; Zhang, H.; Chen, X. Pemetrexed Inhibits Kaposi's Sarcoma-Associated Herpesvirus Replication through Blocking DTMP Synthesis. *Antivir. Res.* **2020**, *180*, 104825. [CrossRef]
148. Xu, B.; Wang, L.; González-Molleda, L.; Wang, Y.; Xu, J.; Yuan, Y. Antiviral Activity of (+)-Rutamarin against Kaposi's Sarcoma-Associated Herpesvirus by Inhibition of the Catalytic Activity of Human Topoisomerase II. *Antimicrob. Agents Chemother.* **2013**, *58*, 563–573. [CrossRef]
149. Davis, D.A.; Rinderknecht, A.S.; Zoeteweij, J.P.; Aoki, Y.; Read-Connole, E.L.; Tosato, G.; Blauvelt, A.; Yarchoan, R. Hypoxia Induces Lytic Replication of Kaposi Sarcoma–Associated Herpesvirus. *Blood* **2001**, *97*, 3244–3250. [CrossRef]
150. Haque, M.; Davis, D.A.; Wang, V.; Widmer, I.; Yarchoan, R. Kaposi's Sarcoma-Associated Herpesvirus (Human Herpesvirus 8) Contains Hypoxia Response Elements: Relevance to Lytic Induction by Hypoxia. *J. Virol.* **2003**, *77*, 6761–6768. [CrossRef]
151. Haque, M.; Wang, V.; Davis, D.A.; Zheng, Z.-M.; Yarchoan, R. Genetic Organization and Hypoxic Activation of the Kaposi's Sarcoma-Associated Herpesvirus ORF34-37 Gene Cluster. *J. Virol.* **2006**, *80*, 7037–7051. [CrossRef]
152. Shrestha, P.; Davis, D.A.; Veeranna, R.P.; Carey, R.F.; Viollet, C.; Yarchoan, R. Hypoxia-inducible factor-1 alpha as a therapeutic target for primary effusion lymphoma. *PLoS Pathog.* **2017**, *13*, e1006628. [CrossRef]
153. He, M.; Tan, B.; Vasan, K.; Yuan, H.; Cheng, F.; da Silva, S.R.; Lu, C.; Gao, S.-J. SIRT1 and AMPK pathways are essential for the proliferation and survival of primary effusion lymphoma cells. *J. Pathol.* **2017**, *242*, 309–321. [CrossRef] [PubMed]
154. Dai, L.; Qiao, J.; Nguyen, D.; Struckhoff, A.P.; Doyle, L.; Bonstaff, K.; Del Valle, L.; Parsons, C.; Toole, B.P.; Renne, R.; et al. Role of heme oxygenase-1 in the pathogenesis and tumorigenicity of Kaposi's sarcoma-associated herpesvirus. *Oncotarget* **2016**, *7*, 10459–10471. [CrossRef] [PubMed]
155. Uldrick, T.S.; Wyvill, K.M.; Kumar, P.; O'Mahony, D.; Bernstein, W.; Aleman, K.; Polizzotto, M.; Steinberg, S.M.; Pittaluga, S.; Marshall, V.; et al. Phase II Study of Bevacizumab in Patients With HIV-Associated Kaposi's Sarcoma Receiving Antiretroviral Therapy. *J. Clin. Oncol.* **2012**, *30*, 1476–1483. [CrossRef] [PubMed]
156. Ramaswami, R.; Uldrick, T.S.; Polizzotto, M.; Wyvill, K.M.; Goncalves, P.; Widell, A.; Lurain, K.; Steinberg, S.M.; Figg, W.D.; Tosato, G.; et al. A Pilot Study of Liposomal Doxorubicin Combined with Bevacizumab followed by Bevacizumab Monotherapy in Patients with Advanced Kaposi Sarcoma. *Clin. Cancer Res.* **2019**, *25*, 4238–4247. [CrossRef] [PubMed]
157. Uldrick, T.S.; Polizzotto, M.; Aleman, K.; Wyvill, K.M.; Marshall, V.; Whitby, D.; Wang, V.; Pittaluga, S.; O'Mahony, D.; Steinberg, S.M.; et al. Rituximab plus liposomal doxorubicin in HIV-infected patients with KSHV-associated multicentric Castleman disease. *Blood* **2014**, *124*, 3544–3552. [CrossRef]
158. Marcelin, A.-G.; Aaron, L.; Mateus, C.; Gyan, E.; Gorin, I.; Viard, J.-P.; Calvez, V.; Dupin, N. Rituximab therapy for HIV-associated Castleman disease. *Blood* **2003**, *102*, 2786–2788. [CrossRef]
159. Neuville, S.; Agbalika, F.; Rabian, C.; Brière, J.; Molina, J.-M. Failure of rituximab in human immunodeficiency virus-associated multicentric Castleman disease. *Am. J. Hematol.* **2005**, *79*, 337–339. [CrossRef] [PubMed]
160. Nagao, A.; Nakazawa, S.; Hanabusa, H. Short-Term Efficacy of the IL6 Receptor Antibody Tocilizumab in Patients with HIV-Associated Multicentric Castleman Disease: Report of Two Cases. *J. Hematol. Oncol.* **2014**, *7*, 10. [CrossRef]
161. Aita, T.; Hamaguchi, S.; Shimotani, Y.; Nakamoto, Y. Idiopathic Multicentric Castleman Disease Preceded by Cutaneous Plasmacytosis Successfully Treated by Tocilizumab. *BMJ Case Rep.* **2020**, *13*, e236283. [CrossRef]
162. Ramaswami, R.; Lurain, K.; Peer, C.J.; Serquiña, A.; Wang, V.Y.; Widell, A.; Goncalves, P.; Steinberg, S.M.; Marshall, V.; George, J.; et al. Tocilizumab in patients with symptomatic Kaposi sarcoma herpesvirus–associated multicentric Castleman disease. *Blood* **2020**, *135*, 2316–2319. [CrossRef]
163. Moodad, S.; El Hajj, R.; Hleihel, R.; Hajjar, L.; Tawil, N.; Karam, M.; Hamie, M.; Merhi, R.A.; El Sabban, M.; El Hajj, H. Lenalidomide in Combination with Arsenic Trioxide: An Effective Therapy for Primary Effusion Lymphoma. *Cancers* **2020**, *12*, 2483. [CrossRef]
164. Shrestha, P.; Davis, D.A.; Jaeger, H.K.; Stream, A.; Aisabor, A.I.; Yarchoan, R. Pomalidomide restores immune recognition of primary effusion lymphoma through upregulation of ICAM-1 and B7-2. *PLoS Pathog.* **2021**, *17*, e1009091. [CrossRef]
165. Polizzotto, M.; Uldrick, T.S.; Wyvill, K.M.; Aleman, K.; Peer, C.J.; Bevans, M.; Sereti, I.; Maldarelli, F.; Whitby, D.; Marshall, V.; et al. Pomalidomide for Symptomatic Kaposi's Sarcoma in People With and Without HIV Infection: A Phase I/II Study. *J. Clin. Oncol.* **2016**, *34*, 4125–4131. [CrossRef]

166. Neil, R.; Halaby, T.; Weverling, G.J.; Dukers, N.H.T.M.; Simpson, G.R.; Coutinho, R.A.; Lange, J.M.A.; Schulz, T.F.; Goudsmit, J. Seroconversion for Human Herpesvirus 8 during HIV Infection Is Highly Predictive of Kaposi's Sarcoma. *AIDS* **1998**, *12*, 2481–2488.
167. Blasig, C.; Zietz, C.; Haar, B.; Neipel, F.; Esser, S.; Brockmeyer, N.H.; Tschachler, E.; Colombini, S.; Ensoli, B.; Stürzl, M. Monocytes in Kaposi's Sarcoma Lesions Are Productively Infected by Human Herpesvirus 8. *J. Virol.* **1997**, *71*, 7963–7968. [CrossRef]
168. Boshoff, C.; Schulz, T.F.; Kennedy, M.M.; Graham, A.K.; Fisher, C.; Thomas, A.; McGee, J.O.; Weiss, R.A.; O'Leary, J.J. Kaposi's Sarcoma-Associated Herpesvirus Infects Endothelial and Spindle Cells. *Nat. Med.* **1995**, *1*, 1274–1278. [CrossRef] [PubMed]
169. Flore, O.; Rafii, S.; Ely, S.; O'Leary, J.J.; Hyjek, E.M.; Cesarman, E. Transformation of primary human endothelial cells by Kaposi's sarcoma-associated herpesvirus. *Nature* **1998**, *394*, 588–592. [CrossRef] [PubMed]
170. Diamond, C.; Brodie, S.J.; Krieger, J.N.; Huang, M.-L.; Koelle, D.M.; Diem, K.; Muthui, D.; Corey, L. Human Herpesvirus 8 in the Prostate Glands of Men with Kaposi's Sarcoma. *J. Virol.* **1998**, *72*, 6223–6227. [CrossRef] [PubMed]
171. Moses, A.V.; Fish, K.N.; Ruhl, R.; Smith, P.P.; Strussenberg, J.G.; Zhu, L.; Chandran, B.; Nelson, J.A. Long-Term Infection and Transformation of Dermal Microvascular Endothelial Cells by Human Herpesvirus 8. *J. Virol.* **1999**, *73*, 6892–6902. [CrossRef]
172. Blackbourn, D.J.; Lennette, E.; Klencke, B.; Moses, A.; Chandran, B.; Weinstein, M.; Glogau, R.G.; Levy, J.A. The Restricted Cellular Host Range of Human Herpesvirus 8. *AIDS* **2000**, *14*, 1123–1133. [CrossRef]
173. Chandran, B.; Hutt-Fletcher, L. Gammaherpesviruses entry and early events during infection. In *Human Herpesviruses: Biology, Therapy, and Immunoprophylaxis*; Arvin, A., Campadelli-Fiume, G., Mocarski, E., Moore, P.S., Roizman, B., Whitley, R., Eds.; Cambridge University Press: Cambridge, UK, 2007.
174. Bechtel, J.T.; Liang, Y.; Hvidding, J.; Ganem, D. Host Range of Kaposi's Sarcoma-Associated Herpesvirus in Cultured Cells. *J. Virol.* **2003**, *77*, 6474–6481. [CrossRef]
175. Ojala, P.M.; Schulz, T. Manipulation of endothelial cells by KSHV: Implications for angiogenesis and aberrant vascular differentiation. *Semin. Cancer Biol.* **2014**, *26*, 69–77. [CrossRef]
176. Dubich, T.; Dittrich, A.; Bousset, K.; Geffers, R.; Büsche, G.; Köster, M.; Hauser, H.; Schulz, T.F.; Wirth, D. 3D culture conditions support Kaposi's sarcoma herpesvirus (KSHV) maintenance and viral spread in endothelial cells. *J. Mol. Med.* **2021**, *99*, 425–438. [CrossRef]
177. Fujiwara, S.; Nakamura, H. Animal Models for Gammaherpesvirus Infections: Recent Development in the Analysis of Virus-Induced Pathogenesis. *Pathogens* **2020**, *9*, 116. [CrossRef] [PubMed]
178. Chang, H.; Wachtman, L.M.; Pearson, C.B.; Lee, J.-S.; Lee, H.-R.; Lee, S.H.; Vieira, J.; Mansfield, K.G.; Jung, J.U. Non-Human Primate Model of Kaposi's Sarcoma-Associated Herpesvirus Infection. *PLoS Pathog.* **2009**, *5*, e1000606. [CrossRef]
179. Orzechowska, B.; Powers, M.F.; Sprague, J.; Li, H.; Yen, B.; Searles, R.P.; Axthelm, M.K.; Wong, S.W. Rhesus macaque rhadinovirus-associated non-Hodgkin lymphoma: Animal model for KSHV-associated malignancies. *Blood* **2008**, *112*, 4227–4234. [CrossRef]
180. Jung, J.U.; Choi, J.-K.; Ensser, A.; Biesinger, B. Herpesvirus saimiri as a model for gammaherpesvirus oncogenesis. *Semin. Cancer Biol.* **1999**, *9*, 231–239. [CrossRef]
181. Efstathiou, S.; Ho, Y.M.; Minson, A.C. Cloning and molecular characterization of the murine herpesvirus 68 genome. *J. Gen. Virol.* **1990**, *71*, 1355–1364. [CrossRef] [PubMed]
182. Virgin, H.; Latreille, P.; Wamsley, P.; Hallsworth, K.; Weck, E.K.; Canto, A.J.D.; Speck, S.H. Complete sequence and genomic analysis of murine gammaherpesvirus 68. *J. Virol.* **1997**, *71*, 5894–5904. [CrossRef]
183. Louna, K.; Houshaymi, B.; Abdel-Samad, R.; Jaafar, M.; Halloum, I.; Pisano, C.; Neipel, F.; Darwiche, N.; Merhi, R.A. Antitumor Activity of the Synthetic Retinoid ST1926 on Primary Effusion Lymphoma in Vitro and in Vivo Models. *Oncol. Rep.* **2018**, *39*, 721–730. [CrossRef]
184. McHugh, D.; Caduff, N.; Barros, M.H.M.; Rämer, P.C.; Raykova, A.; Murer, A.; Landtwing, V.; Quast, I.; Styles, C.; Spohn, M.; et al. Persistent KSHV Infection Increases EBV-Associated Tumor Formation In Vivo via Enhanced EBV Lytic Gene Expression. *Cell Host Microbe* **2017**, *22*, 61–73.e7. [CrossRef] [PubMed]

viruses MDPI

Article

Peptide Inhibitor of Complement C1, RLS-0071, Reduces Zosteriform Spread of Herpes Simplex Virus Type 1 Skin Infection and Promotes Survival in Infected Mice

Maimoona S. Bhutta [1], Daniel G. Sausen [1], Kirstin M. Reed [1], Elisa S. Gallo [2], Pamela S. Hair [3], Brittany P. Lassiter [3], Neel K. Krishna [3], Kenji M. Cunnion [1,3,4,5,6] and Ronen Borenstein [1,*]

1 Department of Microbiology and Molecular Cell Biology, Eastern Virginia Medical School, Norfolk, VA 23507, USA; BhuttaM@EVMS.EDU (M.S.B.); SausenDG@EVMS.EDU (D.G.S.); ReedKM@EVMS.EDU (K.M.R.); cunniokm@EVMS.EDU (K.M.C.)
2 Board-Certified Dermatologist and Independent Researcher, Norfolk, VA 23507, USA
3 ReAlta Life Sciences, Inc., Norfolk, VA 23502, USA; phair@realtals.com (P.S.H.); blassiter@realtals.com (B.P.L.); nkrishna@realtals.com (N.K.K.)
4 Department of Pediatrics, Eastern Virginia Medical School, Norfolk, VA 23507, USA
5 Children's Specialty Group, 811 Redgate Avenue, Norfolk, VA 23507, USA
6 Children's Hospital of The King's Daughters, Norfolk, VA 23507, USA
* Correspondence: borensR@evms.edu

Citation: Bhutta, M.S.; Sausen, D.G.; Reed, K.M.; Gallo, E.S.; Hair, P.S.; Lassiter, B.P.; Krishna, N.K.; Cunnion, K.M.; Borenstein, R. Peptide Inhibitor of Complement C1, RLS-0071, Reduces Zosteriform Spread of Herpes Simplex Virus Type 1 Skin Infection and Promotes Survival in Infected Mice. *Viruses* **2021**, *13*, 1422. https://doi.org/10.3390/v13081422

Academic Editor: Barry J. Margulies

Received: 7 June 2021
Accepted: 17 July 2021
Published: 22 July 2021

Publisher's Note: MDPI stays neutral with regard to jurisdictional claims in published maps and institutional affiliations.

Abstract: Herpes simplex virus type 1 (HSV-1) is a prevalent human pathogen primarily transmitted through skin-to-skin contact, especially on and around mucosal surfaces where there is contact with contaminated saliva during periods of viral shedding. It is estimated that 90% of adults worldwide have HSV-1 antibodies. Cutaneous HSV-1 infections are characterized by a sensation of tingling or numbness at the initial infection site followed by an eruption of vesicles and then painful ulcers with crusting. These symptoms can take ten days to several weeks to heal, leading to significant morbidity. Histologically, infections cause ballooning degeneration of keratinocytes and formation of multinucleated giant cells, ultimately resulting in a localized immune response. Commonly prescribed treatments against HSV-1 infections are nucleoside analogs, such as acyclovir (ACV). However, the emergence of ACV-resistant HSV (ACV^R-HSV) clinical isolates has created an urgent need for the development of compounds to control symptoms of cutaneous infections. RLS-0071, also known as peptide inhibitor of complement C1 (PIC1), is a 15-amino-acid anti-inflammatory peptide that inhibits classical complement pathway activation and modulates neutrophil activation. It has been previously shown to aid in the healing of chronic diabetic wounds by inhibiting the excessive activation of complement component C1 and infiltration of leukocytes. Here, we report that treatment of cutaneous infections of HSV-1 and ACV^R-HSV-1 in BALB/cJ mice with RLS-0071 significantly reduced the rate of mortality, decreased zosteriform spread, and enhanced the healing of the infection-associated lesions compared to control-treated animals. Therefore, RLS-0071 may work synergistically with other antiviral drugs to aid in wound healing of HSV-1 cutaneous infection and may potentially aid in rapid wound healing of other pathology not limited to HSV-1.

Keywords: RLS-0071; PIC1; antiviral; herpes simplex type 1; acyclovir-resistance; zosteriform infection; anti-inflammatory; complement; neutrophil; wound healing

1. Introduction

An estimated 3.7 billion individuals live with herpes simplex virus 1 (HSV-1) infection worldwide [1]. HSV-1 primarily infects the mucosal epithelial cells, causing the formation of painful, vesicular lesions [2]. Primary infection in the epithelium occurs as HSV-1 targets the basal keratinocytes, spreading into the supra-basal layers [3,4]. Cellular entry of HSV-1 requires the interaction of envelope glycoproteins and cell surface receptors. Glycoprotein D (gD) receptors, herpesvirus entry mediator (HVEM), nectin-1/nectin-2, and 3-O-sulfotransferase-generated heparan sulfate mediate viral entry in murine and human models of infection [3,5].

Murine models have been widely used to investigate cutaneous HSV-1 infection, as they contain HVEM and nectin-1 receptor homologs that support viral entry [3]. In addition, cutaneous or zosteriform scarification models are utilized to infect mice efficiently. In the latter, HSV-1 is scratched onto the skin to expose the epidermal cells to the virus, and as the virus spreads to the innervating sensory neurons, it travels to the dorsal root ganglia. A retrograde spread of infection is seen following viral reactivation, as HSV-1 travels from the spinal cord back to the skin, causing the formation of zosteriform lesions along the dermatome of the nerve [6,7]. Commonly prescribed antiviral agents against HSV are nucleoside analogues, including acyclovir (ACV), which acts as a competitive inhibitor of viral DNA polymerase to block viral replication [8]. ACV-resistant (ACV^R)-HSV strains have been isolated at an increasing rate from immunocompromised patients and stem-cell transplant recipients [9]. Due to the growing population of HSV-1 infected individuals, the emergence of resistant viral strains has generated a need to develop new antiviral agents.

Complement pathways regulate the clearance of necrotic/apoptotic cells, inflammation, and tissue regeneration in response to injury. The complement system is activated by classical, lectin, or alternative pathways and regulates the activation/migration of immune cells, such as neutrophils. Notably, previous research has reported that keratinocytes contain abundant innate immune mediators, complement receptors, and regulatory proteins [10,11]. However, elevated levels of complement factors (C3, C5, and membrane attack complex (MAC)) have been reported to cause excessive inflammation, thus delaying the process of healing and leading to the formation of chronic wounds [10,11]. Therefore, inhibition of complement activation may improve the healing process.

Peptide inhibitor of complement C1 (RLS-0071) is a 15-amino-acid peptide with a monodisperse 24-mer polyethylene glycol (PEG) on its C terminus (IALILEPICCQERAA-dPEG24) that inhibits the activation of C1 and the classical complement pathway and modulates neutrophil activation via inhibition of myeloperoxidase activity and neutrophil extracellular trap formation [12–15]. RLS-0071 was previously reported to bind to C1q and mannose-binding lectin (MBL), displacing the serine protease complex and preventing C1 cleavage [12]. Recently, direct topical application of RLS-0071 was shown to reduce inflammation associated with diabetic wounds of db/db mice, suggesting that this compound may play a role in reducing complement system activation and infiltration of immune cells in the wounded skin [16].

In this paper, we report that RLS-0071 has beneficial activity against HSV-1 skin infection in BALB/cJ mice. Although RLS-0071 did not show direct in vitro HSV-1 inhibition, RLS-0071 formulated in 2.5% hydroxyethyl cellulose (HEC) gel resulted in a significant reduction in mortality and infection scores compared to vehicle-control of HSV-1 and ACV^R-HSV-1 skin infection in BALB/cJ mice. Furthermore, we propose that RLS-0071 inhibits the activation of C1 in surface wounds of BALB/cJ mice, thus reducing inflammation and promoting wound healing.

2. Materials and Methods

2.1. Cells and Animals

GFP-HSV-1 strain 17+ (a generous gift from Dr. Peter O'Hare [17]), was propagated in Vero cells (CCL-81, ATCC) in Dulbecco's Modified Eagle Medium (DMEM, Cat# sc-224478, Ultra-Cruz, Dallas, TX, USA) supplemented with 5% heat-inactivated fetal bovine serum (FBS, Cat# 10082-147, Gibco, Waltham, MA, USA) and 1% penicillin and streptomycin (P/S, Cat# 15140-122, Gibco, Waltham, USA), DMEM/5%. Acyclovir-resistant GFP-HSV-1 (ACV^R-HSV-1) mutant strain was generated in laboratory [18]. Female BALB/cJ mice (5–6 weeks old; Jackson Laboratory, Bar Harbor, ME, USA) were housed in biosafety level 2 (BSL-2) animal facility. Following infections, all mice were single-housed in sterile cages and kept on a 12:12 light-dark cycle. Eastern Virginia Medical School's Institutional Animal Care and Use Committee approved all in vivo procedures under protocol #18-012.

2.2. Sequencing ACV^R-HSV-1 17+

Vero cells were infected with 1MOI of ACV^R-HSV-1 in medium 199 (1X) (Cat# 11150-059, Gibco), supplemented with 1% FBS (Cat# 10082-147, Gibco) and 1% P/S (Cat# 15140-122, Gibco), referred to as 199V, for 1 h at 37 °C. The infected media was removed, fresh DMEM/5% was added to the cells, and the cells were incubated at 37 °C for 20 h. The infected cells were then harvested and collected using low centrifugation (3000 rpm for 5 min). Viral DNA was extracted from the cells using QIAamp DSP DNA Mini Kit (Cat# 61304, Qiagen, MD, USA) according to the manufacturer's instructions. The desired thymidine kinase (TK) primers (Table 1) were generated using ApE Software (ApE- A plasmid Editor, version 3.0.3, Multiplatform DNA editing software, Salt Lake City, UT, USA) and human herpesvirus 1 strain 17, complete genome (NCBI Reference Sequence: NC_001806.2).

Table 1. Thymidine kinase (TK) primers used with their respective sequences and melting temperatures.

Name	Melting Temperature	Sequences
Forward	54.3 °C	5′- CTT AAC AGC GTC AAC AGC G -3′
Reverse	54.5 °C	5′- CAC CCG TGC GTT TTA TTC TG -3′

The forward primer was located at nucleotides 47,886-47,868 of HSV-1 strain 17+ genome (NCBI Reference Sequence: NC_001806.2), 83 nucleotides upstream to the ORF of the TK gene. The reverse primer was located at nucleotides 46,598-46,617 of HSV-1 strain 17+ genome (NCBI Reference Sequence: NC_001806.2), 75 nucleotides upstream to the ORF of the TK gene. The entire TK gene (1131 bp plus the additional 83 bp and 75 bp) was amplified using Herculase II PCR Fusion Polymerase Kit (Cat# 600675, Agilent Technologies Inc., Santa Clara, CA, USA) according to the manufacturer's instructions. The cycling program consisted of initial denaturing for 3 min at 95 °C, followed by 34 cycles of 30 s at 95 °C, 30 s at 51 °C, and 1.5 min at 72 °C, with a final extension of 5 min at 72 °C. The PCR product was purified using GeneJet PCR Purification kit (Cat# K0701, Thermo Fisher Scientific, Waltham, MA, USA) according to the manufacturer's instructions. The purified PCR product was sequenced, using the primers in Table 1, in forward and reverse directions by the Molecular Core Facility at Eastern Virginia Medical School (Norfolk, VA, USA).

2.3. Plaque Assay

The virus titer of GFP-HSV-1 (6.0×10^7 PFU/mL) was determined by standard plaque assays, as previously described by our lab [18,19]. The antiviral and virucidal activity of RLS-0071, following GFP-HSV-1 infection, was assessed in in vitro cell culture before in vivo experiments. The Vero cell monolayer in a 6-well plate was pretreated with 0-to-5 mM of RLS-0071 or 0.05 M Histidine Buffer (HIS buffer) for 1 h. The cells were then infected with 0.1 MOI of GFP-HSV-1 17+ in 199 media, supplemented with 1% FBS and 1% P/S (199V), for 1 h at 37 °C. After incubation, Vero cells were washed twice with DPBS 1× and replaced with 199V media containing the respective treatments for 16 h. To test the virucidal activity of RLS-0071, 0.1 MOI cell-free GFP-HSV-1 17+ virus was incubated with increasing concentrations of RLS-0071 or HIS buffer for 1 h. The treated virus was then used to infect Vero cell monolayer in 6-well plates in 199V media for 1 h at 37 °C. After incubation, the Vero cells were washed twice with DPBS 1×, and fresh 199V was added to the monolayer for 16 h. The infected culture was collected, and the viral titer was measured using plaque assays, as previously described [18,19].

2.4. Zosteriform Infection Model and Treatments

Prior to infection, the right flank skin of female BALB/cJ mice was chemically denuded using Nair cream (Nair™, Ewing, NJ, USA) under gas anesthesia. Following 24 h with no signs of chemical irritation, BALB/cJ mice were anesthetized with intraperitoneal injections of ketamine/xylazine (120 mg/kg; 12 mg/kg), and the shaved skin was scratch-inoculated with 6×10^4 PFU of GFP-HSV-1 strain 17+ or 2.0×10^5 PFU of ACV^R-HSV-1 [18], using the pointed-side of a 27-gauge needle. The epidermal scarification-zosteriform model was used as previously described [6].

RLS-0071 was a generous gift from ReAlta Life Sciences (Norfolk, VA, USA) and was solubilized in 0.05M Histidine buffer (HIS buffer) (pH 6.5). To ascertain there was no vehicle effect, a control study was conducted wherein mice (N = 5/treatment) were initially treated with 40% HIS buffer in 2.5% hydroxyethyl cellulose (HEC) gel (Cat# 09368, Sigma-Aldrich, St. Louis, MO, USA) and compared with animals treated with 10% DMSO (Cat#D2650-5X10mL, Sigma-Aldrich, MO, USA) in 2.5% HEC gel.

The treatment studies, following infections with GFP-HSV-1 17+ or ACV^R-HSV-1, were designed to treat the inoculated site with 10% DMSO (acyclovir vehicle control) and 40% HIS buffer formulated in 2.5% HEC gel, 14.4 mM RLS-0071 (40 mg/mL) in 2.5% HEC gel, or 10 mM ACV (2.25 mg/mL; Cat#2513, Tocris, MN, USA; control for the standard of care) with 40% HIS buffer in 2.5% HEC gel. The treatment schedule started 1-h post-infection and continued twice daily (at 12-h intervals) for 14 days. Signs of disease at the inoculation site were scored by the appearance of vesicles and erosions, as previously outlined [18]. Table 2 outlines the infection grading scales utilized in this study.

Table 2. Zosteriform infection grading scale.

Grade	Skin Outcomes
0	no lesions
1, 2	local site lesions
3, 4, 5	distant site zosteriform lesions along the dermatome
6	progression to severely compromised health
7	mortality (succumbed to infection)

2.5. Statistical Analyses

Prism Graph Pad version 9.0.0 (GraphPad Software, San Diego, CA, USA) was used to analyze survivability by Kaplan–Meier analysis and Log-rank (Mantel–Cox) test. Changes in infections scores were analyzed using one-way ANOVA (with independent *t*-tests) or mixed-model ANOVAs (with multiple comparisons).

3. Results

3.1. RLS-0071 Has No In Vitro Antiviral Activity

RLS-0071 has been previously reported to have antimicrobial activity against Pseudomonas aeruginosa, Staphylococcus aureus, Klebsiella pneumoniae, Neisseria meningitidis, Neisseria gonorrhoeae, Gardnerella vaginalis, and Prevotella bivia bacteria [20]. We began by investigating whether RLS-0071 possesses antiviral or virucidal activity against HSV-1 in vitro. To test the antiviral activity of RLS-0071, 80–85% confluent Vero cells were pretreated with varying concentrations of RLS-0071 or HIS buffer (control) and then infected with 0.1 MOI of GFP-HSV-1 17+. The infected media was replaced with fresh 199V media and incubated for an additional 16 h. The viral titer (PFU/mL) was determined through plaque assay. RLS-0071 did not exhibit a reduction in viral titer when compared to HIS Buffer-treated cells (Table S1). Following this, we examined whether RLS-0071 possesses virucidal activity against HSV-1. 0.1 MOI of GFP-HSV-1 cell-free virus, pre-incubated with varying concentrations of RLS-0071 or HIS buffer for 1 h prior to infecting Vero cells. Vero cells were infected with the cell-free virus for 1 h before the infected media was replaced with fresh 199V media. The infected cells were incubated for an additional 16 h, and the viral titer was determined by plaque assay. RLS-0071 did not exhibit a reduction in viral titer when compared to control-treated Vero cells; thus, virucidal effect could not be concluded in vitro (Table S2).

3.2. Histidine Buffer and DMSO Are Neutral for HSV-1 Cutaneous Infection

To demonstrate that the RLS-0071 and the ACV carriers have no effect on the infection, 0.05 M histidine buffer (HIS buffer), in which RLS-0071 is soluble, was compared with

DMSO, in which ACV is soluble. The inoculated site of BALB/cJ mice was treated with 10% DMSO (control) in 2.5% HEC gel or 40% HIS Buffer (formulation ratio for RLS-0071) in 2.5% HEC gel. The infection scores of the animals were averaged each day across 14 days and analyzed. Our results indicate that there was no significant difference between both control treatments, as they demonstrated a 0% survivability rate within 14 days and a median survival for 9 days ($p = 0.6630$). No observed significance was recorded, as both DMSO-treated and HIS Buffer-treated animals exhibited a significant increase in the severity of HSV-1 infection, reaching the study endpoint (score 7) by day 9 (Figure S1). We concluded that the subsequent observed effects of the treatments would be unaffected by the addition of their respective solvents.

3.3. RLS-0071 Formulated in HEC Gel Protects BALB/cJ Mice Against GFP-HSV-1 Zosteriform Infection

RLS-0071 has previously demonstrated chronic-wound-healing capabilities in db/db mice [16] via inhibition of complement activation and neutrophil extracellular trap (NET) formation in a dose-dependent manner [14]. Thus, we examined the effect of RLS-0071 in healing of infectious wounds in BALB/cJ mice.

Five- to six-week-old female BALB/cJ mice (15 mice in each group) were used to analyze the efficacy of RLS-0071 against zosteriform infection. Cutaneous GFP-HSV-1 infections were conducted using the epidermal scarification-zosteriform model, as previously described by Goel et al. [6]. For topical treatments, we formulated 14.4 mM RLS-0071 (40 mg/mL) in 2.5% hydroxyethyl cellulose (HEC) gel, which does not have active microbicidal activity and has been adopted as a placebo in many clinical trials of microbicides [21,22]. All animals were inoculated with 6.0×10^4 PFU GFP-HSV-1 17+, as previously established [18].

Following GFP-HSV-1 infection, the inoculation site was treated with 10% DMSO (vehicle control) formulated in 2.5% HEC gel, 14.4 mM RLS-0071 in 2.5% HEC gel, or 10 mM acyclovir (ACV) in 2.5% HEC gel (control for the standard of care). Each treatment was administered 1-h post-infection (p.i.) and continued b.i.d. at 12-h intervals for 14 days. Animals were monitored daily for any signs of physical deterioration. Disease at the inoculation site was scored by the appearance of vesicles and erosions.

Our results indicate that vehicle DMSO-treated animals exhibited a 0% survival rate within 14 days (Figure 1A). RLS-0071-treated animals showed a 53.3% rate of survivability p.i. compared to the vehicle-treated control animals across 14 days ($p < 0.0001$ indicated by Log-rank (Mantel–Cox) test). The DMSO-treated animals exhibited significantly increased infection severity and severely compromised health (Figure 1B,C). In addition, RLS-0071-treated animals demonstrated a significant reduction in the vesicle formation compared to control animals on days 9–14 p.i. ($p < 0.01$ and $p < 0.001$, multiple comparisons tests). We also observed healing of the lesions on the skin flank of animals treated with RLS-0071 post day nine (Figure 1B). As expected, animals treated with ACV did not exhibit severe infection and demonstrated 100% survivability p.i. (Figure 1B,C). Analyzing the distribution of infection scores averaged per day for each group indicated that treatment with RLS-0071 significantly reduces infection severity across 14 days ($p < 0.0001$) compared with the DMSO-treated mice for which the infection scores peaked around day nine (Figure 1D).

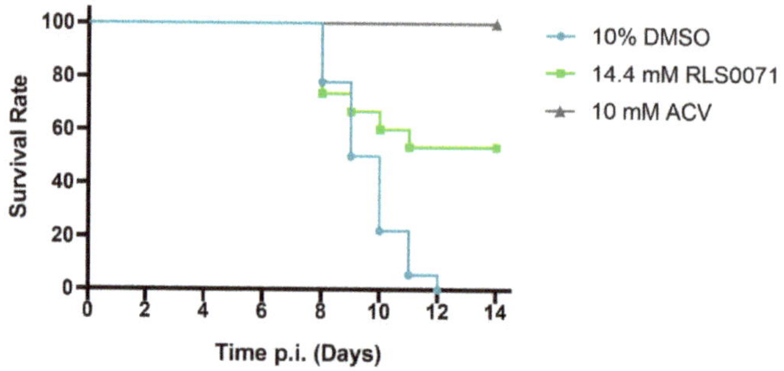

(**A**)

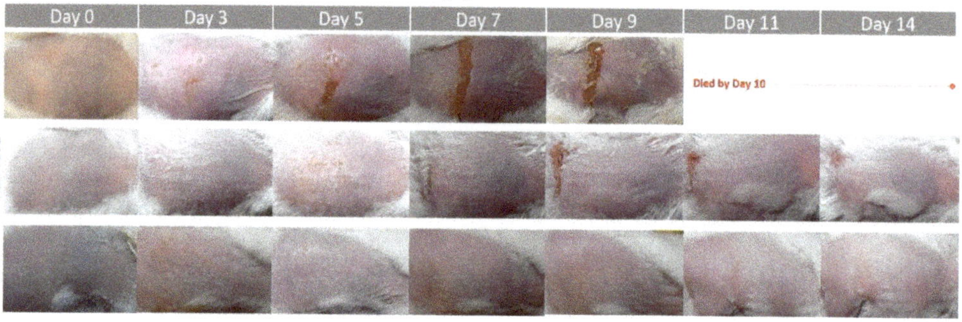

(**B**)

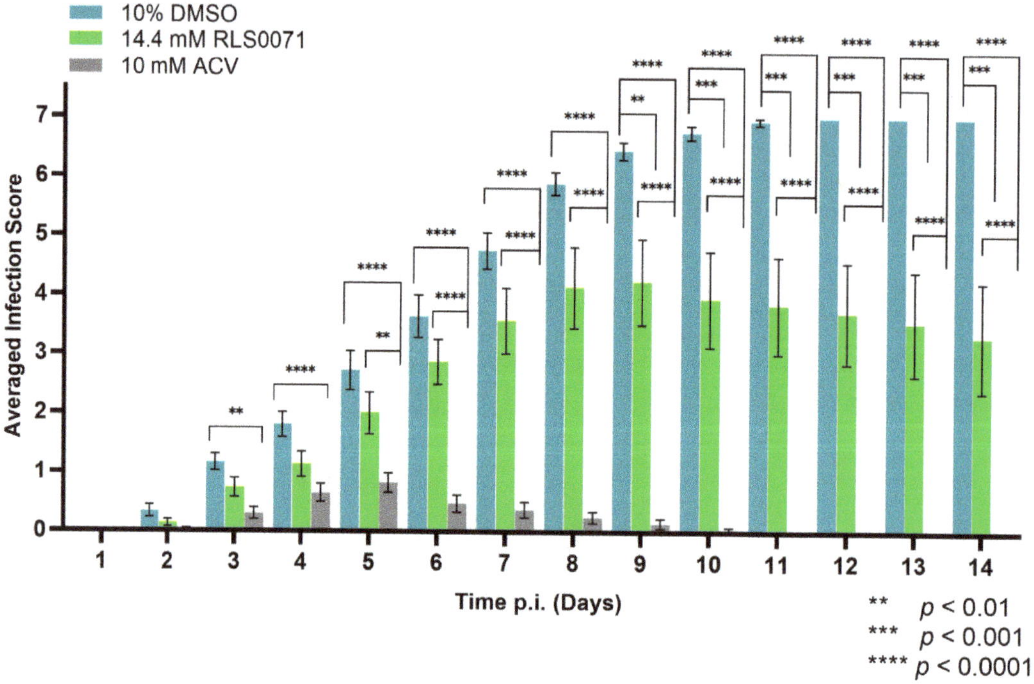

(**C**)

Figure 1. *Cont.*

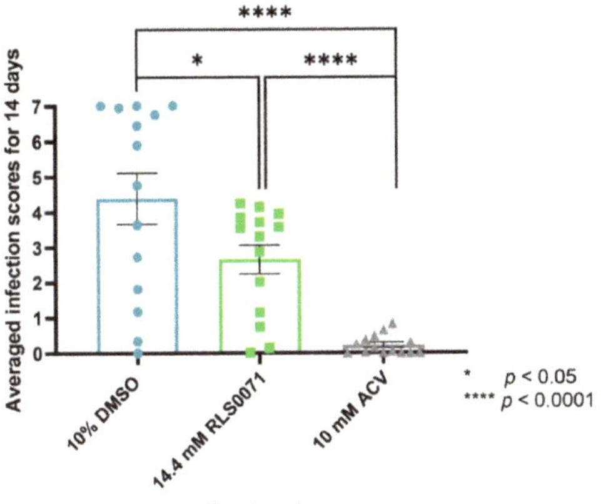

(D)

Figure 1. GFP-HSV-1 zosteriform infections in BALB/cJ mice, following the application of 10% DMSO, 14.4 mM RLS-0071, or 10 mM ACV in 2.5% hydroxyethyl cellulose (HEC) gel. (**A**) Age- and weight-matched BALB/cJ mice were inoculated with 6×10^4 PFU of GFP-HSV-1 and received their respective treatments. Animals were monitored for survival for 14 days. (**B**) Representative images of female BALB/cJ mice in an epidermal scarification-zosteriform model receiving respective treatments across varying time points of the study. (**C**) Averaged infection scores of animals were analyzed for each treatment group across 14 days. (**D**) Distribution of averaged infection score of all animals per day for 14 days. RLS-0071-treated animals demonstrated a significant reduction in the appearance of vesicles and erosions on the skin of BALB/cJ mice compared to control animals. (**C**) Mixed-model ANOVA and multiple comparison tests (Interaction (Time*Treatment): ($p < 0.0001$); Treatments (DMSO/RLS0071/ACV): ($p < 0.0001$); and Time (days): ($p < 0.0001$)) and (**D**) one-way ANOVA ($p < 0.0001$) and independent t-tests (DMSO-RLS0071: $p = 0.0465$; DMSO-ACV: $p < 0.0001$; ACV-RLS0071: $p < 0.0001$); * $p < 0.05$, ** $p < 0.01$, *** $p < 0.001$, **** $p < 0.0001$. All error bars represent SEM.

3.4. Sequencing of ACV^R-HSV-1 Thymidine Kinase, UL23, Gene

Mutations leading to the acquisition of acyclovir-resistance have been found in HSV-1 thymidine kinase gene, (UL23), which accounts for 95% of clinical isolates, or in polymerase gene (UL30), which accounts for 5% of clinical isolates [8,9,23]. Single nucleotide insertions, deletions, or substitutions cause a frameshift mutation resulting in the synthesis of non-functional/truncated thymidine kinase (TK). ACV^R-HSV-1 strain 17+ was previously generated and verified in our laboratory [18].

The TK gene in our ACV^R-HSV-1 strain 17+ was sequenced to reveal possible mutations that cause drug resistance. The isolated viral TK sequence was compared to wild-type HSV-1 strain 17+ (NCBI Reference Sequence: NC_001806.2) using PubMed BLASTn and BLASTx (Figure S2). Our laboratory-generated ACV^R-HSV-1 demonstrated a single-base nucleotide mutation in the viral UL23 gene from cytosine (C) to thymine (T) at nucleotide 860 within one of the highly conserved regions of TK [24,25]. This was reflected by a substitution mutation from threonine at amino acid (aa) 287 (T287) to methionine (T287M), resulting in a substitution mutation in the viral thymidine kinase gene (Figure 2).

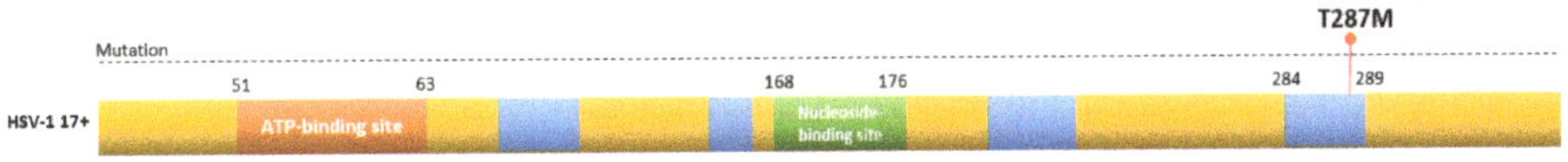

Figure 2. Schematic overview of conserved/active domains of viral thymidine kinase (TK). TK has 6 major conserved regions, an ATP-binding pocket (aa 51–63) composed of glycine-rich loop (red), a nucleoside-binding region (aa 168–177; green), and multiple highly conserved regions (blue), including aa 284–289. The viral TK gene of our ACV^R-HSV-1 had a mutation at nt860 (cytosine to thymine), leading to a substitution mutation at aa 287 within the conserved region (threonine to methionine).

3.5. RLS-0071 Protects BALB/cJ Mice against Cutaneous ACV^R-HSV-1 Strain 17+ Infection

Due to the ongoing battle against drug-resistant HSV, we tested the effect of RLS-0071 against acyclovir-resistant infections. Female BALB/cJ mice (N = 8/treatment) were inoculated with 2.0×10^5 PFU of ACV^R-HSV-1 previously established in our laboratory [18]. The infected skin was treated with 10% DMSO, 14.4 mM RLS-0071, or 10 mM ACV formulated in 2.5% HEC gel. Each treatment was administered 1 h p.i. and continued twice daily (at 12-h intervals) for 14 days. The signs of disease at the inoculation site were scored per the appearance of vesicles.

Our results indicated 100% survivability of all animals regardless of treatment. This was expected because ACV-resistant mutants have been shown to have reduced pathogenicity in BALB/cJ mice, as judged by animal survival following infection [18,26]. Analyzing the interactions between BALB/cJ mice receiving DMSO or ACV revealed similar levels of infection, as no statistical significance was observed between the respective two treatment groups ($p = 0.4655$). On the other hand, RLS-0071-treated animals demonstrated a significant reduction in the formation of vesicles and erosions compared to DMSO-treated animals on days 3, 4, and 8-to-12 ($p < 0.05$, $p < 0.01$, and $p < 0.001$, indicated by multiple comparison tests). RLS-0071-treated mice also demonstrated a significant decrease in the vesicle formation compared to ACV-treated animals from days 7-to-12 ($p < 0.05$, $p < 0.01$, and $p < 0.001$, indicated by multiple comparison tests) (Figure 3). We observed that the infected vesicles on the skin of RLS-0071-treated mice healed completely by day 12. These results indicate that RLS-0071 exhibits efficacious effects on healing of the skin following ACV^R infection.

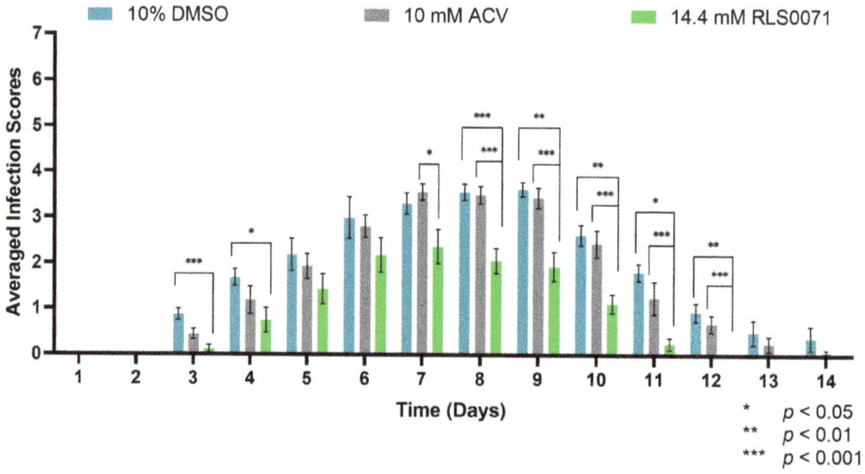

Figure 3. ACV^R-HSV-1 infection scores of BALB/cJ mice following the application of 10% DMSO, 14.4 mM RLS-0071, or 10 mM ACV in 2.5% HEC gel (N = 8/group). Age-matched BALB/cJ mice were inoculated with 2.0×10^5 PFU of ACV^R-HSV-1 and treated. The mice were monitored for 14 days, and the averaged infection scores of animals in each treatment group were recorded. RLS-0071-treated BALB/cJ mice demonstrated a significant reduction in the appearance of vesicles compared to DMSO-treated animals. Mixed-model ANOVA and multiple comparison tests (Interactions (Time*Treatment): ($p = 0.0017$); Treatments (DMSO/RLS0071/ACV): ($p < 0.0001$); and Time (days): ($p < 0.0001$)); * $p < 0.05$; ** $p < 0.01$; *** $p < 0.001$. All error bars represent SEM.

4. Discussion

In this study, we demonstrated that RLS-0071 significantly reduces the appearance of vesicles and erosions on the skin of GFP-HSV-1-infected BALB/cJ mice and significantly improves survivability when compared to HSV-1-infected animals receiving the control treatment. Infection scores in RLS-0071 animals were significantly lower compared to control-treated mice. The infection scores of BALB/cJ mice began decreasing around day nine, and healing of the infected sites was observed. Whereas infection scores of the control DMSO-treated mice continued to increase, by day 12, all control-treated animals succumbed. In contrast, HSV-1-infected animals receiving 10 mM of ACV did not demonstrate formation of infected vesicles, which is consistent with the effect of ACV seen in previous studies [18]. This effect of RLS-0071 is also consistent with our observations in animals infected with ACV-resistant HSV-1 strain 17+. RLS-0071-treated BALB/cJ mice demonstrated a significant reduction in the appearance of infected vesicles when compared to animals receiving control or ACV treatment across 14 days. The infection score of ACV^R-infected animals treated with DMSO and ACV peaked around days seven to eight p.i., whereas the infection score for RLS-0071 did not peak, but rather, lesions healed completely by day 11 p.i.

The first phase of acute cutaneous infection caused by HSV-1 occurs in keratinocytes at the site of infection. As the virus enters the sensory neurons, it travels to the dorsal root ganglia (DRG), where it replicates. Following replication, the virus travels in an anterograde manner from the DRG back to the skin, inducing the second phase of viral growth, which results in zosteriform infection across the dermatome [6,27]. The role of neutrophils has been studied during viral infection, specifically their recruitment to skin flanks at the peak of infection [28,29]. Infected or damaged cells release pathogen-associated molecular patterns (PAMP), which trigger the release of inflammatory chemokines (Cxcl1/2/3) by resident macrophages and mast cells, leading to the recruitment of neutrophils to the infected sites [29,30]. The innate immune system is activated when pattern-recognition receptors detect viral PAMPs. The role of toll-like receptors (TLRs) in recognizing three classes of HSV PAMPs, such as viral proteins, DNA, and RNA, has been extensively reviewed [30–32]. At the cell surface, TLR2 senses viral glycoproteins B (gB) and gH/L, which activate nuclear factor κB pathway to induce expression of chemokines (C-X-C chemokine ligands) and pro-inflammatory cytokines (TNF-α, IL-6, IL-12). After entering the cell, endosomal TLR3/9 are activated by HSV nucleic acids, and PRRs (NOD-like receptors, melanoma differentiation-associated gene 5, interferon-inducible protein 16, and several helicases) recognize viral DNA and RNA in the cytoplasm. As a result, type I and III interferon (IFN) signaling is activated in human keratinocytes and infiltrating monocytes [31,32]. Previous studies have shown neutrophil accumulation below the infected epidermal layer; however, only a small number of neutrophils can migrate to the draining lymph nodes after T-cell priming five to seven days post infection, which is consistently seen within HSV-1-infected keratinocytes [33]. Hung et al. reported that although neutrophils in circulation undergo apoptosis within 24–36 h, HSV-1 can still be detected in neutrophils 36 h post exposure [34]. As the neutrophils are broken into apoptotic bodies, they are engulfed by macrophages. Live HSV-1 viruses within the engulfed apoptotic bodies can survive, evading the immune system and facilitating the spread of infection [34]. Thus, targeting the excessive infiltration of immune cells at the site of infection may reduce the site inflammation, thereby decreasing the appearance of surface vesicles and erosions. As we report in this paper, RLS-0071 has shown significant reduction in the appearance of vesicles on the skin of infected mice. We attributed the reduction of lesions to RLS-0071's similar success in healing chronic diabetic wounds [16]. Cunnion et al. reported that RLS-0071 reduced inflammation, as observed by a reduction in activation of the complement system and leukocyte infiltration, after applied directly onto the skin of diabetic C57BL/Ks db/db male mice or when saturated in an acellular skin scaffold [16]. Hair et al. reported that within systemic lupus erythematosus (SLE) pathogenesis, RLS-0071 not only inhibited immune complex-initiated complement activation but also inhibited neutrophil extracellular trap (NET) formation in a dose-dependent fashion [14]. The inhibition of NET formation was suggested to occur following the inhibition of myeloperoxidase (MPO), which mediates NET formation by generating hypochlorous acid from hydrogen peroxide and chloride ions [14,15]. This would suggest that RLS-0071 may decrease excessive immune complex-initiated complement activation and accumulation of neutrophils by inhibiting NET formation on the skin of mice with wild-type and drug-resistant HSV-1 infection, thereby aiding in the healing process.

It was previously reported that a higher proportion of mutations causing resistance to acyclovir normally occur within the conserved regions of the ATP-binding site and or the nucleoside-binding site [25,35]. However, conserved amino acid regions spanning loci of aa 83–88, aa 216–222, aa 162–164, and aa 284–289 are not as affected [32]. Interestingly, sequencing our laboratory-generated, acyclovir-resistant HSV-1 strain 17+ revealed a single-base substitution mutation in the conserved region of thymidine kinase (TK) gene occurring at nucleotide 860, which resulted in a nucleotide change from cytosine of the wild-type HSV-1 17+ to thymine in the ACV^R-HSV-1 strain 17+. Studies investigating ACV-resistance have often reported that 50% of HSV-1 drug resistance is attributable to a frameshift mutation in TK, whereas the majority of the mutations are triggered by amino acid substitutions following changes in a nucleotide that occurs in a non-conserved region (64.9%) as opposed to a conserved region (5.2%) [25]. We reported that the single-base nucleotide change in viral TK of ACV^R-HSV-1 caused the substitution of threonine (T287) to methionine (T287M) in a conserved region of TK. A substitution mutation of T287M has also been previously reported by Sauerbrei et al. to occur in ACV-resistant clinical isolates of HSV-1 [24].

In conclusion, we report that RLS-0071 demonstrates the ability to decrease the appearance of vesicle formation on the flank of infected BALB/cJ mice. We propose that RLS-0071 may decrease excessive infiltration of leukocytes and complement activation at the site of infection, thereby promoting healing of lesions. Given these findings, RLS-0071 may have utility in conjunction with antiviral or virucidal compounds to aid in rapid wound healing of HSV-1 skin infections and potentially other pathology not limited to HSV-1 infection.

Supplementary Materials: The following are available online at https://www.mdpi.com/article/10.3390/v13081422/s1, Table S1: Testing the antiviral effect of RLS-0071 using plaque assays, Table S2: Testing the virucidal effect of RLS-0071 using plaque assay, Figure S1: GFP-HSV-1 zosteriform infection scores of BALB/cJ mice (N = 5/treatment) following the application of 10% DMSO or 40% HIS buffer in 2.5% hydroxyethyl cellulose (HEC) gel, Figure S2: Analysis of ACV^R-HSV-1 thymidine kinase gene sequence using PubMed BLASTn and BLASTx.

Author Contributions: Conceptualization, R.B., M.S.B., E.S.G., N.K.K. and K.M.C.; methodology, M.S.B. and R.B.; resources, R.B., B.P.L., P.S.H., N.K.K. and K.M.C.; statistical analysis, M.S.B.; validation, R.B. and M.S.B.; in vitro data curation, M.S.B.; in vivo data curation, M.S.B., D.G.S. and K.M.R.; formal analysis M.S.B. and R.B.; writing—original draft preparation, M.S.B., R.B. and E.S.G.; writing—review and editing, R.B., M.S.B., D.G.S., K.M.R., E.S.G., N.K.K. and K.M.C.; supervision/project, R.B.; administration/funding acquisition, R.B. All authors have read and agreed to the published version of the manuscript.

Funding: This research received no external funding.

Institutional Review Board Statement: Not applicable.

Informed Consent Statement: Not applicable.

Data Availability Statement: The data presented in this study are available upon request from the corresponding author.

Acknowledgments: We would like to sincerely acknowledge the kind technical support of EVMS Comparative Medicine's attending veterinarian, Mario Rodriguez, DVM, and veterinarian technicians Sarah Pisani Martin, Josiah Hamilton, and Jason A. Ekins. We would also like to acknowledge the kind support of Julia Sharp, director of Eastern Virginia Medical School's Molecular Core Facility.

Conflicts of Interest: Pam Hair, Brittany Lassiter, Kenji Cunnion, and Neel Krishna are employees of ReAlta Life Sciences, Inc., an entity that is pursuing therapeutic development of the Peptide Inhibitors of Complement C1 (EPICC molecules) for various clinical applications. https://urldefense.com/v3/__https://realtalifesciences.com/__;!!Aeua5Q!DjwQxwpAcCfdbMwAsJI2Caa3GCLg_OZqcpkI5-ekA2pFVz3yTqLWBRVVgY2CYAc$. ReAlta Life Sciences provided the molecule RLS-0071 for these studies but provided no other financial support for this work. Pam Hair, Brittany Lassiter, Kenji Cunnion, and Neel Krishna are employed by ReAlta, but they did not participate in the actual performance of the experiments or data collection. Other than the named authors, no other members of ReAlta participated in study design, data collection, and analysis, the decision to publish, or the preparation of the manuscript. Neel Krishna and Kenji Cunnion have ownership of ReAlta shares, and Kenji Cunnion serves as on the Board of Directors of ReAlta Life Sciences. Neel K Krishna and Kenji M Cunnion are listed as inventors on patents that describe PIC1 molecules, which includes RLS-0071. The authors would like to declare the following patents/patent applications associated with this research: 8,241,843 methods for regulating complement cascade proteins using astrovirus coat protein and derivatives thereof, 15/738,786 synthetic peptide compounds and methods of use, 16/400,486 synthetic peptide compounds and methods of use, 8,906,845 peptide compounds to regulate the complement system, 9,422,337 peptide compounds to regulate the complement system, 10,005,818 derivative peptide compounds and methods of use, 9,914,753 peptide compounds to regulate the complement system, 10,414,799 peptide compounds to regulate the complement system, 16/534,200 peptide compounds to regulate the complement system, 16/242,550 PIC1 inhibition of myeloperoxidase oxidative activity in an animal model.

References

1. WHO. Massive Proportion of World's Population Are Living with Herpes Infection. Available online: https://www.who.int/news/item/01-05-2020-massive-proportion-world-population-living-with-herpes-infection#:~{}:text=An%20estimated%203.7%20billion%20people,the%20mouth%20(oral%20herpes) (accessed on 27 May 2021).
2. Waisner, H.; Kalamvoki, M. The ICP0 Protein of Herpes Simplex Virus 1 (HSV-1) Downregulates Major Autophagy Adaptor Proteins Sequestosome 1 and Optineurin during the Early Stages of HSV-1 Infection. *J. Virol.* **2019**, *93*. [CrossRef]
3. Yamamoto, Y.; Yamamoto, T.; Aoyama, Y.; Fujimoto, W. Cell-to-cell transmission of HSV-1 in differentiated keratinocytes promotes multinucleated giant cell formation. *J. Dermatol. Sci.* **2019**, *93*, 14–23. [CrossRef]
4. Rahn, E.; Petermann, P.; Thier, K.; Bloch, W.; Morgner, J.; Wickström, S.A.; Knebel-Mörsdorf, D. Invasion of Herpes Simplex Virus Type 1 into Murine Epidermis: An Ex Vivo Infection Study. *J. Investig. Dermatol.* **2015**, *135*, 3009–3016. [CrossRef]
5. Petermann, P.; Thier, K.; Rahn, E.; Rixon, F.J.; Bloch, W.; Özcelik, S.; Krummenacher, C.; Barron, M.; Dixon, M.J.; Scheu, S.; et al. Entry Mechanisms of Herpes Simplex Virus 1 into Murine Epidermis: Involvement of Nectin-1 and Herpesvirus Entry Mediator as Cellular Receptors. *J. Virol.* **2014**, *89*, 262–274. [CrossRef] [PubMed]
6. Goel, N.; Mao, H.; Rong, Q.; Docherty, J.J.; Zimmerman, D.; Rosenthal, K.S. The ability of an HSV strain to initiate zosteriform spread correlates with its neuroinvasive disease potential. *Arch. Virol.* **2002**, *147*, 763–773. [CrossRef]
7. McGraw, H.M.; Awasthi, S.; Wojcechowskyj, J.A.; Friedman, H.M. Anterograde Spread of Herpes Simplex Virus Type 1 Requires Glycoprotein E and Glycoprotein I but Not Us9. *J. Virol.* **2009**, *83*, 8315–8326. [CrossRef] [PubMed]
8. Frobert, E.; Ooka, T.; Cortay, J.C.; Lina, B.; Thouvenot, D.; Morfin, F. Herpes Simplex Virus Thymidine Kinase Mutations Associated with Resistance to Acyclovir: A Site-Directed Mutagenesis Study. *Antimicrob. Agents Chemother.* **2005**, *49*, 1055–1059. [CrossRef] [PubMed]
9. Piret, J.; Boivin, G. Antiviral resistance in herpes simplex virus and varicella-zoster virus infections. *Curr. Opin. Infect. Dis.* **2016**, *29*, 654–662. [CrossRef]
10. Rafail, S.; Kourtzelis, I.; Foukas, P.G.; Markiewski, M.M.; DeAngelis, R.A.; Guariento, M.; Ricklin, D.; Grice, E.; Lambris, J.D. Complement Deficiency Promotes Cutaneous Wound Healing in Mice. *J. Immunol.* **2015**, *194*, 1285–1291. [CrossRef] [PubMed]
11. Cazander, G.; Jukema, G.N.; Nibbering, P.H. Complement Activation and Inhibition in Wound Healing. *Clin. Dev. Immunol.* **2012**, *2012*, 534291. [CrossRef] [PubMed]
12. Sharp, J.A.; Hair, P.S.; Pallera, H.K.; Kumar, P.S.; Mauriello, C.T.; Nyalwidhe, J.O.; Phelps, C.A.; Park, D.; Thielens, N.M.; Pascal, S.M.; et al. Peptide Inhibitor of Complement C1 (PIC1) Rapidly Inhibits Complement Activation after Intravascular Injection in Rats. *PLoS ONE* **2015**, *10*, e0132446. [CrossRef]
13. Sharp, J.A.; Whitley, P.H.; Cunnion, K.M.; Krishna, N.K. Peptide Inhibitor of Complement C1, a Novel Suppressor of Classical Pathway Activation: Mechanistic Studies and Clinical Potential. *Front. Immunol.* **2014**, *5*, 406. [CrossRef]
14. Hair, P.S.; Enos, A.I.; Krishna, N.K.; Cunnion, K.M. Inhibition of Immune Complex Complement Activation and Neutrophil Extracellular Trap Formation by Peptide Inhibitor of Complement C1. *Front. Immunol.* **2018**, *9*, 558. [CrossRef]
15. Hair, P.S.; Sass, L.A.; Krishna, N.K.; Cunnion, K.M. Inhibition of Myeloperoxidase Activity in Cystic Fibrosis Sputum by Peptide Inhibitor of Complement C1 (PIC1). *PLoS ONE* **2017**, *12*, e0170203. [CrossRef]
16. Cunnion, K.M.; Krishna, N.K.; Pallera, H.K.; Pineros-Fernandez, A.; Rivera, M.G.; Hair, P.S.; Lassiter, B.P.; Huyck, R.; Clements, M.A.; Hood, A.F.; et al. Complement Activation and STAT4 Expression Are Associated with Early Inflammation in Diabetic Wounds. *PLoS ONE* **2017**, *12*, e0170500. [CrossRef] [PubMed]
17. Elliott, G.; O'Hare, P. Live-Cell Analysis of a Green Fluorescent Protein-Tagged Herpes Simplex Virus Infection. *J. Virol.* **1999**, *73*, 4110–4119. [CrossRef]
18. Bhutta, M.S.; Shechter, O.; Gallo, E.S.; Martin, S.D.; Jones, E.; Doncel, G.F.; Borenstein, R. Ginkgolic Acid Inhibits Herpes Simplex Virus Type 1 Skin Infection and Prevents Zosteriform Spread in Mice. *Viruses* **2021**, *13*, 86. [CrossRef] [PubMed]
19. Borenstein, R.; Hanson, B.A.; Markosyan, R.M.; Gallo, E.S.; Narasipura, S.D.; Bhutta, M.; Shechter, O.; Lurain, N.S.; Cohen, F.S.; Al-Harthi, L.; et al. Ginkgolic acid inhibits fusion of enveloped viruses. *Sci. Rep.* **2020**, *10*, 4746. [CrossRef] [PubMed]

20. Hair, P.S.; Rivera, M.G.; Enos, A.I.; Pearsall, S.E.; Sharp, J.A.; Yousefieh, N.; Lattanzio, F.A.; Krishna, N.K.; Cunnion, K.M. Peptide Inhibitor of Complement C1 (PIC1) Inhibits Growth of Pathogenic Bacteria. *Int. J. Pept. Res. Ther.* **2019**, *25*, 83–92. [CrossRef]
21. Karim, Q.A.; Karim, S.A.; Frohlich, J.A.; Grobler, A.; Baxter, C.; Mansoor, L.E.; Kharsany, A.B.M.; Sibeko, S.; Mlisana, K.; Omar, Z.; et al. Effectiveness and Safety of Tenofovir Gel, an Antiretroviral Microbicide, for the Prevention of HIV Infection in Women. *Science* **2010**, *329*, 1168–1174. [CrossRef]
22. Tien, D.; Schnaare, R.L.; Kang, F.; Cohl, G.; McCormick, T.J.; Moench, T.R.; Doncel, G.; Watson, K.; Buckheit, R.W.; Lewis, M.G.; et al. In Vitroandin VivoCharacterization of a Potential Universal Placebo Designed for Use in Vaginal Microbicide Clinical Trials. *AIDS Res. Hum. Retroviruses* **2005**, *21*, 845–853. [CrossRef]
23. Sellar, R.S.; Peggs, K.S. Management of multidrug-resistant viruses in the immunocompromised host. *Br. J. Haematol.* **2011**, *156*, 559–572. [CrossRef]
24. Sauerbrei, A.; Bohn, K.; Heim, A.; Hofmann, J.; Weiβbrich, B.; Schnitzler, P.; Hoffmann, D.; Zell, R.; Jahn, G.; Wutzler, P.; et al. Novel resistance-associated mutations of thymidine kinase and DNA polymerase genes of herpes simplex virus type 1 and type 2. *Antivir. Ther.* **2011**, *16*, 1297–1308. [CrossRef] [PubMed]
25. Sauerbrei, A.; Bohn-Wippert, K.; Kaspar, M.; Krumbholz, A.; Karrasch, M.; Zell, R. Database on natural polymorphisms and resistance-related non-synonymous mutations in thymidine kinase and DNA polymerase genes of herpes simplex virus types 1 and 2. *J. Antimicrob. Chemother.* **2015**, *71*, 6–16. [CrossRef] [PubMed]
26. Betz, U.A.K.; Fischer, R.; Kleymann, G.; Hendrix, M.; Rubsamen-Waigmann, H. Potent in Vivo Antiviral Activity of the Herpes Simplex Virus Primase-Helicase Inhibitor BAY 57-1293. *Antimicrob. Agents Chemother.* **2002**, *46*, 1766–1772. [CrossRef]
27. Filtjens, J.; Roger, A.; Quatrini, L.; Wieduwild, E.; Gouilly, J.; Hoeffel, G.; Rossignol, R.; Daher, C.; Debroas, G.; Henri, S.; et al. Nociceptive sensory neurons promote CD8 T cell responses to HSV-1 infection. *Nat. Commun.* **2021**, *12*, 1–15. [CrossRef] [PubMed]
28. Hor, J.L.; Heath, W.; Mueller, S.N. Neutrophils are dispensable in the modulation of T cell immunity against cutaneous HSV-1 infection. *Sci. Rep.* **2017**, *7*, srep41091. [CrossRef]
29. Stock, A.T.; Smith, J.; Carbone, F.R. Type I IFN suppresses Cxcr2 driven neutrophil recruitment into the sensory ganglia during viral infection. *J. Exp. Med.* **2011**, *11*, 143–154. [CrossRef]
30. Paludan, S.R.; Bowie, A.G.; Horan, K.A.; Fitzgerald, K.A. Recognition of herpesviruses by the innate immune system. *Nat. Rev. Immunol.* **2013**, *11*, 143–154. [CrossRef]
31. Lei, V.; Petty, A.J.; Atwater, A.R.; Wolfe, S.A.; MacLeod, A.S. Skin Viral Infections: Host Antiviral Innate Immunity and Viral Immune Evasion. *Front. Immunol.* **2020**, *11*, 2791. [CrossRef]
32. Wang, L.; Wang, R.; Xu, C.; Zhou, H. Pathogenesis of Herpes Stromal Keratitis: Immune Inflammatory Response Mediated by Inflammatory Regulators. *Front. Immunol.* **2020**, *11*. [CrossRef] [PubMed]
33. Wojtasiak, M.; Pickett, D.L.; Tate, M.D.; Bedoui, S.; Job, E.R.; Whitney, P.G.; Brooks, A.G.; Reading, P.C. Gr-1+ cells, but not neutrophils, limit virus replication and lesion development following flank infection of mice with herpes simplex virus type-1. *Virology* **2010**, *407*, 143–151. [CrossRef] [PubMed]
34. Hung, S.-L.; Chiang, H.-H.; Wu, C.-Y.; Hsu, M.-J.; Chen, Y.-T. Effects of herpes simplex virus type 1 infection on immune functions of human neutrophils. *J. Periodontal Res.* **2012**, *47*, 635–644. [CrossRef] [PubMed]
35. Gaudreau, A.; Hill, E.; Balfour, H.H.; Erice, A.; Boivin, G. Phenotypic and Genotypic Characterization of Acyclovir-Resistant Herpes Simplex Viruses from Immunocompromised Patients. *J. Infect. Dis.* **1998**, *178*, 297–303. [CrossRef] [PubMed]

viruses

MDPI

Article

Arsenicals, the Integrated Stress Response, and Epstein–Barr Virus Lytic Gene Expression

Jaeyeun Lee [1], Jennifer Stone [1], Prashant Desai [1], John G. Kosowicz [1], Jun O. Liu [1,2] and Richard F. Ambinder [1,2,*]

[1] Departments of Oncology, Johns Hopkins University School of Medicine, Baltimore, MD 21287, USA; jannjaeyeun@gmail.com (J.L.); jstone29@jhmi.edu (J.S.); pdesai1@jhmi.edu (P.D.); john.kosowicz@gmail.com (J.G.K.); joliu@jhu.edu (J.O.L.)
[2] Departments of Pharmacology and Molecular Sciences, Johns Hopkins University School of Medicine, Baltimore, MD 21287, USA
* Correspondence: rambind1@jhmi.edu; Tel.: +1-410-955-8839; Fax: +1-410-955-0960

Abstract: Following our observation that clofoctol led to Epstein–Barr virus (EBV) lytic gene expression upon activation of the integrated stress response (ISR), we decided to investigate the impact of As_2O_3 on viral lytic gene expression. As_2O_3 has also been reported to activate the ISR pathway by its activation of the heme-regulated inhibitor (HRI). Our investigations show that As_2O_3 treatment leads to eIF2α phosphorylation, upregulation of ATF4 and TRB3 expression, and an increase of EBV Zta gene expression in lymphoid tumor cell lines as well as in naturally infected epithelial cancer cell lines. However, late lytic gene expression and virion production were blocked after arsenic treatment. In comparison, a small molecule HRI activator also led to increased Zta expression but did not block late lytic gene expression, suggesting that As_2O_3 effects on EBV gene expression are also mediated through other pathways.

Keywords: Epstein–Barr virus; integrated stress response; arsenic

Citation: Lee, J.; Stone, J.; Desai, P.; Kosowicz, J.G.; Liu, J.O.; Ambinder, R.F. Arsenicals, the Integrated Stress Response, and Epstein–Barr Virus Lytic Gene Expression. *Viruses* **2021**, *13*, 812. https://doi.org/10.3390/v13050812

Academic Editor: Barry J. Margulies

Received: 18 March 2021
Accepted: 26 April 2021
Published: 30 April 2021

1. Introduction

The Epstein–Barr virus (EBV), a human gammaherpesvirus, is associated with a variety of malignancies including some lymphomas of B, T, and NK cell origin, and carcinomas including nasopharyngeal and gastric carcinomas [1,2]. In tumors, latency gene expression predominates and there is little or no expression of the viral proteins associated with virion production. While some have argued that lytic gene expression plays an important role in the transformation and maintenance of malignancy, others have argued that pharmacologic induction of viral lytic gene expression might be a therapeutic strategy to treat these cancers [3–5]. EBV reactivation may also be important in a variety of chronic diseases [6].

Arsenic trioxide (As_2O_3) has been reported to activate EBV lytic gene expression in epithelial cells [7,8] but not in Burkitt lymphoma cells [9]. As_2O_3 is used in the clinic in the treatment of promyelocytic leukemia [10]. In that disease which is characterized by a fusion of the PML and RARα genes, As_2O_3 reacts with the RING-finger domain of PML leading to SUMOylation and degradation of the fusion protein [11].

In recent work, we reported that eIF2α phosphorylation, by the protein kinase R (PKR)-like endoplasmic reticulum (ER) kinase (PERK), activated EBV lytic viral transcription [12]. Phosphorylation of eIF2α has been extensively studied in other contexts [13]. A variety of cellular stresses lead to its phosphorylation at Ser51, stalling of translation initiation complexes, and inhibition of global protein synthesis. This pathway is known as the integrated stress response (ISR). Four kinases phosphorylate this eIF2α serine: PERK, heme-regulated inhibitor kinase (HRI), general control nonderepressible 2 (GCN2), and double-stranded RNA-dependent protein kinase (PKR). Homologous in their catalytic domains, the regulatory domains of these kinases respond to different stresses. PERK is activated by endoplasmic reticulum stress associated with the accumulation of unfolded proteins. HRI is expressed at the highest levels in erythroid cells where it is activated by a deficiency in heme. It regulates globin mRNA translation as a function of the availability of heme. PKR is induced by class 1 interferons and activated by binding to highly structured double-stranded RNAs. GCN2 is activated by binding uncharged tRNAs that are associated with amino acid starvation. With the observation that PERK-mediated phosphorylation of eIF2α led to activation of EBV lytic gene expression [12], we were interested in the possibility that the other arms of the ISR might also mediate activation of lytic gene expression, including HRI, which is activated by As_2O_3 (Figure 1A) [14–16].

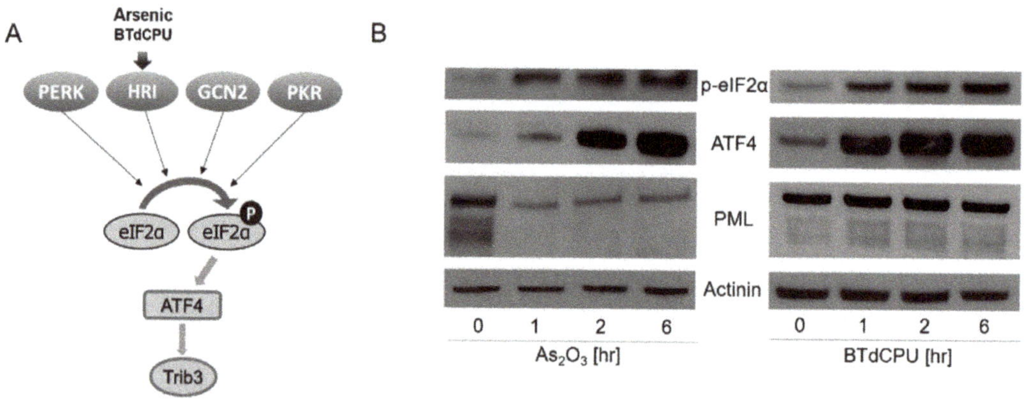

Figure 1. Arsenic and BTdCPU activate the p-eIF2α-ATF4 pathway in a lymphoma cell line. (**A**) A diagram illustrating how arsenic and BTdCPU activate the p-eIF2α-ATF4 pathway. (**B**) BX1-Akata cells were treated with 10 μM As_2O_3 or BTdCPU for the indicated time period, and expression of p-eIF2α, ATF4, and PML protein accumulation were determined by western blot. The cell lysate proteins on the blot were also incubated with actin antibodies.

In the experiments reported here, we sought to better understand the impact of arsenicals and other ISR activators on EBV lytic gene expression.

2. Materials and Methods

2.1. Cell Culture

BX1-Akata, an engineered derivative of the Akata EBV (+) Burkitt lymphoma cell line, which carries a recombinant EBV expressing GFP, was a gift from L. Hutt-Fletcher (Louisiana State University) [17]. Raji is an EBV (+) Burkitt lymphoma cell line. SNU719 is a naturally derived EBV (+) gastric cancer cell line and was a gift from J.M. Lee (Yonsei University) [18]; C666-1 is an EBV (+) nasopharyngeal carcinoma cell line and was a gift from S. Diane Hayward [19]. LCL is an EBV-immortalized lymphoblastoid cell line established in the lab by infecting normal B lymphocytes with EBV strain B95-8. All cell lines were cultured in RPMI 1640, 2 mM L-glutamine, 100 μg/mL streptomycin, 100 IU/mL penicillin, and 10% v/v fetal bovine serum (FBS). Additionally, 500 μg/mL G418 (Geneticin; Gibco™ by Life Technologies, New York, NY, USA) was added for the BX1-Akata cell line.

2.2. Reagents

Arsenic trioxide, sodium arsenite, BTdCPU, and anti-IgG were purchased from MilliporeSigma (Burlington, MA, USA).

2.3. qRT-PCR

RNeasy Mini Kit (QIAGEN, Germantown, MD, USA) was used for RNA extraction, and iScript reverse synthase kit (Bio-Rad, Hercules, CA, USA) was used to reverse-transcribe the RNA into cDNA. SsoFast Evagreen Supermix (Bio-Rad, Hercules, CA,

USA) with 500 nM primers and cDNA corresponding to 20 ng of the RNA were used for each reaction of qPCR. cDNA was amplified at 95 °C for 30 s for 1 cycle and 95 °C for 5 s and 60 °C for 10 s, for a total of 40 cycles in a CFX96 real-time thermocycler. EBV primers used were Zta Forward (5′-ACATCTGCTTCAACAGGAGG-3′), Zta Reverse (5′-AGCAGACATTGGTGTTCCAC-3′), BMRF1 Forward (5′-CTAGCCGTCCTGTCCAAGTGC-3′), BMRF1 Reverse (5′-AGCCAAACGCTCCTTGCCCA-3′), gp350 Forward (5′-GTCAGTACACCATCCAGAGCC-3′), gp350 Reverse (5′-TTGGTAGACAGCCTTCGTATG-3′), gp110 Forward (5′-AACCTTTGACTCGACCATCG-3′), and gp110 Reverse (5′-ACCTGCTCTTCGATGCACTT-3′). Trib3 primers were Forward (5′- CGTGATCTCAAGCTGTGTCG-3′) and Trib3 Reverse (5′- AGCTTCTTCCTCTCACGGTC-3′). GAPDH primers Forward (5′-TCTTTTGCGTCGCCAGCCGA-3′) and GAPDH Reverse (5′-AGTTAAAAGCAGCCCTGGTGACCA-3′) were used as a control. The HRI primer set was purchased from Santa Cruz Biotechnology. The gene expression was normalized to GAPDH expression by using the comparative Ct method and presented as the fold change relative to the untreated control.

2.4. Immunoblots

For protein extractions, 1×10^7 cells were washed in PBS, and the pellets were resuspended in RIPA buffer containing 1× protease/phosphatase inhibitor cocktail (Santa Cruz Biotechnology, Dallas, TX, USA). After 15 min incubation in ice and 15 min of rotation at 4 °C, the proteins were isolated by centrifugation at 13,000 rpm at 4 °C for 5 min and collected from the supernatant. Equal amounts of protein (30 μg) per sample were separated by SDS-PAGE and subsequently transferred to nitrocellulose membranes. Western blotting were performed with antibodies against EBV Zta, BMRF1, ATF4 (Santa Cruz Biotechnology, Dallas, TX, USA), p-eIF2α (Abcam, Cambridge, UK), PML (Novus Biologicals, Littleton, CO, USA), Actinin (Cell Signaling technology, Danvers, MA, USA), and β-actin (Sigma-Aldrich, St. Louis, MO, USA). ECL chemiluminescent detection reagents (GE Healthcare, Chicago, IL, USA) with autoradiography film (Thomas Scientific, Swedesboro, NJ, USA) were used for the detection.

2.5. Immunofluorescence

Next, 1.5×10^5 cells were spun onto microscope slides using a Cytospin centrifuge and fixed using ice-cold methanol for 15 min. After blocking with 5% Bovine serum albumin (BSA) in PBS for 30 min, cells were stained with anti-EBV Zta or gp350 antibody (Santa Cruz, Dallas, TX, USA) for 1 h, washed three times for ten minutes each with 5% BSA, 0.1% Tween-20 in PBS, and incubated with Cy3 goat anti-mouse antibody (Jackson Immunoresearch, West Grove, PA, USA) for 1 h at room temperature. After three final washes, cells were stained with Vectashield mounting media with DAPI (Vector Laboratories, Burlingame, CA, USA), and a ZOE Fluorescent cell imager (Bio-Rad) was used for the fluorescence detection.

2.6. shRNA Knockdown

A pool of lentiviral particles containing 3 different shRNA constructs targeting HRI, a shRNA targeting PML, and control lentiviral particles encoding a scrambled sequence (Santa Cruz Biotechnology, Dallas, TX, USA) were used according to the manufacturer's protocol, and the stable cell lines expressing the shRNA were selected with puromycin.

2.7. Raji Infection Assay

BX1-Akata cells (1.5×10^7) were treated with anti-IgG (10 μg/mL), arsenic trioxide (10 μM), or sodium arsenite (10 μM) and incubated for 4 days. After spinning the cells, the supernatant was passed through a Millex-HV Syringe Filter Unit (0.45 μm, Milli-poreSigma, Burlington, MA, USA), concentrated with a centrifugal filter (Amicon Ultra-15 Centrifugal Filter Unit, MilliporeSigma, Burlington, MA, USA), and 0.2 mL was used to infect Raji cells (2×10^5 in 1 mL medium). TPA (20 ng/mL) and NaB (3 mM) were added 24 h after the infection and the GFP-positive cells were counted the next day using a ZOE Fluorescent cell imager.

3. Results

3.1. Arsenical-Induction of the ISR

We first assessed markers of ISR induction in an EBV (+) Burkitt lymphoma cell line, BX1-Akata, following treatment with As_2O_3. Phosphorylation of eIF2α and increased ATF4 protein accumulation were observed after this treatment (Figure 1B). Parallel results were seen with *N,N′*-diarylurea, BTdCPU (1-(benzo[*d*][1,2,3]thiadiazol-6-yl)-3-(3,4-dichlorophenyl)urea). This small molecule has been previously identified as directly interacting with HRI and inducing eIF2α phosphorylation [15]. As_2O_3 treatment also led to a time- and dose-dependent increase in Trib3 RNA (also known as NIPK and SKIP3) (Figure S1). These results are consistent with As_2O_3-mediating ISR activation [20–22]. We also observed that As_2O_3 treatment leads to degradation of PML, whereas BTdCPU had no effect on PML expression as judged by immunoblot methods (Figure 1B).

3.2. EBV Immediate Early Lytic Gene Expression Is also Activated

BX1-Akata cells were treated with varying doses of As_2O_3 or sodium arsenite ($NaAsO_2$), and EBV Zta RNA levels were examined by qRT-PCR. Zta expression increased in a dose-dependent and time-dependent manner at concentrations of As_2O_3 that are achieved clinically in the treatment of promyelocytic leukemia (2–5 μM) [23] (Figure 2A). Increased Zta expression was also confirmed by immunofluorescence (Figure 2B). We note that the percentage of cells expressing Zta is high and exceeds activation typically seen in comparable experiments with TPA and sodium butyrate. The BX1-Akata cell line carries a recombinant viral genome that expresses green fluorescent protein (GFP) under control of the cytomegalovirus promoter. In the absence of lytic induction, only rare cells are lytic and only rare cells express GFP. With lytic induction, the numbers of cells expressing GFP also increase (Figure 2C). To investigate the relationship of the HRI pathway to activation of Zta expression by arsenicals, we performed a genetic knockdown experiment with a pool of three HRI shRNA constructs. HRI shRNA inhibited HRI RNA expression and substantially blocked arsenical induction of Trib3 and Zta (Figure 3A). Induction of lytic replication as judged by GFP expression was also blocked (Figure 3B). These results are consistent with the interpretation that the effects of arsenicals on Trib3 and Zta expression are mediated by HRI activation of the ISR. When HRI expression is blocked by shRNA constructs, the lytic response to the arsenicals is blocked.

3.3. Lytic Induction in Epithelial Cancer Cell Lines and LCLs

To better assess the generality of the findings with the Akata Burkitt line, we investigated the impact of arsenicals on naturally EBV-infected gastric carcinoma (SNU719) and nasopharyngeal carcinoma (C666-1) cell lines. Similar to the results seen in the Burkitt cell line, Trib3 RNA and Zta RNA increased following As_2O_3 treatment (Figure 4A,B). However, by immunofluorescence Zta protein was only marginally increased in SNU719 cells, and no increase could be detected in C666-1 cells). Zta RNA expression in an EBV lymphoblastoid cell line was activated by arsenic compounds (Figure 4C), but increased Zta protein expression was not observed following arsenical treatment). Thus, we conclude that the effects of arsenicals on Zta RNA were not limited to lymphoma cells—but note that protein levels varied substantially among cell lines.

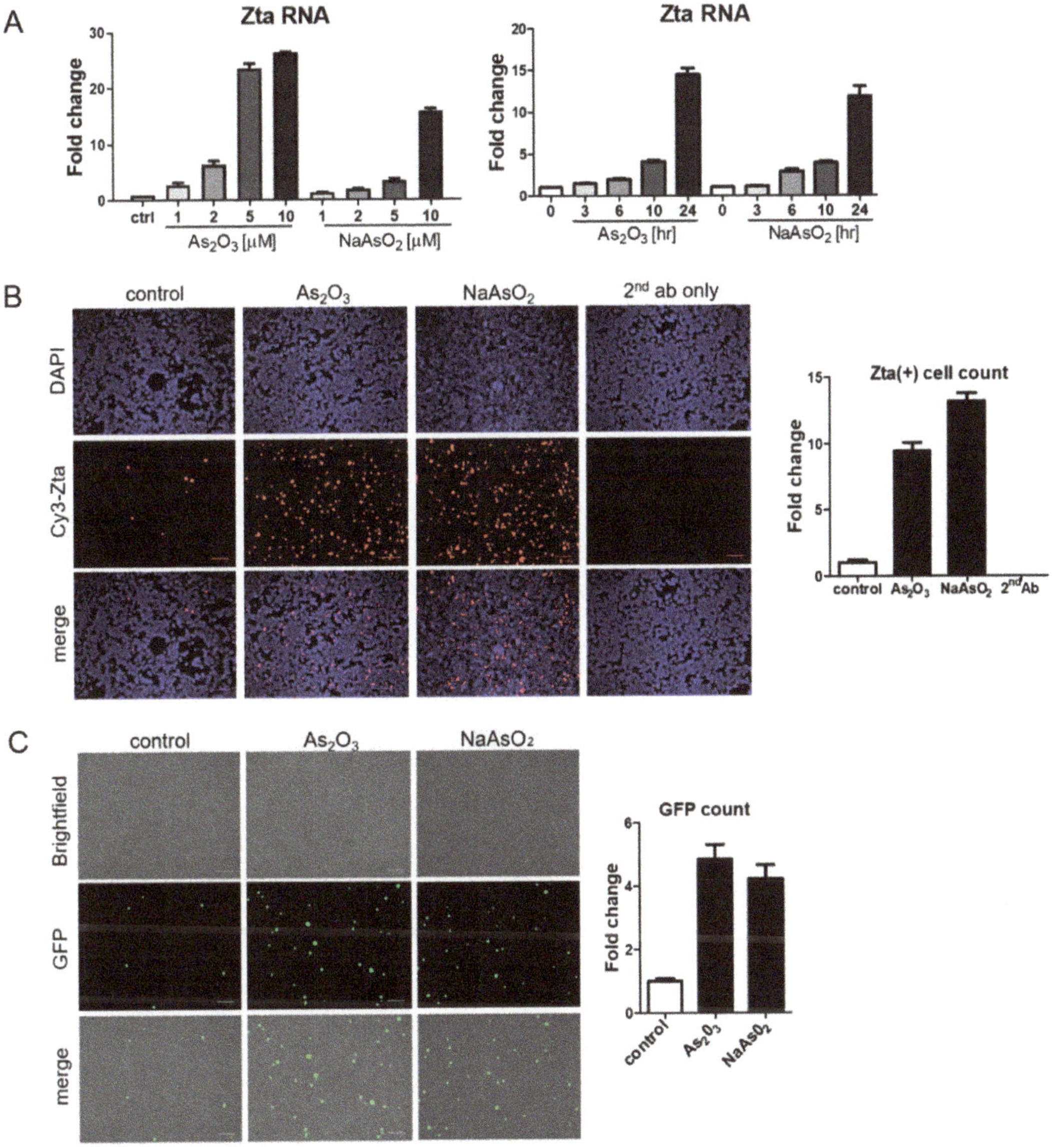

Figure 2. Arsenic induces EBV Zta expression in a lymphoma cell line. (**A**) BX1-Akata cells were treated with the indicated concentrations of As_2O_3 or $NaAsO_2$ for 24 h, and isolated RNA was used for qRT-PCR with Zta primers (Left). BX1-Akata cells were treated with 10 μM As_2O_3 or $NaAsO_2$ for the indicated time periods, and qRT-PCR was performed to detect Zta RNA levels (Right). (**B**,**C**) BX1-Akata cells were treated with 10 μM As_2O_3 or $NaAsO_2$ for 24 h. Fluorescence was used to assess Zta (**B**) and GFP expression (**C**) following treatment. All scale bars on the bottom right represent 100 μm. Fold changes in numbers of positive cells are quantitated in the side panels.

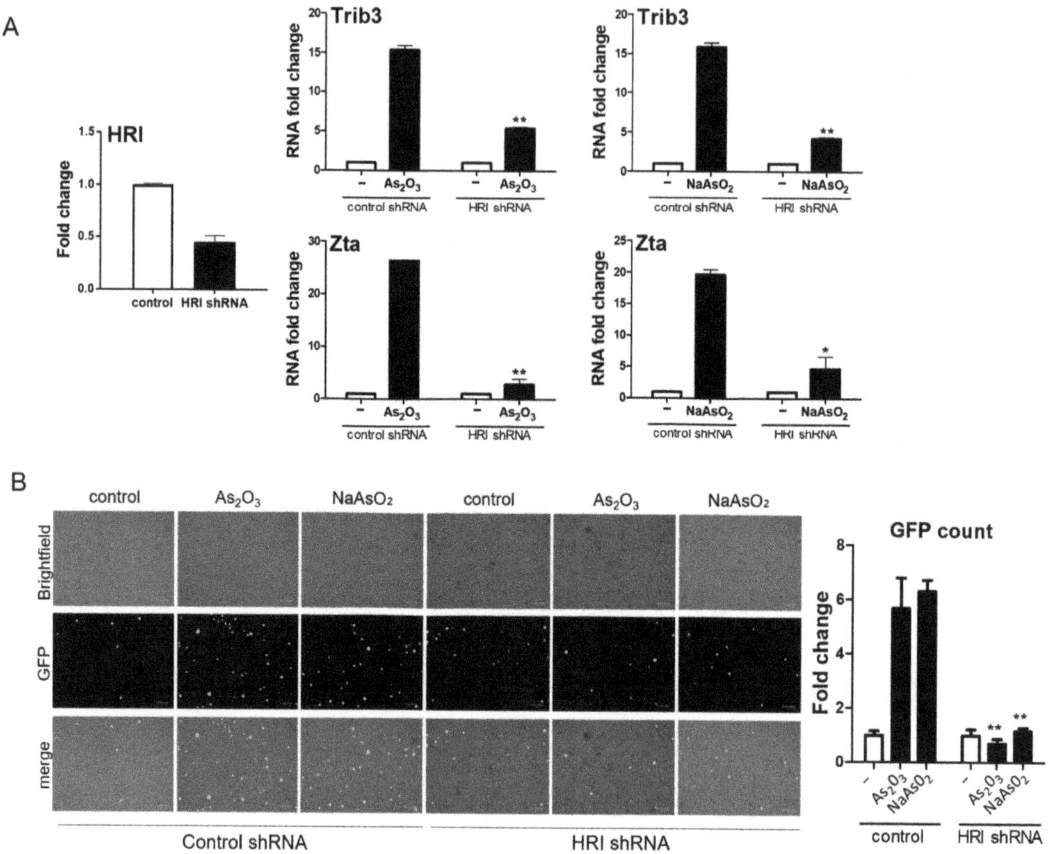

Figure 3. shRNA knockdown of HRI reduces EBV Zta activation by arsenic. BX1-Akata cells were transduced with shRNA lentiviral vectors designed to knockdown HRI gene expression or control shRNA lentiviral vectors. (**A**) HRI knockdown was confirmed by qRT-PCR. The rise in Trib3 and Zta RNA associated with arsenical treatment was blunted by HRI knockdown. (**B**) Fluorescence microscopy showed that HRI knockdown also eliminated any rise in GFP-positive cells after 24 h of arsenic treatment (* $p < 0.05$; ** $p < 0.01$).

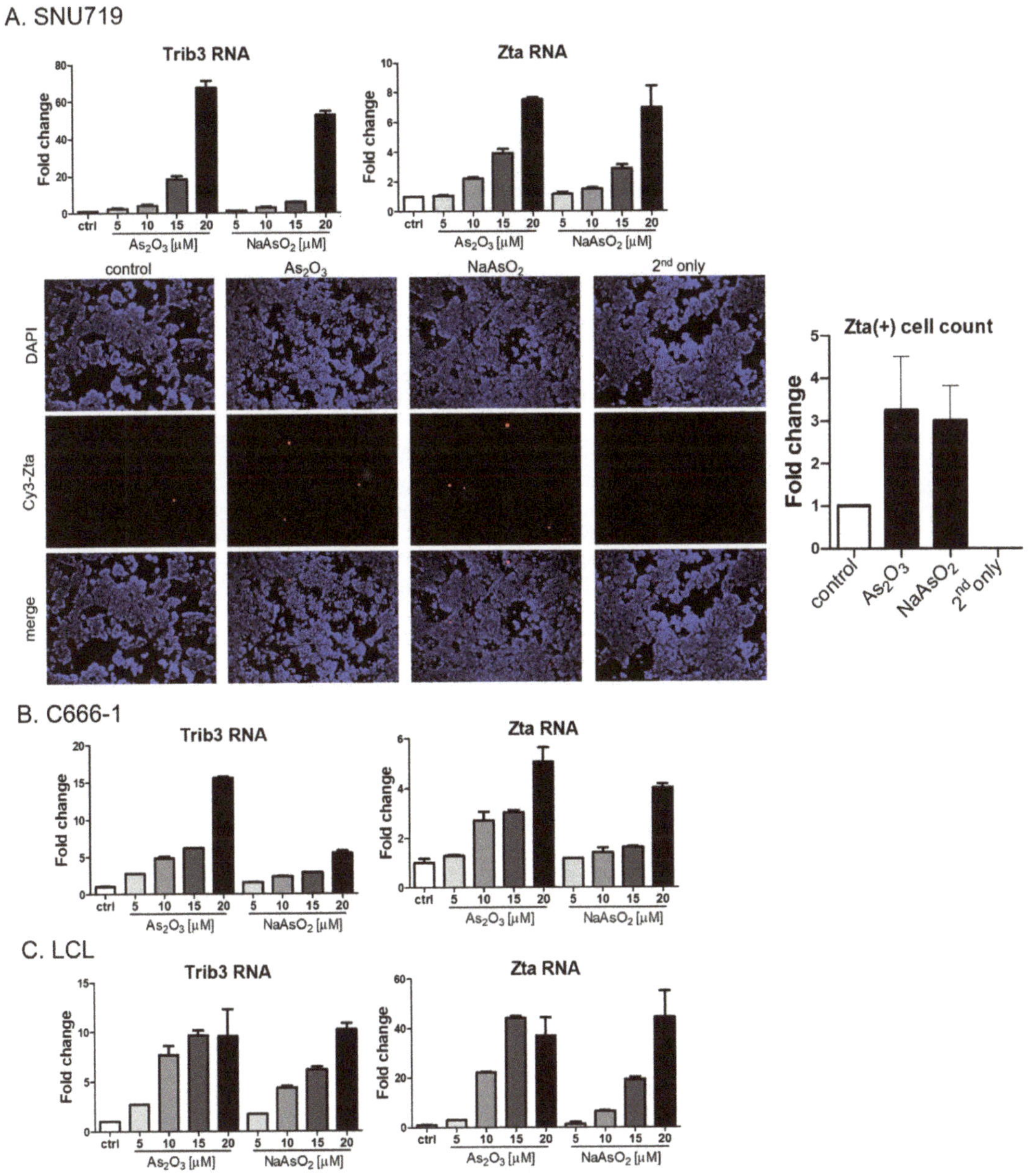

Figure 4. Arsenic activates EBV Zta expression in naturally infected epithelial cells and LCLs. (**A**) SNU719 cells were treated with indicated doses of arsenic for 24 h, and RNA was isolated. Trib3 (left) and Zta (right) RNA levels were determined by qRT-PCR. SNU719 cells were treated with 10 μM As_2O_3 or $NaAsO_2$ for 24 h, and immunofluorescence was performed with an anti-Zta antibody (bottom). Zta-positive cells were quantified and graphed in the right. (**B**,**C**) C666-1 cells (**B**) and LCLs (**C**) were treated with indicated doses of arsenic for 24 h and isolated RNA was used for Trib3 (left) and Zta (right) RNA quantification.

3.4. Arsenicals Have Different Impacts on Expression of a Delayed Early Gene and a Late Gene

Although EBV Zta RNA and protein expression were induced by arsenic treatment, the effects on BMRF1, a delayed early gene, were quite different. RNA levels increased (Figure 5A) whereas protein levels decreased (Figure 5B). RNA and protein levels (as judged by immunofluorescence) of the late lytic gene gp350 did not increase following arsenic treatment (Figure 5C,D). To further evaluate the impact of arsenicals on lytic infection, we assessed virion production. For this purpose, we relied on the Raji infection assay [24,25]. In this assay, virions from BX1-Akata cells that infect Raji cells lead to the induction of the GFP expression in Raji cells. Lytic induction of BX1-Akata cells with anti-IgG yielded a supernatant that induced GFP expression in Raji cells and served as a positive control as can be seen in Figure 5E. In contrast, the supernatant from arsenical-treated BX1-Akata cells yielded no GFP signal. Thus following arsenic treatment, the immediate early Zta RNA and protein were expressed and the delayed early BMRF1 RNA was induced, but the BMRF1 protein was not detected. The late gp350 RNA was not induced and the protein was not detected and was consistent with a block in delayed early and late gene expression; virion production was inhibited (relative to baseline).

3.5. Effects of Direct HRI Activator on EBV Lytic Gene Expression

With the unexpected discordance between the impact of arsenicals on immediate early vs. delayed early and late genes, we were interested in investigating the impact of the small-molecule HRI activator BTdCPU on viral gene expression. As already noted (Figure 1B), BTdCPU led to eIF2α phosphorylation and ATF4 expression, but in contrast to the arsenicals, BTdCPU did not impact PML expression. With regard to viral gene expression, BTdCPU resulted in increased GFP expression in BX1-Akata cells (Figure 6A). When BX1-Akata cells were treated with As_2O_3, BTdCPU, or the combination, both drugs increased Trib3 RNA. The combination of As_2O_3 and BTdCPU markedly increased Zta RNA. In contrast, while both drugs individually increased BMRF1 RNA, the combination didn't lead to further increase. For the late lytic genes, gp110 and gp350, As_2O_3 did not lead to an increase in RNA, but BTdCPU did. Used in combination, As_2O_3 inhibited BTdCPU-induction of late lytic gene expression (Figure 6B).

The comparison and the use of the two agents in combination made clear that the effects of As_2O_3 on late lytic gene expression were not strictly limited to effects mediated by eIF2α phosphorylation. One explanation might be that degradation of PML protein following As_2O_3 might account for the difference. In order to investigate whether the impact of As_2O_3 could be mimicked by BTdCPU in combination with a PML knockdown, we used a target-specific PML shRNA construct (Figure 6C). As shown in Figure 6D, knockdown of PML expression was not sufficient to block gp110 and gp350 RNA expression induced by BTdCPU treatment. Thus, it would appear that As_2O_3 effects cannot be entirely explained by effects on HRI or PML.

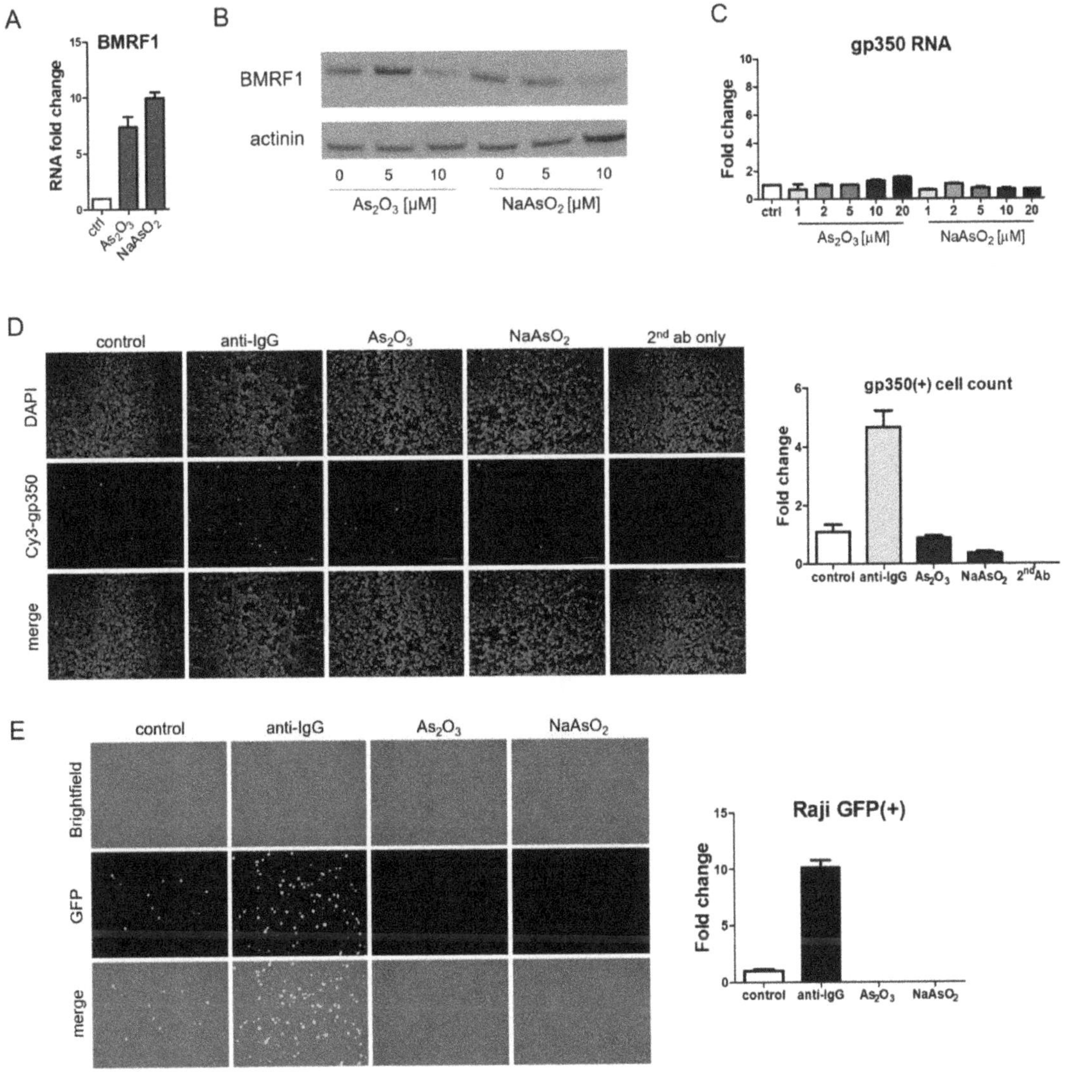

Figure 5. Arsenic does not induce late lytic gene expression and inhibits virion production. (**A**) BX1-Akata cells were treated with 10 μM As_2O_3 or $NaAsO_2$ for 24 h, and BMRF1 RNA was measured by qRT-PCR. (**B**) BX1-Akata cells were treated with indicated doses of As_2O_3 or $NaAsO_2$ for 24 h, and immunoblot was performed to detect BMRF1 protein expression. (**C**) BX1-Akata cells were treated with indicated doses of As_2O_3 or $NaAsO_2$ for 24 h, and gp350 RNA was measured by qRT-PCR. (**D**) BX1-Akata cells were treated with either anti-IgG, 10 μM As_2O_3, or $NaAsO_2$ for 24 h, and immunofluorescence was performed to detect gp350 protein level. (**E**) BX1-Akata cells were treated with either anti-IgG, 10 μM As_2O_3, or $NaAsO_2$ for 4 days, and Raji cell infection assay was performed to determine infectious viral titers.

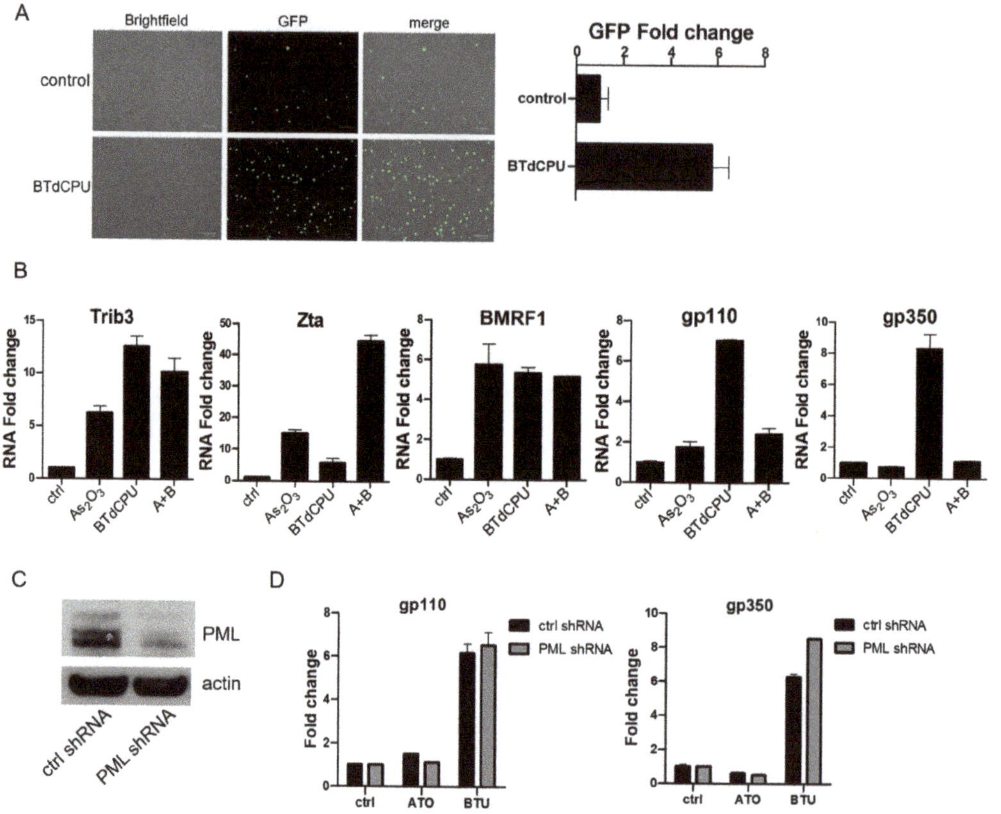

Figure 6. BTdCPU induces EBV lytic gene expression. (**A**) BX1-Aakta cells were treated with 10 µM BTdCPU, and fluorescence microscopy was used for detecting GFP positive cells after 24 h of treatment. (**B**) BX1-Akata cells were treated with either As_2O_3, BTdCPU, or in combination (**A+B**) for 24 h, and qRT-PCR was performed. (**C,D**) BX1-Akata cells were transduced with lentiviral particles designed to knockdown PML, and cells were selected by puromycin. Immunoblot was performed to detect PML expression (**C**), and qRT-PCR was performed 24 h after As_2O_3 or BTdCPU treatment (**D**).

4. Discussion

These investigations confirm that HRI activation of the ISR is associated with upregulation of immediate early, early, and late EBV RNA expression and that As_2O_3 activates the ISR pathway. However, As_2O_3 activation of EBV genes is complex. While stimulating Zta and BMRF1 RNA expression as well as Zta protein expression, As_2O_3 inhibits BMRF1 protein expression and does not lead to an increase in late gp110 or gp350 RNA expression.

We have used GFP expression by the BX1 cell line as an indicator of lytic gene expression in this and several previous investigations [12,26]. GFP expression is appreciated in only a small percentage of cells under basal conditions. This percentage increases with lytic activation. Thus, as in this report, we typically see Zta protein expression in a larger percentage of cells than we see GFP expression. Similarly, others have used BX1 virus to superinfect the Raji EBV BL cell line and only appreciate GFP signal after lytic induction with TPA [27]. GFP expression in these cell lines is not marking the presence of the viral genome but lytic induction.

Previous investigators have studied the impact of arsenicals on EBV gene expression [7–9,28]. Sides et al. reported activation of Zta and BMRF1 RNA expression in epithelial cells [8]. Yin et al. studied EBV-positive lymphoma cell lines treated with As_2O_3

at nanomolar concentrations for three days or longer. They reported decreased cell viability and reduced expression of Zta and BMRF1 [9]. Our results parallel those in the previous reports in some regards but differ in others, possibly reflecting differences in particular cell lines studied or in the duration of drug treatment. Our investigations also differ insofar as we report on the ISR pathway and HRI and studied BTdCPU, a direct activator of HRI.

Study of As_2O_3 and BTdCPU made clear that some effects of As_2O_3 are easily explained by the effect on HRI, while other effects must be mediated by other pathways. As_2O_3 effects on PML protein and fusion proteins have been investigated in great detail, as these effects underlie its therapeutic effect in the promyelocytic leukemia [11,29,30]. PML shRNA knockdown in combination with BTdCPU did not replicate the effects of As_2O_3 on late viral genes, so other pathways are likely involved. We note that As_2O_3 has been shown to induce oxidative stress, DNA damage, and mitochondrial stress, and these pathways may be important for the effects on late viral gene expression [31,32]. We should note that several EBV lytic genes (BZLF1, BRLF1, BGLF4) disrupt PML nuclear bodies through PML dispersal [33,34].

As has been true with other lytic activators, we found that activation of Burkitt cell lines was stronger than naturally infected epithelial cell lines [12,35]. However, although the extent of activation varied, activation of Zta was seen in all cell lines studied.

Differential effects of As_2O_3 and $NaAsO_2$ at increasing BZLF1 transcription in a lymphoblastoid cell line were previously reported [28]. However, our findings did not show any differences between As_2O_3 and $NaAsO_2$.

The effects of As_2O_3 we report are at levels achieved in leukemia patients with As_2O_3 [23]. The abortive lytic infection is of interest because activation of immediate early proteins may allow EBV-specific T cells (either a patient's own or the result of adoptive immunotherapy) to more readily target tumor cells. At the same time, the blockade of delayed early and late lytic protein expression may protect against unwanted effects of lytic activation that some have hypothesized might help drive tumorigenesis or have other adverse effects.

Supplementary Materials: The following are available online at https://www.mdpi.com/article/10.3390/v13050812/s1, Figure S1: Arsenic leads to ATF4 and Trib3 expression.

Author Contributions: Conceptualization, R.F.A. and J.L.; methodology, R.F.A., J.L., J.S., P.D., J.G.K., and J.O.L.; writing—original draft preparation, J.L. and R.F.A.; writing—review and editing, all authors. All authors have read and agreed to the published version of the manuscript.

Funding: This research was funded by National Cancer Institute, grant number P30CA06973.

Institutional Review Board Statement: Not applicable.

Informed Consent Statement: Not applicable.

Data Availability Statement: Data is contained within the article or Supplementary Materials.

Conflicts of Interest: The authors declare no conflict of interest.

References

1. Longnecker, R.M.; Kieff, E.; Cohen, J.I. Epstein-barr virus. In *Fields Virology*, 6th ed.; Wolters Kluwer Health Adis (ESP): Philadelphia, PA, USA, 2013.
2. Shannon-Lowe, C.; Rickinson, A.B.; Bell, A.I. Epstein-Barr virus-associated lymphomas. *Philos. Trans. R. Soc. Lond. B Biol. Sci.* **2017**, *372*, 20160271. [CrossRef]
3. Yiu, S.P.T.; Dorothea, M.; Hui, K.F.; Chiang, A.K.S. Lytic Induction Therapy against Epstein–Barr Virus-Associated Malignancies: Past, Present, and Future. *Cancers* **2020**, *12*, 2142. [CrossRef]
4. Bristol, J.A.; Djavadian, R.; Albright, E.R.; Coleman, C.B.; Ohashi, M.; Hayes, M.; Romero-Masters, J.C.; Barlow, E.A.; Farrell, P.J.; Rochford, R.; et al. A cancer-associated Epstein-Barr virus BZLF1 promoter variant enhances lytic infection. *PLoS Pathog.* **2018**, *14*, e1007179. [CrossRef] [PubMed]
5. Munz, C. Latency and lytic replication in Epstein-Barr virus-associated oncogenesis. *Nat. Rev. Microbiol.* **2019**, *17*, 691–700. [CrossRef] [PubMed]
6. Kerr, J.R. Epstein-Barr virus (EBV) reactivation and therapeutic inhibitors. *J. Clin. Pathol.* **2019**, *72*, 651–658. [CrossRef]

7. Sides, M.D.; Sosulski, M.L.; Luo, F.; Lin, Z.; Flemington, E.K.; Lasky, J.A. Co-treatment with arsenic trioxide and ganciclovir reduces tumor volume in a murine xenograft model of nasopharyngeal carcinoma. *Virol. J.* **2013**, *10*, 152. [CrossRef]
8. Sides, M.D.; Block, G.J.; Shan, B.; Esteves, K.C.; Lin, Z.; Flemington, E.K.; Lasky, J.A. Arsenic mediated disruption of promyelocytic leukemia protein nuclear bodies induces ganciclovir susceptibility in Epstein-Barr positive epithelial cells. *Virology* **2011**, *416*, 86–97. [CrossRef] [PubMed]
9. Yin, Q.; Sides, M.; Parsons, C.H.; Flemington, E.K.; Lasky, J.A. Arsenic trioxide inhibits EBV reactivation and promotes cell death in EBV-positive lymphoma cells. *Virol. J.* **2017**, *14*, 121. [CrossRef]
10. McCulloch, D.; Brown, C.; Iland, H. Retinoic acid and arsenic trioxide in the treatment of acute promyelocytic leukemia: Current perspectives. *OncoTargets Ther.* **2017**, *10*, 1585. [CrossRef] [PubMed]
11. Kaiming, C.; Sheng, Y.; Zheng, S.; Yuan, S.; Huang, G.; Liu, Y. Arsenic trioxide preferentially binds to the ring finger protein PML: Understanding target selection of the drug. *Metallomics* **2018**, *10*, 1564–1569. [CrossRef] [PubMed]
12. Lee, J.; Kosowicz, J.G.; Hayward, S.D.; Desai, P.; Stone, J.; Lee, J.M.; Liu, J.O.; Ambinder, R.F. Pharmacologic Activation of Lytic Epstein-Barr Virus Gene Expression Without Virion Production. *J. Virol.* **2019**, *93*, e00998-19. [CrossRef]
13. Kashiwagi, K.; Yokoyama, T.; Nishimoto, M.; Takahashi, M.; Sakamoto, A.; Yonemochi, M.; Shirouzu, M.; Ito, T. Structural basis for eIF2B inhibition in integrated stress response. *Science* **2019**, *364*, 495–499. [CrossRef] [PubMed]
14. McEwen, E.; Kedersha, N.; Song, B.; Scheuner, D.; Gilks, N.; Han, A.; Chen, J.-J.; Anderson, P.; Kaufman, R.J. Heme-regulated inhibitor kinase-mediated phosphorylation of eukaryotic translation initiation factor 2 inhibits translation, induces stress granule formation, and mediates survival upon arsenite exposure. *J. Biol. Chem.* **2005**, *280*, 16925–16933. [CrossRef] [PubMed]
15. Chen, T.; Ozel, D.; Qiao, Y.; Harbinski, F.; Chen, L.; Denoyelle, S.; He, X.; Zvereva, N.; Supko, J.G.; Chorev, M.; et al. Chemical genetics identify eIF2alpha kinase heme-regulated inhibitor as an anticancer target. *Nat. Chem. Biol.* **2011**, *7*, 610–616. [CrossRef] [PubMed]
16. Lu, L.; Han, A.P.; Chen, J.J. Translation initiation control by heme-regulated eukaryotic initiation factor 2alpha kinase in erythroid cells under cytoplasmic stresses. *Mol. Cell. Biol.* **2001**, *21*, 7971–7980. [CrossRef] [PubMed]
17. Molesworth, S.J.; Lake, C.M.; Borza, C.M.; Turk, S.M.; Hutt-Fletcher, L.M. Epstein-Barr virus gH is essential for penetration of B cells but also plays a role in attachment of virus to epithelial cells. *J. Virol.* **2000**, *74*, 6324–6332. [CrossRef] [PubMed]
18. Park, J.G.; Yang, H.K.; Kim, W.H.; Chung, J.K.; Kang, M.S.; Lee, J.H.; Oh, J.H.; Park, H.S.; Yeo, K.S.; Kang, S.H.; et al. Establishment and characterization of human gastric carcinoma cell lines. *Int. J. Cancer* **1997**, *70*, 443–449. [CrossRef]
19. Cheung, S.T.; Huang, D.P.; Hui, A.B.Y.; Lo, K.W.; Ko, C.W.; Tsang, Y.S.; Wong, N.; Whitney, B.M.; Lee, J.C.K. Nasopharyngeal carcinoma cell line (C666-1) consistently harbouring Epstein-Barr virus. *Int. J. Cancer* **1999**, *83*, 121–126. [CrossRef]
20. Ohoka, N.; Yoshii, S.; Hattori, T.; Onozaki, K.; Hayashi, H. TRB3, a novel ER stress-inducible gene, is induced via ATF4-CHOP pathway and is involved in cell death. *EMBO J.* **2005**, *24*, 1243–1255. [CrossRef] [PubMed]
21. Ord, D.; Ord, T. Characterization of human NIPK (TRB3, SKIP3) gene activation in stressful conditions. *Biochem. Biophys. Res. Commun.* **2005**, *330*, 210–218. [CrossRef] [PubMed]
22. Ord, T.; Ord, D.; Kõivomägi, M.; Juhkam, K.; Ord, T. Human TRB3 is upregulated in stressed cells by the induction of translationally efficient mRNA containing a truncated 5′-UTR. *Gene* **2009**, *444*, 24–32. [CrossRef] [PubMed]
23. Hayashi, T.; Hideshima, T.; Akiyama, M.; Richardson, P.; Schlossman, R.L.; Chauhan, D.; Munshi, N.C.; Waxman, S.; Anderson, K.C. Arsenic trioxide inhibits growth of human multiple myeloma cells in the bone marrow microenvironment. *Mol. Cancer Ther.* **2002**, *1*, 851–860. [PubMed]
24. Meng, Q.; Hagemeier, S.R.; Fingeroth, J.D.; Gershburg, E.; Pagano, J.S.; Kenney, S.C. The Epstein-Barr virus (EBV)-encoded protein kinase, EBV-PK, but not the thymidine kinase (EBV-TK), is required for ganciclovir and acyclovir inhibition of lytic viral production. *J. Virol.* **2010**, *84*, 4534–4542. [CrossRef]
25. Li, R.; Zhu, J.; Xie, Z.; Liao, G.; Liu, J.; Chen, M.-R.; Hu, S.; Woodard, C.; Lin, J.; Taverna, S.D.; et al. Conserved herpesvirus kinases target the DNA damage response pathway and TIP60 histone acetyltransferase to promote virus replication. *Cell Host Microbe* **2011**, *10*, 390–400. [CrossRef] [PubMed]
26. Kosowicz, J.G.; Lee, J.; Peiffer, B.; Guo, Z.; Chen, J.; Liao, G.; Hayward, S.D.; Liu, J.O.; Ambinder, R.F. Drug Modulators of B Cell Signaling Pathways and Epstein-Barr Virus Lytic Activation. *J. Virol.* **2017**, *91*, e00747-17. [CrossRef]
27. Zhang, K.; Lv, D.-W.; Li, R. Conserved herpesvirus protein kinases target SAMHD1 to facilitate virus replication. *Cell Rep.* **2019**, *28*, 449–459.e5. [CrossRef]
28. Zebboudj, A.; Maroui, M.A.; Dutrieux, J.; Touil-Boukoffa, C.; Bourouba, M.; Chelbi-Alix, M.K.; Nisole, S. Sodium arsenite induces apoptosis and Epstein-Barr virus reactivation in lymphoblastoid cells. *Biochimie* **2014**, *107*, 247–256. [CrossRef]
29. Jeanne, M.; Lallemand-Breitenbach, V.; Ferhi, O.; Koken, M.; Le Bras, M.; Duffort, S.; Peres, L.; Berthier, C.; Soilihi, H.; Raught, B.; et al. PML/RARA oxidation and arsenic binding initiate the antileukemia response of As_2O_3. *Cancer Cell* **2010**, *18*, 88–98. [CrossRef] [PubMed]
30. Zhang, X.-W.; Yan, X.-J.; Zhou, Z.-R.; Yang, F.-F.; Wu, Z.Y.; Sun, H.-B.; Liang, W.-X.; Song, A.-X.; Lallemand-Breitenbach, V.; Jeanne, M.; et al. Arsenic trioxide controls the fate of the PML-RARalpha oncoprotein by directly binding PML. *Science* **2010**, *328*, 240–243. [CrossRef] [PubMed]
31. Kumar, S.; Yedjou, C.G.; Tchounwou, P.B. Arsenic trioxide induces oxidative stress, DNA damage, and mitochondrial pathway of apoptosis in human leukemia (HL-60) cells. *J. Exp. Clin. Cancer Res.* **2014**, *33*, 42. [CrossRef] [PubMed]

32. Baysan, A.; Yel, L.; Gollapudi, S.; Su, H.; Gupta, S. Arsenic trioxide induces apoptosis via the mitochondrial pathway by upregulating the expression of Bax and Bim in human B cells. *Int. J. Oncol.* **2007**, *30*, 313–318. [PubMed]
33. Bell, P.; Lieberman, P.M.; Maul, G.G. Lytic but not latent replication of Epstein-Barr virus is associated with PML and induces sequential release of nuclear domain 10 proteins. *J. Virol.* **2000**, *74*, 11800–11810. [CrossRef]
34. Frappier, L. Manipulation of PML Nuclear Bodies and DNA Damage Responses by DNA Viruses. In *The Functional Nucleus*; Springer: Berlin/Heidelberg, Germany, 2016; pp. 283–312.
35. Shirley, C.M.; Chen, J.; Shamay, M.; Li, H.; Zahnow, C.A.; Hayward, S.D.; Ambinder, R.F. Bortezomib induction of C/EBPbeta mediates Epstein-Barr virus lytic activation in Burkitt lymphoma. *Blood* **2011**, *117*, 6297–6303. [CrossRef] [PubMed]

viruses

MDPI

Article

The Synthesis and Anti-Cytomegalovirus Activity of Piperidine-4-Carboxamides

Xin Guo [1,†], Ayan Kumar Ghosh [1,†], Robert F. Keyes [2], Francis Peterson [2], Michael Forman [3], David J. Meyers [4,*] and Ravit Arav-Boger [1,*]

1 Department of Pediatrics, Division of Infectious Disease, Medical College of Wisconsin, Milwaukee, WI 53226, USA; xinyuanlian@163.com (X.G.); aghosh@mcw.edu (A.K.G.)
2 Department of Biochemistry, Medical College of Wisconsin, Milwaukee, WI 53226, USA; rkeyes@mcw.edu (R.F.K.); fpeterso@mcw.edu (F.P.)
3 Department of Pathology, Johns Hopkins University School of Medicine, Baltimore, MD 21287, USA; mformaa@jhmi.edu
4 Department of Pharmacology and Molecular Sciences, Johns Hopkins University School of Medicine, Baltimore, MD 21205, USA
* Correspondence: dmeyers7@jhmi.edu (D.J.M.); rboger@mcw.edu (R.A.-B.); Tel.:+1-414-337-7070 (D.J.M.); +1-410-502-4804 (R.A.-B.); Fax: +414-337-7093 (D.J.M.); +410-955-3023 (R.A.-B.)
† These authors contributed equally to this work.

Abstract: Treatment options for human cytomegalovirus (CMV) remain limited and are associated with significant adverse effects and the selection of resistant CMV strains in transplant recipients and congenitally infected infants. Although most approved drugs target and inhibit the CMV DNA polymerase, additional agents with distinct mechanisms of action are needed for the treatment and prevention of CMV. In a large high throughput screen using our CMV-luciferase reporter Towne, we identified several unique inhibitors of CMV replication. Here, we synthesize and test in vitro 13 analogs of the original NCGC2955 hit (**1**). Analogs with no activity against the CMV-luciferase at 10 μM and 30 μM (**2–6, 10–14**) were removed from further analysis. Three analogs (**7–9**) inhibited CMV replication in infected human foreskin fibroblasts. The EC_{50} of (**1**) was 1.7 ± 0.6 μM and 1.99 ± 0.15 μM, based on luciferase and plaque assay, respectively. Compounds **7**, **8**, and **9** showed similar activities: the EC_{50} values of **7** were 0.21 ± 0.06 μM (luciferase) and 0.55 ± 0.06 (plaque), of **8**: 0.28 ± 0.06 μM and 0.42 ± 0.07, and of **9**: 0.30 ± 0.05 μM (luciferase) and 0.35 ± 0.07 (plaque). The CC_{50} for **7**, **8**, and **9** in non-infected human foreskin fibroblasts was >500 μM, yielding a selectivity index of >1500. Compounds **1**, **7**, and **8** were also tested in CMV-infected primary human hepatocytes and showed a dose–response against CMV by luciferase activity and viral protein expression. None of the active compounds inhibited herpes simplex virus 1 or 2. Compounds **7** and **8** inhibited mouse CMV replication in vitro. Both inhibited CMV at late stages of replication; **7** reduced virus yield at all late time points, although not to the same degree as letermovir. Finally, the activity of analog **8** was additive with newly identified CMV inhibitors (MLS8969, NFU1827, MSL8554, and MSL8091) and with ganciclovir. Further structural activity development should provide promising anti-CMV agents for use in clinical studies.

Keywords: cytomegalovirus; mouse cytomegalovirus; piperidine-4-carboxamides; add-on removal

Citation: Guo, X.; Ghosh, A.K.; Keyes, R.F.; Peterson, F.; Forman, M.; Meyers, D.J.; Arav-Boger, R. The Synthesis and Anti-Cytomegalovirus Activity of Piperidine-4-Carboxamides. *Viruses* **2022**, *14*, 234. https://doi.org/10.3390/v14020234

Academic Editor: Barry J. Margulies

Received: 31 December 2021
Accepted: 21 January 2022
Published: 25 January 2022

1. Introduction

Infection with human cytomegalovirus (CMV), a member of the herpesvirus family, is common in humans. The seroprevalence rates increase with age, reaching 90% in individuals older than 80 years [1]. CMV establishes lifelong persistent infection, and patients typically remain asymptomatic. In immunocompromised hosts, including transplant recipients and patients with AIDS, CMV causes significant morbidity and mortality [2–5].

CMV is the most common congenital infection worldwide [6–8]. It is the leading infectious cause of hearing loss and central nervous system damage in children.

Most of the systemic anti-CMV drugs target the viral DNA polymerase [9–12]. Their use is associated with considerable toxicities to the bone marrow (ganciclovir (GCV)) and kidneys (foscarnet and cidofovir), and the emergence of resistant viruses [9–12]. A phase III clinical trial documented the prevention of hearing loss in congenitally infected children treated with intravenous GCV, paving the way for the treatment of congenital CMV with central nervous system involvement [13]. A follow-up phase III clinical trial of oral valganciclovir (the valyl-ester prodrug of GCV) suggested modest neurobehavioral benefit for six months, compared to six weeks of therapy [14]. A six-weeks course of valganciclovir may not prevent the development of long-term hearing loss, but it needs to be determined whether longer courses may have an effect on hearing preservation [15], and how common GCV-resistant mutants are identified in these children.

The widespread use of a limited number of drugs often leads to the development of drug-resistant CMV strains [16,17]. Letermovir, a terminase inhibitor, is approved for CMV prophylaxis after hematopoietic stem cell transplantation [18,19], and resistance has already been reported [20]. Maribavir targets the viral UL97 kinase and showed promising results [21,22]. A phase II clinical trial of maribavir showed ~65% response across all doses. There were no major safety issues and no bone marrow suppression, but CMV recurrences occurred in 35% of the participants [23]. In a phase III clinical trial, maribavir was superior to conventional antiviral therapy for resistant/refractory CMV. This led to the FDA approval of maribavir for adults and children (12 years of age and older) with CMV infection/disease that is refractory to treatment with ganciclovir, valganciclovir, cidofovir or foscarnet. The overall problems of toxicity, resistance, oral-bioavailability, and high-cost drive CMV drug discovery. We recently reported on a successful completion of the largest high-throughput screen (HTS) of ~400,000 compounds that resulted in the identification of five structurally unique CMV inhibitors, active at low μM concentrations [24]. One of these compounds was NCGC2955, which was selected for further development against CMV. Structurally related compounds to NCGC2955, which all contained the piperidine-4-carboxamide motif (see purple rectangle for Compound **1**, Table 1), were reported to inhibit neurotropic alphaviruses (RNA viruses) [25,26]. Here, we report structure-activity relationship (SAR) studies to further characterize the anti-CMV activities of the parental NCGC2955 (**1**) and several structurally related analogs.

Table 1. Chemical structure of compounds **1–14**. Provided are the EC_{50} values for pp28-luciferase CMV, TB40, and the CC_{50} measured in non-infected HFFs. All concentrations are in μM. Comp—compound number.

Comp	Structure	EC_{50} pp28-Luciferase	EC_{50} TB40	CC_{50}	Comp	Structure	EC_{50} pp28-Luciferase	EC_{50} TB40	CC_{50}
1	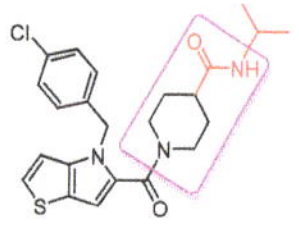	1.7 ± 0.6	1.99 ± 0.15	>200	8	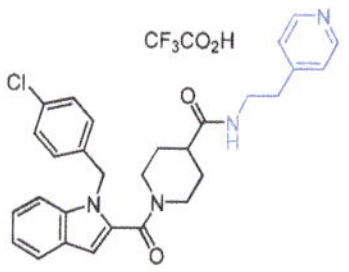	0.28 ± 0.06	0.42 ± 0.07	500
2	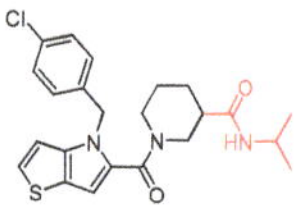	>30			9	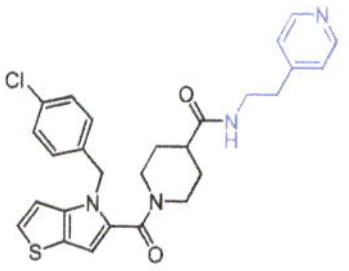	0.3 ± 0.05	0.35 ± 0.07	>500
3	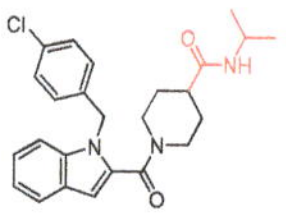	>30			10	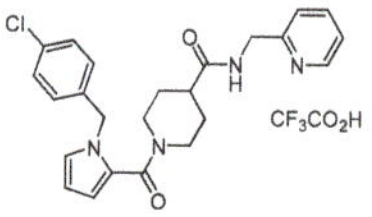	>30		

Table 1. *Cont.*

Comp	Structure	EC_{50} pp28-Luciferase	EC_{50} TB40	CC_{50}	Comp	Structure	EC_{50} pp28-Luciferase	EC_{50} TB40	CC_{50}
4	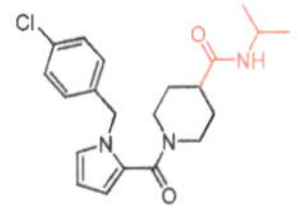	>30			11	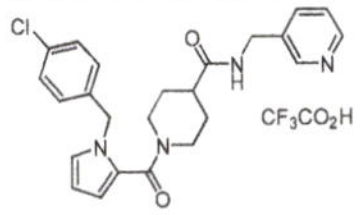	>30		
5	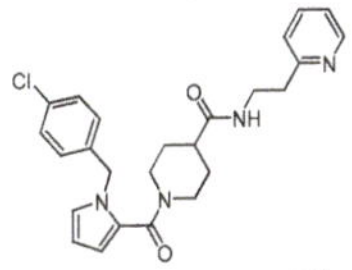	>30			12	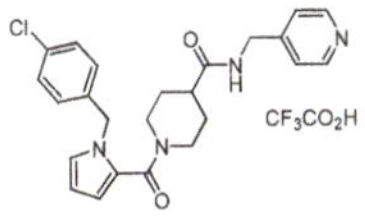	>30		
6	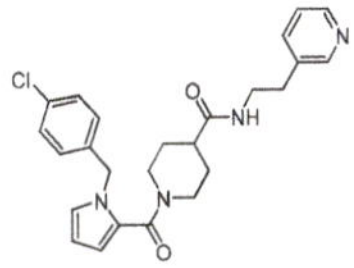	>30			13	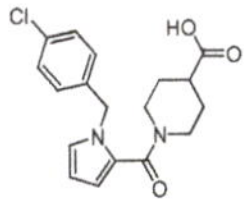	>30		
7	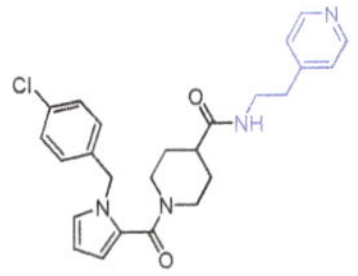	0.21 ± 0.06	0.55 ± 0.06	>500	14	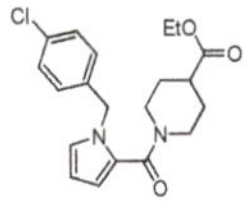	>30		

2. Materials and Methods

2.1. Compounds

Compound synthesis and characterization is detailed in the Supplementary Material. The purities of all the synthesized compounds used in the bioassays were determined by HPLC using either a Phenomenex Luna C18 3.0 × 75 mm column with a 7 min gradient of 4–100% ACN in H_2O with 0.05% *v*/*v* TFA, or a Higgins Analytical, Inc. Targa C18 5 µm 4.6 × 150 mm column with a 30 min gradient of 0–100% ACN in H_2O with 0.01% TFA, and either the absorbance detection at 254 nm or evaporative light scattering detection. All the compounds used in the bioassays exhibited NMR and MS data consistent with their structures and purities of >98% as determined by RP-HPLC.

2.2. Viruses

A pp28-luciferase recombinant Towne CMV strain was used in the luciferase assays. The virus expressed luciferase under the control of the UL99 (pp28) late promoter, and was reported to provide a sensitive and reproducible reporter for drug screening [27]. CMV Towne (VR-977) was used for the Western blots. The CMV UL32-EGFP-TB40 [28] (VR-1578) was obtained from ATCC (VR-1578). Clinical isolates of Human Herpesvirus 1 and 2 (HSV1, HSV2) were collected from the Johns Hopkins Microbiology laboratory without identifiers that could link them to a specific patient. Mouse embryonic fibroblasts (MEFs; ATCC, CRL-1658) were used for infection with the MCMV Smith strain (ATCC VR-1399).

2.3. Cell Culture, Virus Infection, and Anti-Viral Assays

Human foreskin fibroblasts (HFFs), passage 12 to 16 (ATCC, CRL-2088), were grown in Dulbecco's modified Eagle medium (DMEM), containing 10% fetal bovine serum (FBS) (Gibco, Carlsbad, CA, USA) in a 5% CO_2 incubator at 37 °C. Vero cells (Vervet monkey kidney epithelial cells) were from ATCC, CCL-81. Virus infection and anti-viral assays followed previously reported protocols for the lab [24]. Infection was carried out at a multiplicity of 1 plaque forming unit (PFU)/cell (MOI = 1 PFU/cell), unless otherwise noted. Following 90 min adsorption, media containing the virus was removed and replaced by DMEM with 4% FBS (Gibco) in the presence or absence of compounds. Infected or infected-treated HFFs were collected at specific time points depending on the assay used. In the luciferase assay, cell lysates were collected at 72 hpi and the luciferase activity was measured using the Glomax-Multi + Detection System (Promega, Madison, WI, USA), as previously described [27]. For plaque assays, HFFs were seeded into 12-well plates (2×10^5 cells/well) and infected with CMV TB40 at approximately 150 plaques/well. After 90 min, media were aspirated, and DMEM containing 0.5% carboxymethyl-cellulose (CMC), 4% fetal bovine serum (FBS), and compounds were added into duplicate wells. Following incubation at 37 °C for 7–10 days, the overlay was removed and plaques were counted after crystal violet staining. For HSV1 and HSV2 replication in Vero cells (100 plaques/well), the adsorption time was 60 min and plaques were counted after 48 h. For MCMV replication in MEFs (100 plaques/well), the adsorption time was 90 min and plaques were counted after 72 h.

Primary human hepatocytes (PHHs, PXB-cells) isolated by the collagenase perfusion method from chimeric urokinase-type plasminogen activator/severe combined immunodeficiency (uPA/SCID) mice with humanized livers that were obtained from PhoenixBio (Hiroshima, Japan). The cells were seeded on type I collagen-coated 96-well plates or in 24-well plates at a density of 6.8×10^4 and 4×10^5 cells/well. The cells were washed with dHCGM media substituted with 10% FBS and allowed to recover in the complete media for 24 h. For the maintenance of the PHHs, the dHCGM media (10% FBS) was changed every 3–4 days. The PHHs in the 96-well plates were infected with pp28-luciferase CMV or CMV Towne at MOI = 1 PFU/cell for 90 min in serum-free dHCGM media. After infection, the cells were washed once and incubated with several concentrations of GCV, Compounds **1**, **7**, and **8** diluted in dHCGM media containing 10% FBS for 96 h. The cells were lysed in a cell culture lysis buffer (Promega) containing protease inhibitors and the luciferase activity was measured. Lysates from the 96-well plate were also used for the analysis of viral protein expression by Western blot.

2.4. Toxicity Assays

A 3-(4,5-dimethyl-2-thiazolyl)-2,5-diphenyl-2H-tetrazolium bromide (MTT) assay was performed according to the manufacturer's instructions (Millipore Sigma). Non-infected cells were treated with NCGC2955, **7**, **8**, **9** for 72 h, and 20 µL/well of MTT ([3-(4,5-Dimethyl-2-thiazolyl)-2,5-diphenyl-2H-tetrazolium bromide]), 5 mg/mL in phosphate-buffered saline (PBS) was added to each well. After shaking at 150 rpm for 5 min, the plates were incubated at 37 °C for 2–3 h. The conversion of the yellow solution to dark blue formazan by mitochondrial dehydrogenases of living cells was quantified by measuring the absorbance at 560 nm.

2.5. SDS-PAGE and Immunoblot Analysis

The cell lysates containing an equal amount of protein were mixed with an equal volume of sample buffer (125 mM Tris-HCl, pH 6.8, 4% SDS, 20% glycerol, and 5% β-mercaptoethanol) and heated for 10 min at 100 °C. Denatured proteins were resolved by tris-glycine polyacrylamide gels (8–10%) and transferred to polyvinylidine difluoride (PVDF) membranes (Bio-Rad Laboratories, Hercules, CA, USA) by electroblotting. Membranes were incubated in blocking buffer (5% *w*/*v* non-fat dry milk and 0.1% Tween-20 in PBS (PBST)) for 1 h, washed with PBST, and incubated with primary antibodies at 4 °C overnight. Membranes were washed with PBST and incubated with horseradish peroxidase-conjugated secondary antibodies in PBST for 1 h at room temperature. Following washing with PBST, protein bands were visualized by chemiluminescence using SuperSignal West Dura and Pico reagents (Pierce Chemical, Rockford, IL, USA). The following antibodies were used: mouse monoclonal anti-CMV IE1 and IE2 (MAB810, Millipore, Billerica, MA, USA); mouse monoclonal anti-CMV UL83 (pp65, Vector Laboratories Inc., Burlingame, CA, USA); mouse monoclonal anti-CMV UL84; and mouse anti-β-actin anti-mouse IgG (Santa Cruz Biotechnology, Santa Cruz, CA, USA). Horseradish peroxidase (HRP)-conjugated anti-mouse IgG was from GE Healthcare (Waukesha, WI, USA).

2.6. DNA Isolation and Quantitative Real-Time (qPCR)

Total DNA was isolated from non-infected and CMV-infected HFFs using the Wizard SV genomic DNA isolation kit (Promega, Madison, WI, USA). To determine the viral load in the supernatant, total DNA was isolated from supernatants using automated DNA extraction on a BioRobot M48 instrument (Qiagen, Valencia, CA, USA). A US17 real-time PCR assay that targets 151-bp from the highly conserved US17 region of the CMV genome was used [29]. The primers and probe used for US17 were: forward 5′-GCGTGCTTTTTAGCCTCTGCA-3′, reverse 5′-AAAAGTTTGTGCCCCAACGGTA-3′, and US17 probe FAM-5′ TGATCGGGCGTTATCGCGTTCT-3′.

2.7. Add-On and Removal Assays

In the add-on group, compounds were added to infected HFFs at 0, 6, 24, and 48 hpi, and the luciferase activity was measured at 72 hpi. In the removal group, compounds were added immediately after virus infection and were subsequently removed after 0, 6, 24, and 48 h; luciferase was measured at 72 hpi.

2.8. Combination Assays

These experiments were performed as previously reported [30]. The combination of Compound **8** and each compound was tested using the pp28-luciferase CMV. Briefly, 2×10^6 HFFs/plate were seeded in 96-well plates and infected with the pp28-luciferase CMV strain (MOI = 1 PFU/cell). First, a dose–response curve was generated for each compound individually to determine its EC_{50} value. Then, the compounds were combined at twice their EC_{50} values, diluted in DMEM with 4% FBS, followed by serial dilution, and added in combination after infection. The luciferase activity of each compound individually and in combination was quantified at 72 hpi. The Bliss model was used to calculate the effect of each drug combination on pp28-luciferase activity (Kapoor/Ghosh JMC). In this model, synergistic compounds will yield a ratio > 1 of the observed fold inhibition divided by the expected fold inhibition. Antagonistic compounds will yield a ratio < 1. Additive compounds will yield a ratio = 1.

2.9. Statistical Analysis

Dose-response curves were generated as previously described [30]. The EC_{50} and CC_{50} values were calculated using GraphPad Prism software using the non-linear curve fitting and the exponential form of the median effect equation, where the percent inhibition = 1/[1 + (CC_{50} or EC_{50}/drug concentration)m], where m is a parameter that reflects the slope of the concentration-response curve. The statistical significance between two groups was analyzed by the two-tailed Student's *t*-test, and the asterisks indicate the statistical significance: *, $p < 0.05$; **, $p < 0.01$; and *** $p < 0.001$. All experiments were performed at least twice.

3. Results

3.1. CMV Inhibition by NCGC2955 Analogs

We first investigated the importance of the isopropyl carboxamide found in NCGC2955 1, (Table 1). Moving the isopropyl carboxamide from the 4-position of the piperidine found in Compound **1** to the 3-position of the piperidine in Compound 2 (isopropyl carboxamide in red) resulted in the loss of anti-CMV activity (Table 1). Since the synthesis of the thieno[3,2-b]pyrrole heterocycle found in **1** required the synthesis of potentially explosive azido precursors on gram scale, we opted to test the more readily available truncated pyrrole **4** or indole **3** replacements. Both modifications (Compounds **3** and **4**) resulted in a loss of anti-CMV activity even at 30 μM (Table 1).

The compounds with structural similarity to **1** were reported as inhibitors of neurotropic alphaviruses (RNA viruses) [25,31,32], therefore the pyrrole 4-(2-aminoethyl)pyridine **7** [26] was resynthesized (4-(2-aminoethyl)pyridine colored blue). Three analogs of Compound **1** (**5–7**) were initially tested. Compounds **5** and **6** did not inhibit the pp28-luciferase CMV at concentrations ranging from 3–30 μM (Table 1). However, compound **7** exhibited the inhibition of pp28-luciferase CMV in a dose-dependent manner, with EC_{50} of 0.21 ± 0.06 μM (Figure 1A). In a plaque assay using the CMV TB40 strain, **7** also displayed dose-dependent activity, with EC_{50} of 0.55 ± 0.06 μM (Figure 1B). A Western blot analysis performed on cell lysates collected at 72 h post infection (hpi) with CMV Towne, showed no reduction in the level of pp65, UL84, or IE1/2 after treatment with analogs **5** and **6** (10 μM), while treatment with **7** and NCGC2955 resulted in a significant inhibition of protein expression. GCV treatment (5 μM), as expected, reduced the level of CMV proteins (Figure 1C). The activity of NCGC2955 **1** was measured in the same set of experiments and revealed an EC_{50} of 1.7 ± 0.6 μM, and 1.99 ± 0.15 μM for luciferase inhibition and plaque reduction, respectively (Figure 1D,E).

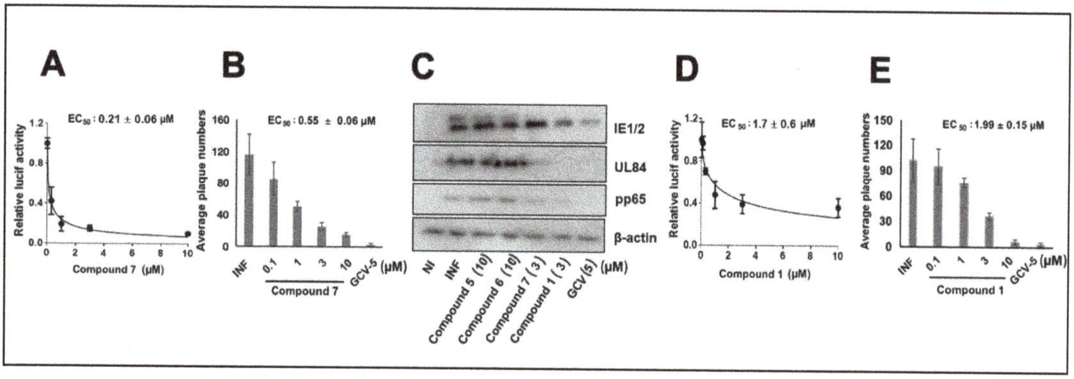

Figure 1. CMV inhibition with Compounds 1 and 7 in HFFs. (**A**) HFFs were infected with pp28-luciferase CMV (MOI = 1 PFU/cell) and treated with the indicated concentrations of Compound **7**. Luciferase activity was measured in cell lysates at 72 hpi. The data represent mean values (±SD) of triplicate determinations from two independent experiments. (**B**) HFFs were infected with CMV TB40 (150 PFU/well) and treated with the indicated concentrations of **7**. Plaques were stained and counted at day 7 post infection. The data represent mean values (±SD) of the triplicate determinations from two independent experiments. (**C**) HFFs were infected with CMV Towne and treated with Compounds **1**, **5**, **6**, **7**, and GCV at the indicated concentrations in parentheses. An immunoblot was performed for the detection of viral proteins at 72 hpi. The experiment was repeated three times, and data from a single representative experiment are shown. (**D**) HFFs were infected with pp28-luciferase CMV and treated with the indicated concentrations of Compound **1**. Luciferase activity was measured in cell lysates at 72 hpi. The data represent mean values (±SD) of triplicate determinations from two independent experiments. (**E**) HFFs were infected with CMV TB40 (150 PFU/well) and treated with the indicated concentrations of Compound **1**. Plaques were stained and counted at day 7 post infection.

The overall anti-CMV activity of **7**, which contains a 4-(2-aminoethyl) pyridine amide, was improved compared to **1**, which contains an isopropyl amide. Compound **7** differed from **5** and **6** only in the position of nitrogen in the pyridine ring, suggesting that the nitrogen in Compound **7** forms a specific interaction with its target. Truncated analogs of **7** (Compounds **10–12**), which differ by the removal of one methylene spacer also lost anti-CMV activity, suggesting that an optimal distance between the 4-carboxy piperidine and the 4-pyridine is required for CMV inhibition (Table 1). A close analog of **7**, Compound **9**, also showed anti-CMV activity in both luciferase and plaque assay (Figure 2, Table 1), EC_{50} 0.3 ± 0.05 μM and 0.35 ± 0.07 μM, respectively, suggesting that the replacement of the pyrrole with thienopyrrole has little effect on CMV inhibition. The CC_{50} of Compounds **7** and **9** was >500 μM, yielding a selectivity index of >1500.

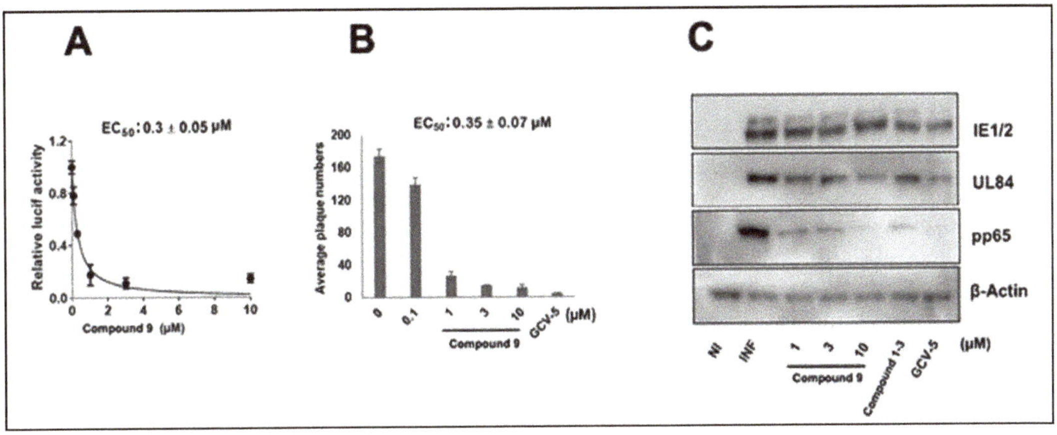

Figure 2. Anti-CMV activity of Compound **9** in HFFs. (**A**) HFFs were infected with pp28-luciferase CMV (MOI = 1 PFU/cell) and Compound **9** was added at the indicated concentrations after infection. Luciferase activity was measured in cell lysates at 72 hpi. The data represent mean values (±SD) of triplicate determinations from two independent experiments. (**B**) HFFs were infected with CMV TB40 (150 PFU/well) and treated with the indicated concentrations of Compound **9**. Plaques were stained and counted at day 7 post infection. The data represent mean values (±SD) of the triplicate determinations from two experiments. (**C**) HFFs were infected with CMV Towne and treated with Compound **9** or GCV at the indicated concentration. The level of viral proteins was measure by Western blot at 72 hpi. The experiment was repeated three times, and data from a single representative experiment are shown. NI—noninfected, I—Infected, and GCV—ganciclovir.

The data represent mean values (±SD) of the triplicate determinations from two independent experiments. NI—noninfected, I—Infected, and GCV—ganciclovir.

3.2. CMV Inhibition by Pyridine Analogs of NCGC2955

Several pyridine analogs were next tested against CMV. Compound **8** showed dose-dependent activity against CMV, $EC_{50}{}^{-}$ 0.28 ± 0.06 (luciferase, Figure 3A), and 0.42 ± 0.07 (plaque, Figure 3B), while Compound **3** had no activity against CMV in pp28- luciferase assay. Similarly, the viral proteins UL84 and pp65 were reduced following treatment with Compound **8** and the original Compound **1** (3 μM), while Compound **3** showed no inhibitory activity at 10 μM (Figure 3C). GCV (5 μM) inhibited IE2, UL84, and pp65 to a higher degree than Compound **1** and analog **8**, suggesting the activity of these compounds may occur at a later stage of CMV replication.

3.3. NCGC2955 Analogs Inhibit CMV in Primary Human Hepatocytes

To expand our studies to another clinically relevant cell line, the activity of Compounds **1**, **7**, **8** was tested in CMV-infected primary human hepatocytes. The pp28-luciferase CMV was used for infection, and luciferase activity was measured at 72 hpi. All three compounds showed dose-dependent activity with a similar EC_{50} of ~3 μM (Figure 4A–C). Viral proteins were also reduced with the three compounds (Figure 4D).

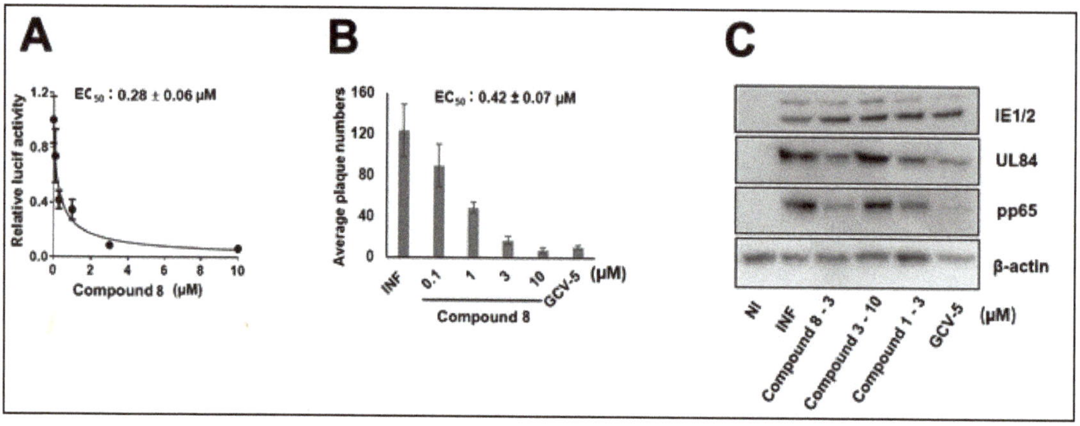

Figure 3. CMV inhibition with Compound **8** in HFFs. (**A**) HFFs were infected with pp28-luciferase CMV, and the indicated concentrations of Compound **8** were added after infection. Luciferase activity was measured in cell lysates at 72 hpi. The data represent mean values (±SD) of the triplicate determinations from two independent experiments. (**B**) HFFs were infected with CMV TB40 (150 PFU/well) and treated with the indicated concentrations of Compound **8**. Plaques were stained and counted at day 7 post infection. The data represent mean values (±SD) of triplicate determinations from two independent experiments. (**C**) HFFs were infected with CMV Towne and treated with Compounds **1**, **8**, **3**, and GCV at the indicated concentrations. The expression of viral proteins was determined by Western blot at 72 hpi. The experiment was repeated three times, and data from a single representative experiment are shown. NI—noninfected, I—Infected, and GCV—ganciclovir.

3.4. NCGC2955 Analogs Inhibit Mouse CMV (MCMV) but Not Herpes Simplex Virus 1 or 2 (HSV1 or 2)

To evaluate the antiviral activity of these compounds for future in vivo studies, and to determine whether other herpesviruses were inhibited, Compounds **7** and **8** were tested against MCMV and HSV1/2, respectively. Both analogs inhibited MCMV in vitro at submicromolar concentrations, and the EC50 values were 0.6 ± 0.34 μM and 0.73 ± 0.32 μM, respectively (Figure 5A,B). None of the analogs tested showed any activity against HSV1 or HSV2, similar to the NCGC2955 (Figure 5C,D) [24]. GCV (5 μM), used as a positive control, showed complete inhibition of HSV1 and HSV2.

3.5. NCGC2955 Analogs Are Late Inhibitors of CMV Replication

The timing of activity of analogs **7** and **8** was evaluated by Western blot (Figure 6A,B) and compound addition or removal at different times during infection (Figure 6C,D). The effect of GCV on reducing the level of viral proteins was similar to but more significant than **7** (Figure 6A,B). Analogs **7** and **8** were tested when added or removed at 6, 10, 24, and 48 hpi. Although the timing of maximal CMV inhibition of **7** and **8** overlapped with that of GCV, since a difference was observed in the viral protein expression, experiments at later time points of the infection were performed.

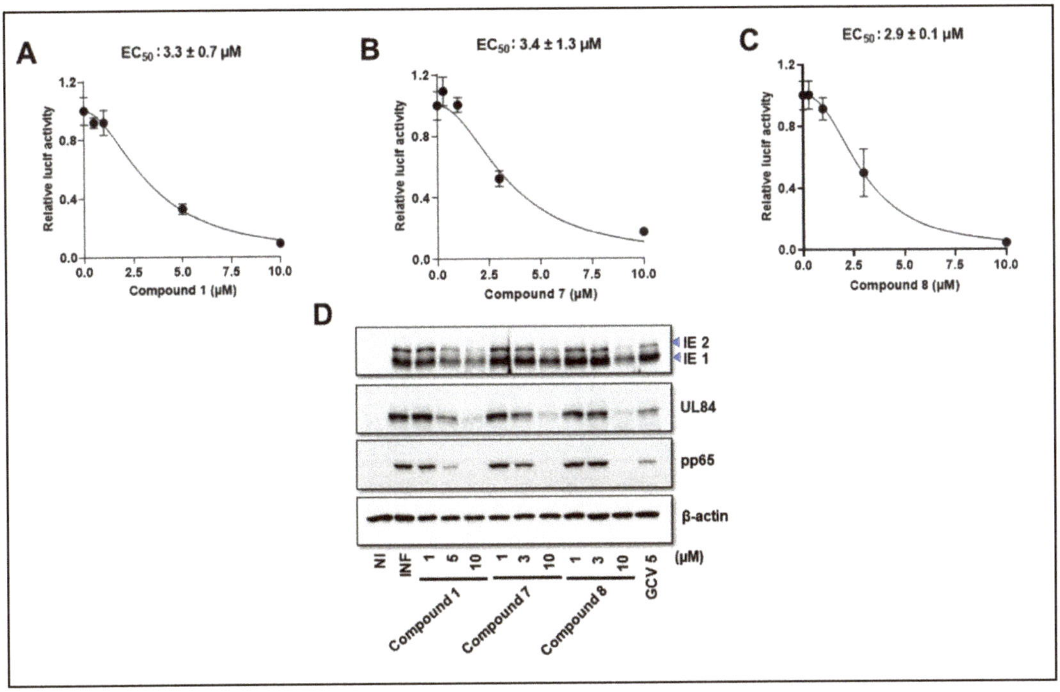

Figure 4. Activity of Compounds **1**, **7**, **8** in CMV-infected primary human hepatocytes. (**A–C**) Primary human hepatocytes (PXB-cells) were infected with pp28-luciferase CMV (MOI =1 PFU/cell) and treated with the indicated concentrations of Compounds **1**, **7**, and **8**. Luciferase activity was measured in cell lysates at 72 hpi. The data represent mean values (±SD) of the triplicate determinations from two independent experiments. (**D**) Primary human hepatocytes were infected with CMV Towne and treated with Compounds **1**, **7**, **8**, and GCV at the indicated concentrations. An immunoblot was performed for the detection of viral proteins at 72 hpi. Data from a single experiment are shown. NI—noninfected, I—Infected, and GCV—ganciclovir.

3.6. NCGC2955 Analogs Reduce CMV Yield

To better define the timing of CMV inhibition by the new analogs, HFFs were infected with CMV TB40 and treated with Compounds **1**, **7**, or **8** (all at 3 μM), letermovir (10 nM), and GCV (5 μM). The supernatants from the infected cells were harvested at 72, 96, and 120 h, and titered by plaque assay. The plaques were stained and counted at day 7 post infection. The reduction in viral titer with **7** and **8** was higher than with **1** and overall similar to GCV. Letermovir (LTV) showed the strongest reduction in viral progeny at all time points (Figure 7A). Viral DNA replication was measured in cells and supernatants (Figure 7B,C) by real-time PCR of CMV US17. GCV reduced DNA replication in both cells and supernatants, while LTV reduced viral loads in supernatants. Compounds **1**, **7**, and **8** did not reduce the cellular viral loads, but **7** decreased the viral loads in supernatants at all time points and **8** decreased viral loads at 120 hpi.

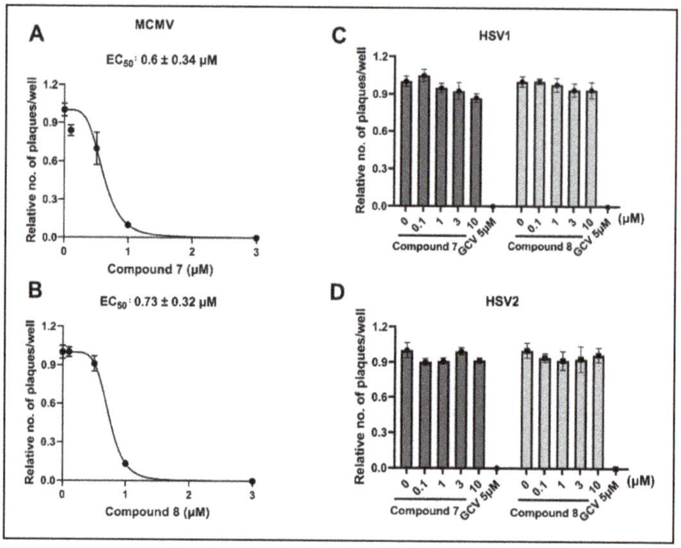

Figure 5. Activity of Compounds **7** and **8** against MCMV, HSV1 and HSV2. (**A**,**B**) Mouse embryonic fibroblasts were infected with MCMV at 100 PFU/well and treated with the indicated concentrations of **7** and **8**. Infected cells were stained, and the viral plaques were counted at 72 hpi. The dose-response curves represent the relative fold inhibition and the data points represent mean ± SD from two independent experiments. (**C**,**D**) Vero cells were infected with HSV1 and HSV2 (100 PFU/well) and treated with the indicated concentrations of Compounds **7** and **8**. Infected cells were stained and the viral plaques were counted at 36 h and 24 h post infection for HSV1 and HSV2, respectively. The data set represent mean ± SD from two independent experiments.

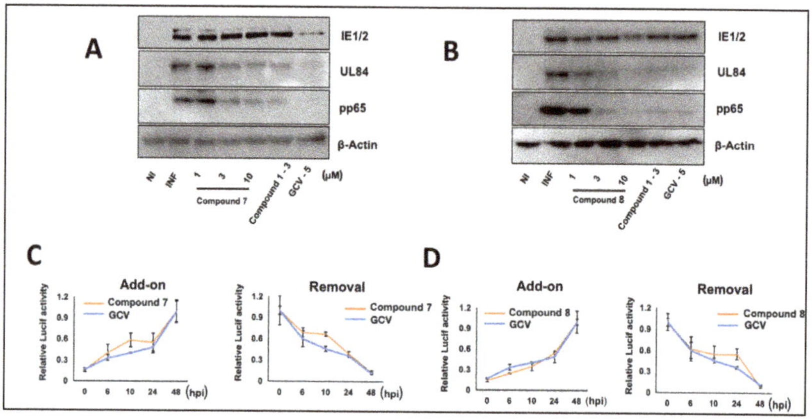

Figure 6. Effect of Compounds **7** and **8** on CMV protein expression and timing of activity. (**A**,**B**) HFFs were infected with CMV Towne (1 PFU/cell) and treated with Compounds **1**, **7**, **8**, and GCV at the indicated concentrations. The expression of viral proteins was determined by Western blot at 72 hpi. The experiment was repeated three times, and data from a single representative experiment are shown. (**C**,**D**) HFFs were infected with pp28-luciferase CMV (MOI = 0.1 PFU/cell). Compounds **7**, **8** (3 μM), or GCV (5 μM) were either added or removed at different times after infection (0, 6, 24, 48, 72 h). Luciferase activity was measured in cell lysates at 72 hpi. Data shown are the average of three independent experiments (average ± SD).

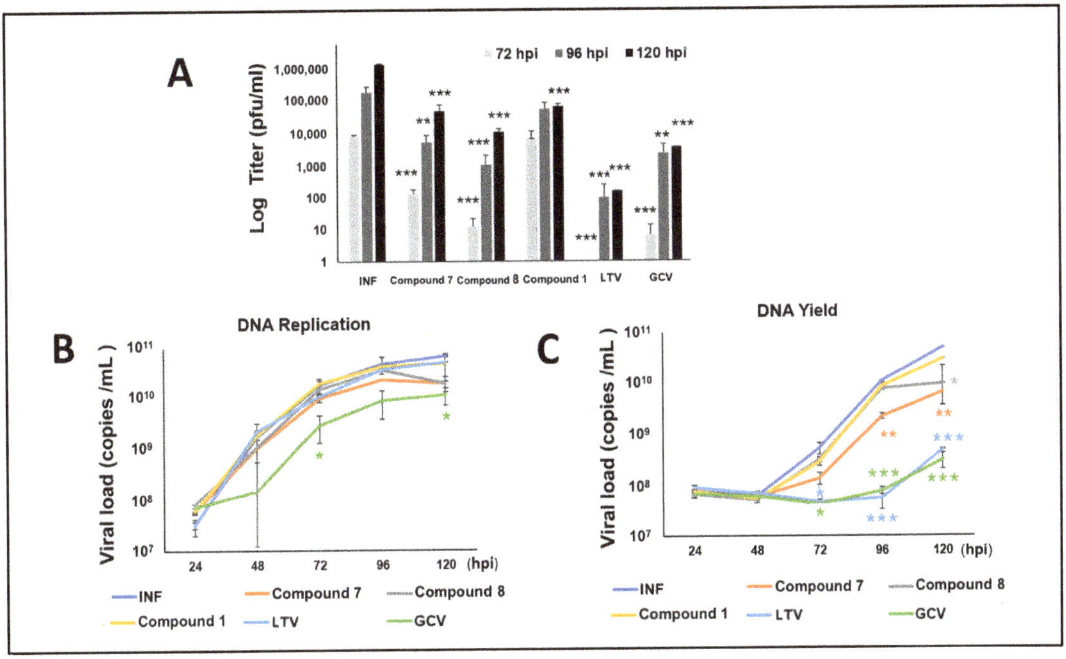

Figure 7. Effect of Compounds **1**, **7**, and **8** on viral progeny, DNA replication (infected cells), and DNA yield (supernatants). HFFs were infected with CMV TB40 (150 PFU/well) and treated with Compounds **1**, **7**, **8** (all at 3 μM), LTV (10 nM), and GCV (5 μM). DNA was isolated from the infected cells, and supernatants were harvested at the indicated time points. (**A**) Titration of supernatants was performed by plaque assay. The plaques were stained and counted at day 7 post infection. The data represent the mean values (±SD) of the triplicate determinations from two independent experiments. (**B**,**C**) Viral DNA replication in cells (**B**) and viral DNA load in the supernatants (**C**) were determined by real-time PCR. Data shown are average ± SD of quadruplicate values from two independent experiments. *, $p < 0.05$; **, $p < 0.01$; and *** $p < 0.001$.

3.7. NCGC2955 Analogs Are Additive with Newly Identified CMV Inhibitors and GCV

Analog **8** was tested in combination with newly identified CMV inhibitors MLS8969, NFU1827, MLS8554, and MLS8091, and GCV [24]. All combination experiments revealed that **8** was additive with all tested compounds with a calculated Bliss coefficient ranging from 1–1.3 (Figure 8, Table 2), suggesting an independent mode of action.

Table 2. EC_{50} of individual compounds and the respective Bliss coefficients.

Compound 1	EC_{50} (μM)	Compound 2	EC_{50} (μM)	Bliss Coefficient
8	0.29 ± 0.1	MLS8969	0.25 ± 0.3	1
8	0.41 ± 0.2	MLS8554	0.55 ± 0.2	1.2
8	0.35 ± 0.07	NFU1827	0.82 ± 0.1	1.2
8	0.27 ± 0.1	MLS8091	0.34 ± 0.1	1.1
8	0.38 ± 0.08	GCV	0.25 ± 0.1	1.3

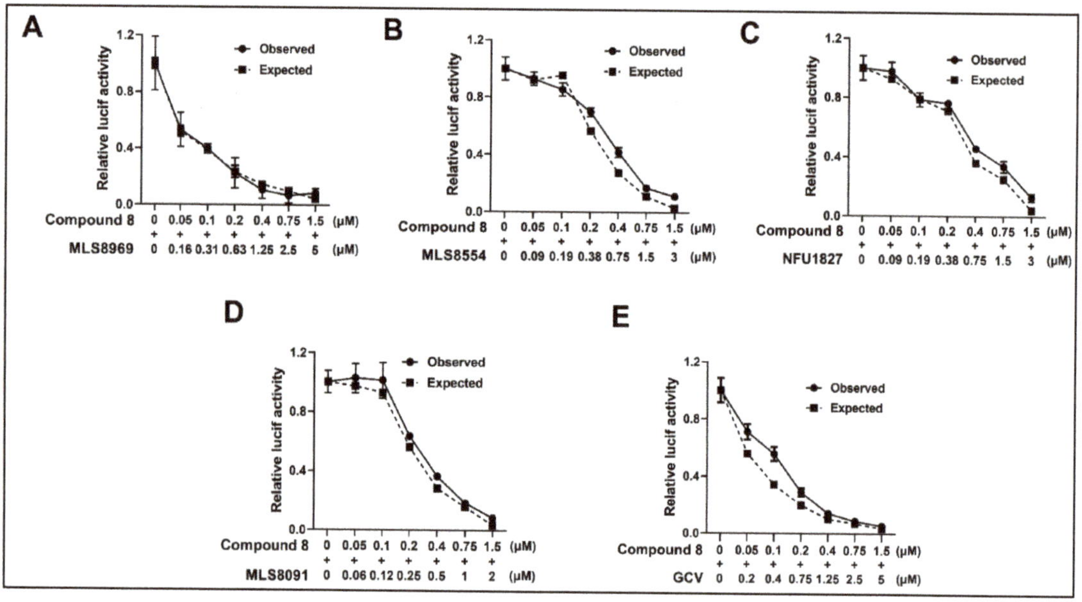

Figure 8. Combination of Compound **8** is an additive with newly identified CMV inhibitors and GCV. (**A**–**E**) HFFs were infected with pp28-luciferase CMV (MOI = 1 PFU/cell) and first treated with each individual compound, followed by a combination of each compound with **8** at different concentrations. In the drug combination experiments, CMV-infected HFFs were treated with an initial drug concentration of twice the EC_{50} value of the individual compound and two-fold serial dilutions. Luciferase activity was measured in cell lysates at 72 hpi and the Bliss model was used to calculate the anti-CMV activity of the compounds in their combination. Solid lines indicate the observed CMV inhibition (dose–response) and dotted lines indicate the expected CMV inhibition at each dose of drug combination. The experiments were repeated twice. Data from a single representative experiment are shown.

4. Discussion

Hit NCGC2955 (Compound **1**) was identified from a recent high-throughput screen (>400,000 compounds) for human CMV inhibitors [24]. It showed in vitro activity against TB40, ganciclovir resistant pp28-luciferase CMV, and mouse CMV at low μM concentrations, but had no activity against HSV1 or 2. The structurally related compounds of Compound **1** were reported to inhibit RNA viruses [25,26]. Piperidine-4-carboxamide analogs were studied in detail in cell-based assays using the Western Equine Encephalitis Virus (WEEV), replicons and showed half-maximal inhibitory concentrations of ~1 μM and selectivity indices of >100. CCG205432, similar to our Compound **8** (the TFA salt of CCG205432), inhibited the infectious virus in cultured human neuronal cells. These compounds showed broad inhibitory activity against RNA viruses in culture, including members of the *Togaviridae*, *Bunyaviridae*, *Picornaviridae*, and *Paramyxoviridae* families. Their mechanism of action was suggested to involve a host factor that modulates cap-dependent translation. CCG205432 did not directly target WEEV RNA-dependent RNA polymerase or other viral enzyme activities that would promote the development of drug-resistant viral mutants. Despite the broad-spectrum antiviral activity, our tested compounds did not inhibit HSV1 or HSV2, suggesting a specific mechanism of action that may involve the host factors required for the efficient replication of several groups of viruses. The interest in host factors that restrict virus replication, such as the electron transport system, cytochrome P450 51, mitochondrial regulatory proteins, and autophagy, led to the identification of agents that could be further developed or repurposed for CMV therapeutics as monotherapy or combination therapy with direct-acting FDA approved antiviral agents [33–37].

Initially, we studied the piperidine-4-carboxamide scaffold. With the synthesis of a handful of compounds, we were able to show that pyrrole, indole, and thienopyrrole are all tolerated when coupled to the 4-(2-aminoethyl)pyridine. The H-bond acceptor in the 4-position appears to be necessary, since CMV inhibition was not observed with the placement of this moiety at the 2- or 3-position. We were also able to demonstrate that CMV inhibition was specific to the position of the pyridine nitrogen atom and spacer between the amide and pyridine.

In addition to testing our compounds in human foreskin fibroblasts, we extended our studies to include primary human hepatocytes as another clinically relevant cell line for infection with CMV. Hepatocytes have rarely been used for CMV infection [38]. These cells were infected with the pp28-luciferase CMV. The three analogs tested revealed similar activity against CMV with EC_{50} values at around 3 μM, although in HFFs their activity was improved. We noted that the variability in antiviral activity was observed in different cell systems. Maribavir showed varied EC_{50} values for CMV inhibition depending on the fibroblasts used, which was attributed to the activity of kinases in different cells [39].

Despite the inhibition of viral progeny by plaque assays and the observed decrease in viral protein levels, the influence of NCGC2955 analogs on viral DNA replication and viral DNA yield was modest (Figure 7), suggesting inhibition via novel mechanisms that do not involve the DNA replication machinery. The terminase complex, targeted by LTV, cleaves DNA to package the viral genome into the capsid [40]. Compared to NCGC2955 analogs, LTV showed a stronger reduction in viral progeny and viral loads in supernatants. These data may suggest the production of CMV DNA containing non-infectious virus that lacks some viral proteins.

Our study is the beginning of structural activity relationship (SARs), following a large high throughput screen for CMV inhibitors. Further studies, including the resistance selection and target identification along with structure-based design, may lead to the identification of novel CMV inhibitors for in vivo studies. Our future goals include increasing the anti-CMV potency and further exploring the SARs, so that a tool compound can be synthesized to aid in the identification of a viral target. This can be approached by varying the H-bond accepting potential of the pyridine. Further SARs will be developed around the chain length. Additionally, the piperidine will be replaced with pyrrolidine and azetidine to fine tune the optimal length and angle of the pyridine's interaction in the active site. The chain length of the 4-chlorobenzyl will also be explored as well as the electronics of the ring. The generation of metabolically stable analogs will assist exploring the in vivo efficacy in animal models.

Conclusion: Piperidine-4-carboxamide analogs inhibit cytomegalovirus with high selectivity and are additive with GCV. Their activity in primary human hepatocytes suggests they may be active in vivo and should be further developed for CMV therapeutics.

Supplementary Materials: The following supporting information can be downloaded at https://www.mdpi.com/article/10.3390/v14020234/s1, File S1: Materials and Methods.

Author Contributions: Conceptualization, R.A.-B. and D.J.M.; methodology, X.G., A.K.G., F.P., M.F., D.J.M. and R.A.-B.; software, X.G. and A.K.G.; validation, F.P. and R.F.K.; formal analysis, X.G., A.K.G., F.P., M.F., D.J.M. and R.A.-B.; investigation, X.G., A.K.G., F.P., M.F., D.J.M. and R.A.-B.; resources, R.A.-B., D.J.M., F.P. and M.F.; data curation, X.G., A.K.G., F.P., M.F., D.J.M. and R.A.-B.; writing—R.A.-B. and D.J.M.; writing—review and editing, R.F.K., M.F., D.J.M. and R.A.-B.; supervision, R.A.-B.; project administration, R.A.-B.; funding acquisition, D.J.M. All authors have read and agreed to the published version of the manuscript.

Funding: D.J.M. acknowledges funding from the Flight Attendant Medical Research Institute (FAMRI) and the Institute for Clinical and Translational Research (UL1TR003098).

Institutional Review Board Statement: Ethical review and approval were waived for this study due to the use of archived human samples that cannot be linked to any specific patient.

Informed Consent Statement: Not applicable.

Acknowledgments: We thank PhoenixBio (Hiroshima, Japan) for providing the primary human hepatocytes (PXB-cells) for this study.

Conflicts of Interest: The authors declare no conflict of interest.

References

1. Staras, S.A.S.; Dollard, S.C.; Radford, K.W.; Flanders, W.D.; Pass, R.; Cannon, M.J. Seroprevalence of Cytomegalovirus Infection in the United States, 1988–1994. *Clin. Infect. Dis.* **2006**, *43*, 1143–1151. [CrossRef] [PubMed]
2. Griffiths, P.D.; Clark, D.A.; Emery, V.C. Betaherpesviruses in transplant recipients. *J. Antimicrob. Chemother.* **2000**, *45*, 29–34. [CrossRef]
3. Jabs, D.A.; Martin, B.K.; Forman, M.S. Mortality Associated with Resistant Cytomegalovirus among Patients with Cytomegalovirus Retinitis and AIDS. *Ophthalmology* **2010**, *117*, 128–132.e2. [CrossRef]
4. Khamduang, W.; Jourdain, G.; Sirirungsi, W.; Layangool, P.; Kanjanavanit, S.; Krittigamas, P.; Pagdi, K.; Somsamai, R.; Sirinontakan, S.; Hinjiranandana, T.; et al. The interrelated transmission of HIV-1 and cytomegalovirus during gestation and delivery in the offspring of HIV-infected mothers. *J. Acquir. Immune Defic. Syndr.* **2011**, *58*, 188–192. [CrossRef] [PubMed]
5. Kovacs, A.; Schluchter, M.; Easley, K.; Demmler, G.; Shearer, W.; La Russa, P.; Pitt, J.; Cooper, E.; Goldfarb, J.; Hodes, D.; et al. Cytomegalovirus Infection and HIV-1 Disease Progression in Infants Born to HIV-1–Infected Women. *N. Engl. J. Med.* **1999**, *341*, 77–84. [CrossRef]
6. Barbi, M.; Binda, S.; Caroppo, S.; Ambrosetti, U.; Corbetta, C.; Sergi, P. A wider role for congenital cytomegalovirus infection in sensorineural hearing loss. *Pediatr. Infect. Dis. J.* **2003**, *22*, 39–42. [CrossRef]
7. Boppana, S.B.; Fowler, K.B.; Britt, W.J.; Stagno, S.; Pass, R.F. Symptomatic Congenital Cytomegalovirus Infection in Infants Born to Mothers with Preexisting Immunity to Cytomegalovirus. *Pediatrics* **1999**, *104*, 55–60. [CrossRef]
8. Demmler, G.J. Infectious Diseases Society of America and Centers for Disease Control: Summary of a Workshop on Surveillance for Congenital Cytomegalovirus Disease. *Clin. Infect. Dis.* **1991**, *13*, 315–329. [CrossRef]
9. Avery, R.K.; Arav-Boger, R.; Marr, K.A.; Kraus, E.; Shoham, S.; Lees, L.; Trollinger, B.; Shah, P.; Ambinder, R.; Neofytos, D.; et al. Outcomes in Transplant Recipients Treated with Foscarnet for Ganciclovir-Resistant or Refractory Cytomegalovirus Infection. *Transplantation* **2016**, *100*, e74–e80. [CrossRef]
10. Chou, S. Cytomegalovirus drug resistance and clinical implications. *Transpl. Infect. Dis.* **2001**, *3*, 20–24. [CrossRef]
11. Schreiber, A.; Härter, G.; Schubert, A.; Bunjes, D.; Mertens, T.; Michel, D. Antiviral treatment of cytomegalovirus infection and resistant strains. *Expert Opin. Pharmacother.* **2009**, *10*, 191–209. [CrossRef] [PubMed]
12. Steininger, C. Novel Therapies for Cytomegalovirus Disease. *Recent Patents Anti-Infect. Drug Discov.* **2007**, *2*, 53–72. [CrossRef] [PubMed]
13. Kimberlin, D.W.; Lin, C.-Y.; Sánchez, P.J.; Demmler, G.J.; Dankner, W.; Shelton, M.; Jacobs, R.F.; Vaudry, W.; Pass, R.F.; Kiell, J.M.; et al. Effect of ganciclovir therapy on hearing in symptomatic congenital cytomegalovirus disease involving the central nervous system: A randomized, controlled trial. *J. Pediatr.* **2003**, *143*, 16–25. [CrossRef]
14. Kimberlin, D.W.; Jester, P.M.; Sánchez, P.J.; Ahmed, A.; Arav-Boger, R.; Michaels, M.G.; Ashouri, N.; Englund, J.A.; Estrada, B.; Jacobs, R.F.; et al. Valganciclovir for Symptomatic Congenital Cytomegalovirus Disease. *N. Engl. J. Med.* **2015**, *372*, 933–943. [CrossRef]
15. Lanzieri, T.M.; Caviness, A.C.; Blum, P.; Demmler-Harrison, G.; Congenital Cytomegalovirus Longitudinal Study Group. Progressive, Long-Term Hearing Loss in Congenital CMV Disease After Ganciclovir Therapy. *J. Pediatric Infect. Dis. Soc.* **2021**. [CrossRef]
16. Chou, S. RapidIn VitroEvolution of Human Cytomegalovirus UL56 Mutations That Confer Letermovir Resistance. *Antimicrob. Agents Chemother.* **2015**, *59*, 6588–6593. [CrossRef]
17. Chou, S.; Ercolani, R.J.; Lanier, E.R. Novel Cytomegalovirus UL54 DNA Polymerase Gene Mutations Selected In Vitro That Confer Brincidofovir Resistance. *Antimicrob. Agents Chemother.* **2016**, *60*, 3845–3848. [CrossRef]
18. Chemaly, R.F.; Ullmann, A.J.; Stoelben, S.; Richard, M.P.; Bornhäuser, M.; Groth, C.; Einsele, H.; Silverman, M.; Mullane, K.M.; Brown, J.; et al. Letermovir for Cytomegalovirus Prophylaxis in Hematopoietic-Cell Transplantation. *N. Engl. J. Med.* **2014**, *370*, 1781–1789. [CrossRef]
19. Marty, F.M.; Ljungman, P.; Chemaly, R.F.; Maertens, J.; Dadwal, S.S.; Duarte, R.F.; Haider, S.; Ullmann, A.J.; Katayama, Y.; Brown, J.; et al. Letermovir Prophylaxis for Cytomegalovirus in Hematopoietic-Cell Transplantation. *N. Engl. J. Med.* **2017**, *377*, 2433–2444. [CrossRef]
20. Frietsch, J.J.; Michel, D.; Stamminger, T.; Hunstig, F.; Birndt, S.; Schnetzke, U.; Scholl, S.; Hochhaus, A.; Hilgendorf, I. In Vivo Emergence of UL56 C325Y Cytomegalovirus Resistance to Letermovir in a Patient with Acute Myeloid Leukemia after Hematopoietic Cell Transplantation. *Mediterr. J. Hematol. Infect. Dis.* **2019**, *11*, e2019001. [CrossRef] [PubMed]
21. Winston, D.J.; Saliba, F.; Blumberg, E.; Abouljoud, M.; Garcia-Diaz, J.B.; Goss, J.A.; Clough, L.; Avery, R.; Limaye, A.P.; Ericzon, B.G.; et al. Efficacy and Safety of Maribavir Dosed at 100 mg Orally Twice Daily for the Prevention of Cytomegalovirus Disease in Liver Transplant Recipients: A Randomized, Double-Blind, Multicenter Controlled Trial. *Arab. Archaeol. Epigr.* **2012**, *12*, 3021–3030. [CrossRef]

22. Winston, D.J.; Young, J.-A.; Pullarkat, V.; Papanicolaou, G.; Vij, R.; Vance, E.; Alangaden, G.J.; Chemaly, R.F.; Petersen, F.; Chao, N.; et al. Maribavir prophylaxis for prevention of cytomegalovirus infection in allogeneic stem cell transplant recipients: A multicenter, randomized, double-blind, placebo-controlled, dose-ranging study. *Blood* **2008**, *111*, 5403–5410. [CrossRef]
23. Papanicolaou, G.A.; Silveira, F.P.; Langston, A.A.; Pereira, M.R.; Avery, R.K.; Uknis, M.; Wijatyk, A.; Wu, J.; Boeckh, M.; Marty, F.; et al. Maribavir for Refractory or Resistant Cytomegalovirus Infections in Hematopoietic-cell or Solid-organ Transplant Recipients: A Randomized, Dose-ranging, Double-blind, Phase 2 Study. *Clin. Infect. Dis.* **2019**, *68*, 1255–1264. [CrossRef]
24. Kapoor, A.; Ghosh, A.K.; Forman, M.; Hu, X.; Ye, W.; Southall, N.; Marugan, J.J.; Keyes, R.F.; Smith, B.C.; Meyers, D.J.; et al. Validation and Characterization of Five Distinct Novel Inhibitors of Human Cytomegalovirus. *J. Med. Chem.* **2020**, *63*, 3896–3907. [CrossRef]
25. Delekta, P.C.; Dobry, C.J.; Sindac, J.A.; Barraza, S.J.; Blakely, P.K.; Xiang, J.; Kirchhoff, P.D.; Keep, R.F.; Irani, D.N.; Larsen, S.D.; et al. Novel Indole-2-Carboxamide Compounds Are Potent Broad-Spectrum Antivirals Active against Western Equine Encephalitis Virus In Vivo. *J. Virol.* **2014**, *88*, 11199–11214. [CrossRef]
26. Sindac, J.A.; Barraza, S.J.; Dobry, C.J.; Xiang, J.; Blakely, P.K.; Irani, D.N.; Keep, R.F.; Miller, D.J.; Larsen, S.D. Optimization of novel indole-2-carboxamide inhibitors of neurotropic alphavirus replication. *J. Med. Chem.* **2013**, *56*, 9222–9241. [CrossRef]
27. He, R.; Sandford, G.; Hayward, G.S.; Burns, W.H.; Posner, G.H.; Forman, M.; Arav-Boger, R. Recombinant luciferase-expressing human cytomegalovirus (CMV) for evaluation of CMV inhibitors. *Virol. J.* **2011**, *8*, 40. [CrossRef]
28. Sampaio, K.L.; Cavignac, Y.; Stierhof, Y.-D.; Sinzger, C. Human Cytomegalovirus Labeled with Green Fluorescent Protein for Live Analysis of Intracellular Particle Movements. *J. Virol.* **2005**, *79*, 2754–2767. [CrossRef]
29. Forman, M.S.; Vaidya, D.; Bolorunduro, O.; Diener-West, M.; Pass, R.; Arav-Boger, R. Cytomegalovirus Kinetics Following Primary Infection in Healthy Women. *J. Infect. Dis.* **2017**, *215*, 1523–1526. [CrossRef]
30. Cai, H.; Kapoor, A.; He, R.; Venkatadri, R.; Forman, M.; Posner, G.H.; Arav-Boger, R. In VitroCombination of Anti-Cytomegalovirus Compounds Acting through Different Targets: Role of the Slope Parameter and Insights into Mechanisms of Action. *Antimicrob. Agents Chemother.* **2014**, *58*, 986–994. [CrossRef]
31. Ching, K.-C.; Kam, Y.-W.; Merits, A.; Ng, L.F.P.; Chai, C.L.L. Trisubstituted Thieno[3,2-b]pyrrole 5-Carboxamides as Potent Inhibitors of Alphaviruses. *J. Med. Chem.* **2015**, *58*, 9196–9213. [CrossRef] [PubMed]
32. Ching, K.-C.; Tran, T.N.Q.; Amrun, S.N.; Kam, Y.-W.; Ng, L.F.P.; Chai, C.L.L. Structural Optimizations of Thieno[3,2-b]pyrrole Derivatives for the Development of Metabolically Stable Inhibitors of Chikungunya Virus. *J. Med. Chem.* **2017**, *60*, 3165–3186. [CrossRef] [PubMed]
33. Clark, A.E.; Sabalza, M.; Gordts, P.L.S.M.; Spector, D.H. Human Cytomegalovirus Replication Is Inhibited by the Autophagy-Inducing Compounds Trehalose and SMER28 through Distinctively Different Mechanisms. *J. Virol.* **2018**, *92*, e02015-17. [CrossRef] [PubMed]
34. Combs, J.A.; Monk, C.H.; Harrison, M.A.A.; Norton, E.B.; Morris, C.A.; Sullivan, D.E.; Zwezdaryk, K.J. Inhibiting cytomegalovirus replication through targeting the host electron transport chain. *Antivir. Res.* **2021**, *194*, 105159. [CrossRef]
35. Hahn, F.; Niesar, A.; Wangen, C.; Wild, M.; Grau, B.; Herrmann, L.; Capci, A.; Adrait, A.; Couté, Y.; Tsogoeva, S.B.; et al. Target verification of artesunate-related antiviral drugs: Assessing the role of mitochondrial and regulatory proteins by click chemistry and fluorescence labeling. *Antivir. Res.* **2020**, *180*, 104861. [CrossRef]
36. Mercorelli, B.; Luganini, A.; Celegato, M.; Palù, G.; Gribaudo, G.; Lepesheva, G.I.; Loregian, A. The Clinically Approved Antifungal Drug Posaconazole Inhibits Human Cytomegalovirus Replication. *Antimicrob. Agents Chemother.* **2020**, *64*, e00056-20. [CrossRef]
37. Mukhopadhyay, R.; Venkatadri, R.; Katsnelson, J.; Arav-Boger, R. Digitoxin Suppresses Human Cytomegalovirus Replication via Na(+), K(+)/ATPase alpha1 Subunit-Dependent AMP-Activated Protein Kinase and Autophagy Activation. *J. Virol.* **2018**, *92*, e01861-17. [CrossRef]
38. Sinzger, C.; Bissinger, A.L.; Viebahn, R.; Oettle, H.; Radke, C.; Schmidt, C.A.; Jahn, G. Hepatocytes are Permissive for Human Cytomegalovirus Infection in Human Liver Cell Culture and In Vivo. *J. Infect. Dis.* **1999**, *180*, 976–986. [CrossRef]
39. Chou, S.; Van Wechel, L.C.; Marousek, G.I. Effect of Cell Culture Conditions on the Anticytomegalovirus Activity of Maribavir. *Antimicrob. Agents Chemother.* **2006**, *50*, 2557–2559. [CrossRef]
40. Ligat, G.; Cazal, R.; Hantz, S.; Alain, S. The human cytomegalovirus terminase complex as an antiviral target: A close-up view. *FEMS Microbiol. Rev.* **2018**, *42*, 137–145. [CrossRef]

viruses

MDPI

Article

Antibodies to Crucial Epitopes on HSV-2 Glycoprotein D as a Guide to Dosing an mRNA Genital Herpes Vaccine

Lauren M. Hook [1], Sita Awasthi [1], Tina M. Cairns [2], Mohamad-Gabriel Alameh [1], Bernard T. Fowler [1], Kevin P. Egan [1], Molly M. H. Sung [3], Drew Weissman [1], Gary H. Cohen [2] and Harvey M. Friedman [1,*]

1 Infectious Disease Division, Department of Medicine, Perelman School of Medicine, University of Pennsylvania, Philadelphia, PA 19104, USA; lhook@pennmedicine.upenn.edu (L.M.H.); sawasthi@pennmedicine.upenn.edu (S.A.); mg.alameh@pennmedicine.upenn.edu (M.-G.A.); bernard.fowler@pennmedicine.upenn.edu (B.T.F.); kevinpe@pennmedicine.upenn.edu (K.P.E.); dreww@pennmedicine.upenn.edu (D.W.)

2 Department of Basic and Translational Sciences, School of Dental Medicine, University of Pennsylvania, Philadelphia, PA 19104, USA; tmcairns@upenn.edu (T.M.C.); ghc@upenn.edu (G.H.C.)

3 Acuitas Therapeutics Inc., Vancouver, BC V6T 1Z3, Canada; msung@acuitastx.com

* Correspondence: hfriedma@pennmedicine.upenn.edu

Abstract: The toxicity of mRNA-lipid nanoparticle (LNP) vaccines depends on the total mRNA-LNP dose. We established that the maximum tolerated dose of our trivalent mRNA-LNP genital herpes vaccine was 10 μg/immunization in mice. We then evaluated one of the mRNAs, gD2 mRNA-LNP, to determine how much of the 10 μg total dose to assign to this immunogen. We immunized mice with 0.3, 1.0, 3.0, or 10 μg of gD2 mRNA-LNP and measured serum IgG ELISA, neutralizing antibodies, and antibodies to six crucial gD2 epitopes involved in virus entry and spread. Antibodies to crucial gD2 epitopes peaked at 1 μg, while ELISA and neutralizing titers continued to increase at higher doses. The epitope results suggested no immunologic benefit above 1 μg of gD2 mRNA-LNP, while ELISA and neutralizing titers indicated higher doses may be useful. We challenged the gD2 mRNA-immunized mice intravaginally with HSV-2. The 1-μg dose provided total protection, confirming the epitope studies, and supported assigning less than one-third of the trivalent vaccine maximum dose of 10 μg to gD2 mRNA-LNP. Epitope mapping as performed in mice can also be accomplished in phase 1 human trials to help select the optimum dose of each immunogen in a multivalent vaccine.

Keywords: herpes simplex virus type 2; nucleoside-modified mRNA; lipid nanoparticle; glycoprotein D; genital herpes vaccine; IgG ELISA; neutralizing antibodies; epitope mapping; surface plasmon resonance

Citation: Hook, L.M.; Awasthi, S.; Cairns, T.M.; Alameh, M.-G.; Fowler, B.T.; Egan, K.P.; Sung, M.M.H.; Weissman, D.; Cohen, G.H.; Friedman, H.M. Antibodies to Crucial Epitopes on HSV-2 Glycoprotein D as a Guide to Dosing an mRNA Genital Herpes Vaccine. *Viruses* **2022**, *14*, 540. https://doi.org/10.3390/v14030540

Academic Editor: Barry J. Margulies

Received: 30 January 2022
Accepted: 3 March 2022
Published: 5 March 2022

1. Introduction

Nucleoside-modified mRNA-lipid nanoparticle (LNP) vaccines have been highly successful in reducing hospitalizations and deaths from COVID-19 [1]. mRNA vaccines for rabies, influenza, and cytomegalovirus are in human trials (https://clinicaltrials.gov/ct2/show/NCT05085366, accessed on 30 January 2022) [2,3]. Other viral vaccines are likely to follow, possibly including our candidate HSV-2 trivalent vaccine to prevent genital herpes [4–7].

The mRNA-LNP vaccines for COVID-19 demonstrated dose-dependent toxicity in phase 1 human studies [8,9]. An mRNA dose of 30 μg of the Pfizer/BioNTech COVID-19 vaccine was well tolerated, however higher doses had more adverse reactions [9]. The cutoff dose for the Moderna vaccine was 100 μg [9]. These vaccines use different proprietary LNP formulations. The LNP component tends to be the reactogenic constituent in the vaccine, and the LNP content increases proportional to the mRNA dose [10]. The COVID-19 mRNA-LNP vaccine contains a single mRNA encoding the Spike protein [1]. Our genital herpes vaccine contains three mRNAs while the CMV vaccine in phase 3 human trials contains

6 mRNAs [4,5]. Multivalent vaccines need to use lower doses of individual immunogens to keep the total mRNA-LNP content below toxic levels.

Antigen doses for vaccines are often determined in dose escalation phase 1 human trials based on balancing toxicity and immunogenicity. The selected dose is then evaluated for efficacy in much larger and more costly phase 2 and 3 human trials. Here, we evaluated whether measuring antibody responses to crucial epitopes on immunogens in dose escalation (phase 1-like) studies adds value to more established methods, such as serum IgG ELISA and neutralizing antibody assays, in selecting the optimum dose of immunogens to include in larger efficacy studies. We used the mouse model of genital herpes and gD2 mRNA-LNP as the test immunogen to evaluate our hypothesis that epitope mapping will help select the optimal dose of an immunogen to include in a multivalent vaccine.

We previously performed epitope mapping studies using high throughput biosensor technology to measure antibody responses to crucial epitopes on HSV-2 glycoprotein D (gD2) in immunized mice, guinea pigs, and humans [5,11–13]. In the guinea pig HSV-2 genital infection model, antibody responses to crucial gD2 epitopes correlated with vaccine efficacy [11]. The greater the number of crucial gD2 epitopes recognized by the immune serum and the higher the antibody titer, the greater the protection was against the genital disease [11]. Here, we compare the utility of epitope mapping with serum IgG ELISA and neutralizing antibody titers for selecting the lowest effective dose of an mRNA immunogen to include in a multivalent vaccine.

2. Materials and Methods

2.1. Evaluating Trivalent mRNA-LNP Vaccine Toxicity

For toxicity studies, female BALB/c mice (Charles River) age 7–9 weeks were immunized twice 28 days apart intramuscularly (IM) in the hind limb hip muscle with a total dose of 1, 3, or 10 µg in 30 µL containing equal concentrations of gC2, gD2, and gE2 mRNA-LNP, or with sterile saline as a control [5]. The DNA constructs designed to prepare the mRNA and procedures used to generate the mRNA have been described previously [5]. The mRNA was encapsulated in LNP prepared by Acuitas [5]. Mice were evaluated for weight loss and hind limb mobility daily for 6–7 days after the first and second immunizations. Mice received a daily score of 2 for a moderate reduction in hind limb mobility, 1 for a minor reduction, and 0 for no reduction.

2.2. Immunizing with gD2 mRNA-LNP

To determine the lowest effective dose of gD2 mRNA to include in the vaccine, female BALB/c mice were immunized twice at 28-day intervals with gD2 mRNA-LNP at doses of 0.3, 1.0, 3.0, or 10 µg (10 mice/group) diluted in 30 µL of sterile saline. An additional group of 10 mice received two immunizations with 10 µg of Poly(C) RNA-LNP as a control. Serum was obtained just prior to the first immunization and four weeks after the first and second immunizations and stored at −80 °C.

2.3. Serum IgG ELISA and Neutralizing Antibody Titers

Purified baculovirus-derived gD2 was added to 96-well High Binding Costar microtiter plates at 100 ng/well in 50 mM sodium bicarbonate pH 8.5 binding buffer, incubated for 1 h at room temperature then overnight at 4 °C, and blocked for 2 h with 5% (wt/vol) nonfat milk in PBS 0.05% Tween 20 [14]. Serial 2-fold dilutions of serum starting at 1:1000 were added to gD2-coated wells. Bound IgG was detected at an optical density of 405 nm using horseradish peroxidase-conjugated anti-mouse IgG at a 1:2000 dilution followed by 2,2′-azino-bis-3-ethylbenzothiazoline-6-sulfonic acid (ABTS). Endpoint titers were determined by regression analysis as the serum dilution resulting in an OD reading two-fold above background.

Neutralizing titers were measured by incubating 2-fold serial dilutions of mouse sera with 5% human serum as the source of complement obtained from an HSV-1- and HSV-2 seronegative donor and 100 PFU of HSV-2 at 37 °C for 1 h. The remaining virus was determined by plaque assay on Vero cells. The neutralizing titer was defined as the highest serum dilution that reduced plaques by ≥50% [14].

2.4. Biosensor-Based Antibody Competition Assay

Antibody competition assays were performed using the Carterra Microfluidics continuous flow microspotter surface plasmon resonance imaging (CFM/SPRi, Salt Lake City, UT, USA) system [5,11,15]. Monoclonal antibodies (MAb) that recognize gD were amine-coupled to a CDM200M sensor chip (XanTec GmbH, Dusseldorf, Germany). Antibody competition assays were then performed in the surface plasmon resonance imager (IBIS MX96, Salt Lake City, UT, USA) in a pre-mix assay format by saturating soluble gD2(285t) at a concentration of 75 ng/reaction with 2% (1:50 dilution) mouse sera. Each gD2(285t)/mouse serum mix was flowed across the sensor chip spotted with the gD MAbs. gD2 alone was flowed across the chip for the first 2–3 cycles and every 10th cycle to establish the background binding of gD2 compared to gD2 plus mouse serum. Data were recorded as response units (RU). The blocking activity of mouse sera was calculated for each Mab as a percentage using the formula: [1 − (RU gD2(285t) + mouse serum)/(RU gD(285t) alone)] × 100. Occasionally, the (RU gD2(285t) + mouse serum) yielded a negative RU value that was lower than the baseline value of buffer alone, resulting in percent blocking values that exceeded 100%.

2.5. HSV-2 Vaginal Infection and Vaccine Efficacy

Mice were injected subcutaneously with 2 mg of medroxyprogesterone five days prior to infection [16]. The vagina was cleared using a sterile swab moistened with phosphate-buffered saline (PBS), and mice were infected intravaginally five weeks after the second immunization with 5×10^3 PFU (275 LD_{50}) HSV-2 strain MS. Mice were monitored for survival, weight loss, genital disease, and vaginal virus titers on days two and four post-infection, and HSV-2 DNA in dorsal root ganglia (DRG) at the time of humane euthanasia or at the end of the experiment on days 28–32 post-infection. Mice received a daily score of one each for redness/erythema, hair loss, vaginal exudate, and necrosis for a maximum daily score of four for genital disease.

2.6. Vaginal Virus Titers

Vaginal swabs were obtained on days two and four post-infection and placed in 1 mL of complete Dulbecco's modified Eagle's medium supplemented with L-glutamine, HEPES, antibiotics, and 5% fetal bovine serum. Serial 10-fold dilutions were evaluated by plaque assay on Vero cells [5].

2.7. qPCR for HSV-2 DNA Present in the DRG

DRG samples were analyzed in duplicate for HSV-2 genomic DNA [5]. Separate reactions were used to amplify HSV-2 DNA and the mouse adipsin gene. Five microliters of purified DNA (QiaCube HT, Germantown, MD, USA) were amplified via Taqman qPCR (Roche LightCycler 96, Indianapolis, IN, USA). The primers and probe used to amplify the HSV-2 Us9 gene were: Forward, GGCAGAAGCCTACTACTCGGAAAA; Reverse, CCATGCGCACGAGGAAA; and Probe, FAM-CGAGGCCGCCAAC-MGBNFQ. The primers and probe used to amplify the mouse adipsin gene were: Forward, GCAGTCGAAGGTGTGGTTACG; Reverse, GGTATAGACGCCCGGCTTTT; and Probe, FAM-CTGTGGCAATGGC-MGBNFQ. The DRG HSV-2 DNA copy number was expressed as $\log_{10}$ DNA copies per 10^5 adipsin genes. Samples with less than one copy by 40 cycles in duplicate wells were considered negative. If only one of the duplicate wells was positive, the sample was tested in triplicate. The DRG sample was considered positive for HSV-2 DNA if two or more of the triplicates were positive [4].

2.8. Statistical Analysis

Area under the curve (AUC) *p* values for weight loss and leg toxicity were calculated by the Mann–Whitney–Wilcoxon Test with Holm adjustment for multiple comparisons using R Studio Version 1.3.1056 with R software version 4.0.2 (R Core Team, 2020, DE, USA) and the trapezoid rule with function "AUC" from the package "DescTools" version 0.99.44. *p* values comparing endpoint serum IgG ELISA titers after the first and second immunization were calculated by Wilcoxon matched pairs signed rank test. The two-tailed Mann–Whitney test was used to compare gD2 IgG ELISA, neutralizing antibody titers, epitope antibody titers, day two and day four vaginal virus titers, and the HSV-2 DNA copy number in DRG. When multiple comparisons were performed, we used ordinary one-way ANOVA with Sidak's correction. The log-rank (Mantel–Cox) test was used to calculate *p* values for survival. With the exception of AUC, *p* values were calculated using GraphPad Prism version 9.2.0. Results were considered significant at $p < 0.05$.

2.9. Study Approval

The mouse studies were approved by the University of Pennsylvania Institutional Animal Care and Use Committee under protocol 805187.

3. Results

3.1. Experimental Design and Rationale

The study design can be divided into three parts. In experiment 1, we immunized mice with our gC2, gD2, and gE2 trivalent mRNA-LNP vaccine to determine the total mRNA-LNP dose per administration that is safe. These results established the upper limits for the total dose of mRNA-LNPs, however did not define the optimum dose of the individual mRNA-LNP immunogens within that total. In experiment 2, we performed immunology assays as a guide for determining the optimum dose of an individual mRNA-LNP immunogen to include in a multivalent vaccine. We used only one of the immunogens, gD2 mRNA-LNP, to test our hypothesis that measuring antibody responses to crucial, functional epitopes on an antigen adds value to more standard assays, such as serum IgG ELISA and neutralizing antibodies, to define the optimum immunogen dose. Experiment 3 involved infecting the animals to assess vaccine efficacy. The goal was to determine which of the immunology assays best predicted the immunogen dose that protected the animals. Lessons learned about the predictive value of immune responses in preclinical studies will help select immunogen doses of multivalent vaccines in human trials.

3.2. Experiment 1: Toxicity Is Dose Dependent for the Trivalent mRNA-LNP Vaccine

We evaluated vaccine toxicity in mice receiving the trivalent genital herpes vaccine that contains nucleoside-modified gC2, gD2, and gE2 mRNA packaged into LNPs at equivalent concentrations. The goal of experiment 1 was to determine the maximum tolerated dose when all three immunogens were included in the vaccine. BALB/c mice were immunized IM two times 28 days apart with 1, 3, or 10 μg of the trivalent HSV-2 mRNA-LNP vaccine or with sterile PBS as a control. Mice were evaluated after the first and second immunizations for weight loss and reduction in hind limb mobility. By comparing 10 μg of the trivalent mRNA-LNP vaccine with either PBS or the 1-μg dose, it was found that mice receiving the 10-μg dose lost more weight and developed greater loss in mobility of the immunized hind limb after both immunizations (Figure 1). Mice receiving the 3-μg dose had weight loss and decreased hind limb mobility in-between the 1-μg and 10-μg groups. We detected no differences for weight loss or hind limb mobility when comparing the 1-μg group with the PBS group or comparing the first with second immunization. Our mouse studies establish that lower doses of the trivalent mRNA vaccine are better tolerated than higher doses and support choosing the lowest vaccine dose possible that is effective. For the purposes of the current study, we established that the total dose of RNA-LNP immunogens within the vaccine should not exceed 10 μg.

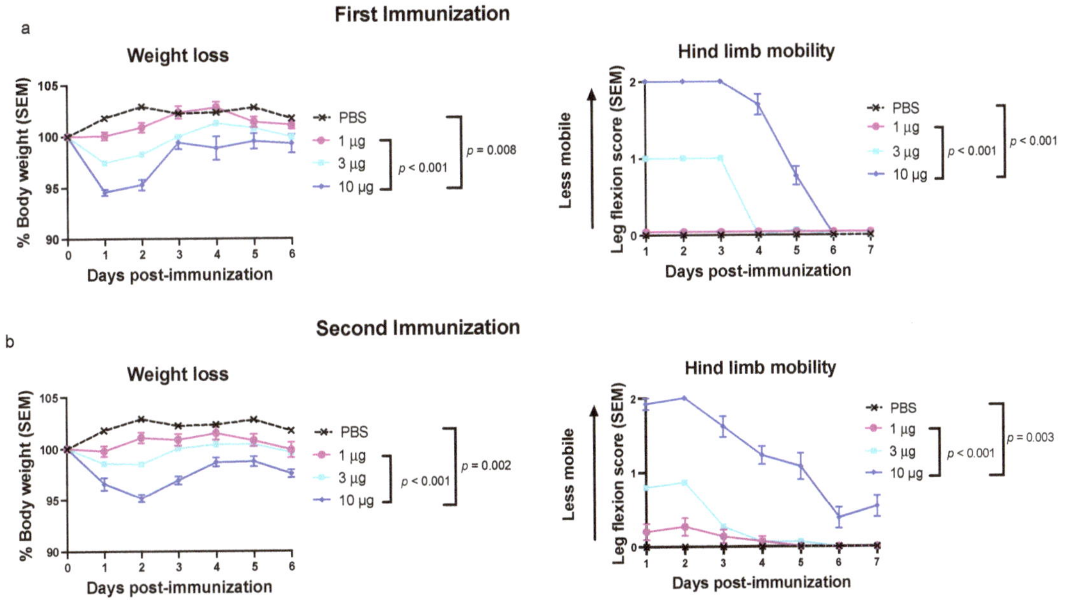

Figure 1. Trivalent mRNA-lipid nanoparticle (LNP) vaccine toxicity is dose dependent. Weight loss and hind limb mobility were assessed after (**a**) the first and (**b**) second immunization. The trivalent mRNA-LNP and phosphate-buffered saline (PBS) vaccination groups were weighed on days 1–6 post-infection and evaluated for mobility in the inoculated hind limb on days 1–7 post-immunization (weight: n = 15 animals in the 1-µg and 3-µg groups, 9 animals in the 10-µg group, and 5 animals in the PBS group; hind limb mobility: n = 15 mice in the 1-µg and 3-µg group, 13 mice in the 10-µg group, and 5 mice in the PBS group). P values were not calculated comparing 3 µg with PBS, 1 µg, or 10 µg. p values were determined by comparing area under the curve (AUC) using the Mann–Whitney–Wilcoxon test with Holm adjustment for multiple comparisons.

3.3. Experiment 2: Dose Escalation Study of gD2 mRNA to Evaluate IgG ELISA Titers, Neutralizing Antibodies, and Antibodies to Crucial gD2 Epitopes

Choosing the lowest effective vaccine dose for each immunogen in a multivalent vaccine is challenging. We established in experiment 1 that the total dose of all three mRNA immunogens should not exceed 10 µg. The issue is whether to include equal concentrations of each mRNA immunogen or increase the concentration of one or more immunogens while decreasing another will improve the outcome without changing the total mRNA-LNP content. We evaluated gD2 mRNA as one of the three immunogens in the trivalent genital herpes vaccine to determine whether measuring antibody responses to crucial gD2 epitopes in a dose escalation study provides useful information beyond that gained from serum gD2 IgG ELISA and neutralizing antibody titers to establish the dose of an immunogen to include in a vaccine [11,15,17].

3.3.1. Serum IgG ELISA Titers

We first evaluated whether gD2 IgG ELISA is helpful when assessing the number of vaccine doses to administer. Mice were immunized twice at one-month intervals with gD2 mRNA-LNP at doses ranging from 0.3 µg to 10.0 µg (33-fold range). Sera were obtained prior to immunization and four weeks after the first and second immunizations. Serum gD2 IgG ELISA titers increased significantly after the second immunization at each gD2 mRNA dose (Figure 2a). Two immunizations at the lowest dose of 0.3 µg significantly exceeded the IgG ELISA titers after a single immunization with 10-µg gD2 (Figure 2a). These results indicate that a major boost in gD2 IgG ELISA titers occurs after the second immunization and demonstrate the value of serum IgG ELISA when selecting dosing frequency.

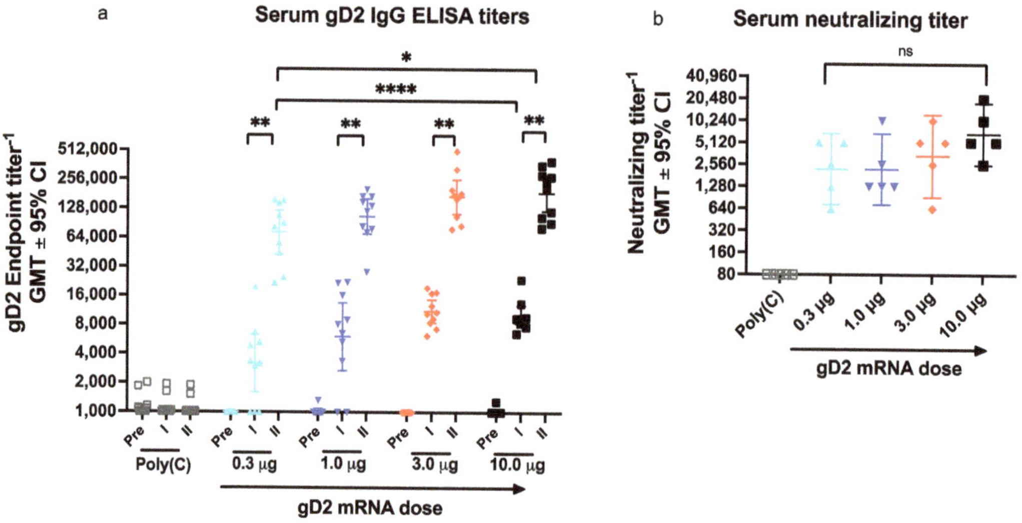

Figure 2. gD2 mRNA-LNP generates serum IgG ELISA and neutralizing antibody responses in a dose-dependent pattern. (**a**) Serum gD2 IgG ELISA titers were evaluated prior to the first immunization and four weeks after the first and second immunization (n = 10 sera/dose) (pre and prior to the first immunization; I and II, sera obtained after the first and second immunizations, respectively). (**b**) Neutralizing antibody titers were determined in the presence of complement (n = 5 sera/dose). p values comparing ELISA IgG titers after the first and second bleeds were calculated by the Wilcoxon matched pairs signed rank test. p values comparing different doses in (**a**,**b**) were calculated by the two-tailed Mann–Whitney test. p value in (**a**) comparing 10.0 µg with 0.3 µg was significantly different, however p values comparing 10.0 µg with 1.0 or 3.0 µg were not statistically different. * $p < 0.05$; ** $p < 0.01$; **** $p < 0.0001$. GMT, geometric mean titer, ns, not significant.

We next evaluated gD2 IgG ELISA titers after the second immunization to determine whether IgG ELISA is useful for selecting the optimal gD2 dose per administration of the vaccine. The serum IgG ELISA titers increased 2.4-fold when comparing 0.3 µg and 10.0 µg doses (Figure 2a). A dose-response pattern is apparent because higher gD2 doses produced higher ELISA titers, although titers changed relatively little over the 33-fold range. Based on the ELISA results, we would likely include gD2 mRNA-LNP at a dose of 3.33 µg in the trivalent vaccine, representing one-third of the maximum tolerated dose of 10 µg for all three immunogens. Our reasoning is that ELISA titers continued to rise with each higher dose, providing no clear guidance whether a dose lower than 3.33 µg would be equally efficacious.

3.3.2. Serum Neutralizing Antibody Titers

We next evaluated neutralizing antibody responses after the second immunization using five sera per group that were selected based on the volume of serum available. We previously reported that neutralizing antibodies in guinea pigs immunized with the trivalent mRNA vaccine correlated with protection against genital infection [4]. Therefore, selecting the gD2 mRNA dose that produces the highest neutralizing titers without toxicity is important for the success of the trivalent mRNA vaccine. Neutralizing antibody titers at the three highest doses followed a dose-response pattern and were highest in the 10-µg group (Figure 2b). Therefore, we would likely choose a dose of 3.33 µg for gD2 mRNA in the trivalent vaccine for similar reasons as stated for ELISA titers.

3.3.3. Antibodies to Crucial gD2 Epitopes

We used high throughput biosensor technology to define epitope-specific antibody responses to six crucial gD2 epitopes [5,11–13,15]. Antibodies that bind to these six gD2 epitopes perform one or more of the following functions: block gD2 binding to the herpesvirus entry mediator (HVEM) receptor, nectin-1 receptor, or both; block gD2 binding to the heterodimer fusion regulator, glycoproteins H/L (gH2/gL2); inhibit cell-to-cell spread; and alter the timing of important gD2 conformational changes [5,11,17].

We evaluated epitope-specific antibody responses to the six gD2 epitopes after the second immunization using five sera per gD2 dose that were selected based on the volume available. Our goal was to determine whether epitope mapping adds useful information to ELISA and neutralizing antibody titers during a phase 1-like dose escalation study to help select the optimum gD2 mRNA-LNP dose for phase 3 efficacy trials. Serum was mixed with purified gD2(285t) and then flowed sequentially over a biosensor chip spotted with multiple MAb [11,15]. Binding of gD2 to the MAb on the chip was measured for each gD2-immune serum mixture and compared to binding when gD2 was mixed with the buffer. A reduction in gD2 binding to a particular MAb when mixed with serum compared to buffer indicates competition and signifies that an antibody is present in the immune serum to an epitope recognized by the MAb on the chip.

MAbs that recognize identical or overlapping epitopes are referred to as a community of MAbs [13]. We spotted multiple MAbs from each community on the chip, and report the results of prototype MAbs for each community [11]. (1) Prototype MAb MC23 blocks gD2 binding to the nectin-1 receptor and to gH2/gL2 [11,15,17]. Titers of blocking antibodies to MC23 were highest in the 10-µg group and were significantly higher than in the 0.3-µg group that had the lowest titers (Figure 3a). (2) We next evaluated prototype MAb 77S, which recognizes an epitope that is involved with binding to HVEM and nectin-1 [11,15]. Similar to MC23, the antibody titers at 10 µg were highest and significantly greater than at 0.3 µg (Figure 3b). (3) We then assessed prototype MAb 1D3, which blocks gD2 binding to the HVEM receptor [11,15]. In contrast to the prior MAbs, the 10-µg group had lower antibody titers than at 1.0 µg, although differences did not achieve statistical significance (Figure 3c). This result suggests that at high doses, other (polyclonal) gD2 antibodies in the immune sera may alter ID3 epitope conformation or interfere with antibodies that bind to this epitope. We again detected the lowest antibody titers in the 0.3-µg group. (4) We next evaluated prototype MAbs MC2, which blocks gD2 activation thereby preventing its interaction with gH2/gL2 [17,18]. The antibody titers to the MC2 epitope followed a similar pattern as ID3 in that the 10-µg group had lower titers than the 1-µg group, suggesting possible changes to epitope conformation or interference by other antibodies in the sera (Figure 3d). (5) We then assessed prototype MAb MC5, which blocks gD2 binding to gH2/gL2 [18]. The antibody titers to MC5 plateaued at doses $\geq$ 1 µg (Figure 3e). (6) The final epitope was one that interacts with gH2/gL2 and mediates cell-to-cell spread and is recognized by prototype MAb MC14 [17,19]. As noted for several other epitopes, the 0.3-µg group had the lowest antibody titers (Figure 3f). We conclude that antibodies were produced to most epitopes at all immunization doses; that for some epitopes a high gD2 dose improved the antibody response, while for others, a high gD2 dose resulted in somewhat reduced antibody titers; and the 0.3-µg group generally produced the lowest antibody titers. No clear pattern emerged for choosing the optimal gD2 mRNA dose when analyzing antibody responses to individual epitopes.

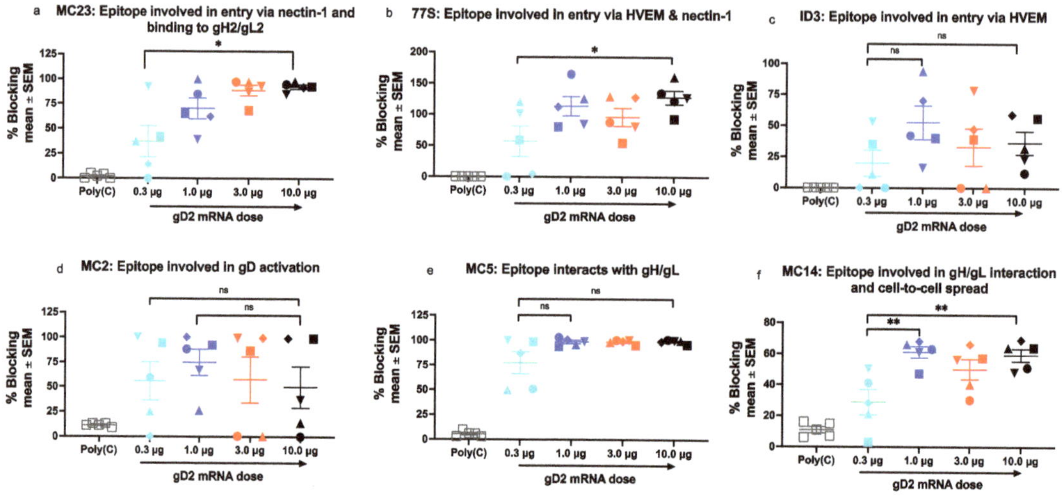

Figure 3. gD2 mRNA-LNP produces antibodies to important functional epitopes. Antibody responses were measured to six functional gD2 epitopes identified by MAb (**a**) MC23, (**b**) 77S, (**c**) ID3, (**d**) MC2, (**e**) MC5, and (**f**) MC14. Sera from five mice were evaluated per vaccine dose. The shape of the symbol identifies individual mice in the gD2 mRNA groups; for example, the animal indicated by a rectangle in (**a**) is also denoted by a rectangle in (**b**–**f**). We calculated p values comparing the highest dose (10 µg) with the lowest dose (0.3 µg), and the dose producing the highest antibody titer with the lowest antibody titer. p values were performed using the two-tailed Mann–Whitney test or ordinary one-way ANOVA with Sidak's correction when multiple comparisons were performed. * $p < 0.05$; ** $p < 0.01$; ns, not significant.

Our prior studies indicated that high titer antibody responses to multiple epitopes are required for protection against genital HSV-2 infection with no individual epitope emerging as dominant [11]. Therefore, we combined the epitope-specific antibody responses into a single graph to demonstrate the polyclonal antibody response to all six epitopes at each gD2 dose (Figure 4). Importantly, we did not observe a dose-response pattern for antibody titers to gD2 epitopes. Instead, we identified a plateau in antibody titers at gD2 doses ≥1 µg with no further increase at higher doses. The plateau at 1 µg distinguishes the epitope antibody titers from IgG ELISA and neutralizing antibody responses that failed to plateau even at 10 µg. The epitope antibody titers suggest that the 1-µg dose is as effective as the higher doses in producing high titers of antibodies to the six crucial epitopes, leaving up to 9 µg available to accommodate the remaining two mRNA immunogens, if needed. In contrast, the IgG ELISA and neutralizing antibody titers supported using 3.33 µg without signaling that lower the gD2 mRNA dose may be equally effective.

3.4. Experiment 3: Vaccine Efficacy in gD2 mRNA Immunized Mice

To evaluate vaccine efficacy, the same mice used for immunology studies in Figures 2–4 were challenged with HSV-2 at 5×10^3 PFU (275 LD_{50}) 35 days after the second immunization (10 mice/group). Nine of ten mice in the control (Poly(C) RNA) group required humane euthanasia, while all 40 gD2 mRNA-immunized animals survived, including those in the lowest dose group of 0.3 µg (Figure 5a). No animal immunized with gD2 mRNA lost weight (Figure 5b), developed genital disease (Figure 5c), or had any other sign of illness, including ruffled fur, hunched posture, abnormal gait, or lethargy.

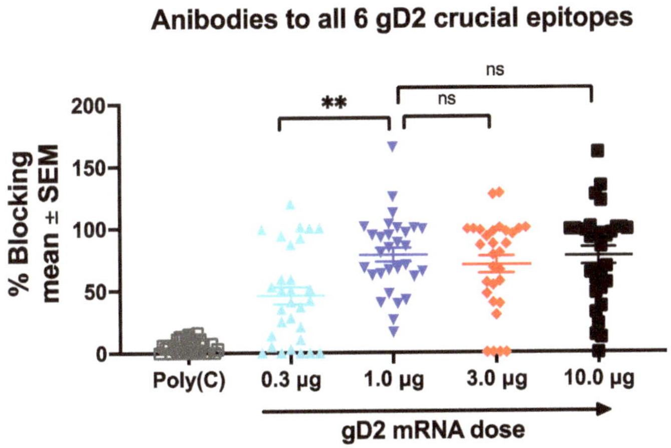

Figure 4. Combined responses to all six epitopes. The antibody titers to all six crucial gD2 epitopes at each immunization dose are displayed on a single graph. p values were calculated by ordinary one-way ANOVA with Sidak's correction for multiple comparisons; $n = 30$ data points at each gD2 dose based on antibody responses to 6 epitopes x 5 sera; ** $p < 0.01$; ns, not significant.

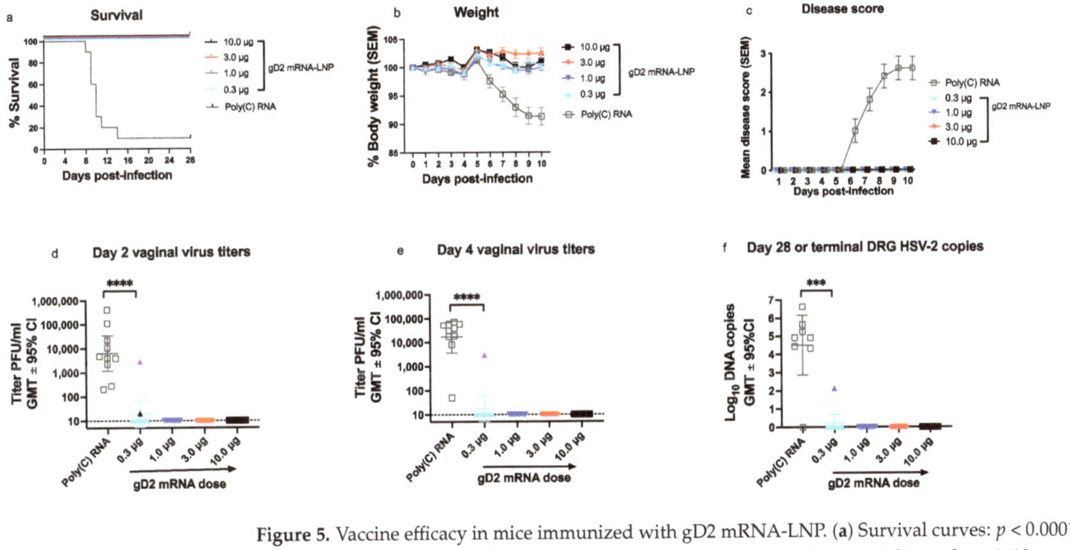

Figure 5. Vaccine efficacy in mice immunized with gD2 mRNA-LNP. (**a**) Survival curves: $p < 0.0001$ comparing the Poly(C) RNA group with all other groups. (**b**) Mean weight on days 1–10 post-infection. (**c**) Mean genital disease scores on days 1–10 post-infection. (**d**) Vaginal swab virus titers on day 2 post-infection (**e**) Vaginal swab virus titers on day 4 post-infection. The purple triangle symbol in (**d**,**e**) indicate that the vaginal virus titer is from the same animal. Dotted line in (**d**,**e**) indicates the assay limit of detection of 10 PFU/mL. (**f**) HSV-2 DNA copy number in dorsal root ganglia (DRG) at the time of euthanasia for the Poly(C) RNA group or at the end of the experiment on days 28–32 for the gD2 mRNA-LNP groups. The dark blue symbol identifies this animal as different from the positive animals in (**d**,**e**). p values in (**a**) were calculated by the log-rank (Mantel–Cox) test, and in (**d**–**f**) by the two-tailed Mann–Whitney test; $n = 10$ mice/group; ***, $p < 0.001$; ****, $p < 0.0001$.

We next evaluated mice for evidence of subclinical infection by measuring virus titers in vaginal swabs obtained on days two and four post-infection and by assaying for HSV-2 DNA copy number in DRG (site of latency) at the time of humane euthanasia or at the end of the experiment on days 28–32. All animals in the Poly(C) group had HSV-2 isolated from vaginal swabs on days two and four post-infection (Figure 5d,e). Only two of forty (5%) animals immunized with gD2 mRNA had positive vaginal virus cultures on day two and one of the same animals (2.5%) had a positive vaginal culture on day four (Figure 5d,e). Both animals with positive vaginal virus cultures were in the 0.3-μg group (Figure 5d,e). Six of seven animals in the Poly(C) group had HSV-2 DNA detected in DRG at the time of humane euthanasia 8–14 days post-infection (Figure 5f). Only one of forty (2.5%) animals immunized with gD2 mRNA was positive for HSV-2 DNA in DRG obtained at the end of the experiment (Figure 5f). This animal was different from the two that had positive vaginal virus cultures on days two or four and was also in the 0.3-μg group. Overall, three of ten (30%) mice in the 0.3-μg group had evidence of subclinical infection compared to 0/30 (0%) at higher doses ($p = 0.0121$ by two-tailed Fisher's exact test). We conclude that the gD2 mRNA-LNP vaccine provided outstanding protection against clinical disease at 1 μg; however, breakthrough subclinical infections occurred when the vaccine dose was 0.3 μg. Only the epitope-specific antibody responses offered a preview that 1 μg was likely sufficient, enabling the inclusion of higher doses of the other immunogens in the vaccine, if needed.

4. Discussion

We included equal concentrations of each mRNA in the gC2, gD2, and gE2 trivalent vaccine in our prior mRNA vaccine publications and the current study to define the maximum tolerated dose [4–7]. The vaccine efficacy could possibly be improved by using lower doses of one antigen and higher doses of another rather than equal doses of each antigen. The Merck nonavalent human papillomavirus vaccine (Gardasil® 9) is an example of a multivalent vaccine that incorporates different doses of protein antigens in the vaccine ranging from 20 μg to 60 μg [20].

We used the murine mouse model of genital herpes to determine if epitope mapping provides useful information beyond IgG ELISA and neutralizing antibody titers during the dose escalation phase of a trial to select immunogen doses for a multivalent vaccine. We evaluated serum IgG binding assays over a 33-fold range of gD2 mRNA-LNP doses. Two immunizations were more immunogenic than one, supporting the value of IgG ELISA in selecting the dosing frequency. However, IgG ELISA was less valuable for deciding the dose per administration to include in the trivalent vaccine. A plateau in ELISA titers did not occur to guide the decision. Instead, antibody titers increased at higher doses with a significantly higher gD2 IgG ELISA titers at 10 μg than at 0.3 μg. We detected a similar dose-response pattern for neutralizing antibody titers. Toxicity studies suggested a maximum tolerated dose of 10 μg for all three mRNA-LNP immunogens. The ELISA and neutralizing antibody titers provided no clues that less than one-third of that total dose was needed for gD2 mRNA-LNP.

We used high throughput biosensor technology to evaluate antibody responses to crucial gD2 epitopes. We made four important observations. First, antibody responses to crucial gD2 epitopes plateaued at doses ≥1 μg, suggesting little benefit of using higher doses, distinguishing the epitope responses from ELISA and neutralizing antibody titers. Second, antibody responses to some gD2 epitopes were lower at 10 μg than 1 μg, indicating that using too high a dose may be detrimental from both an immunology and toxicity perspective. Third, combining antibody responses to all six crucial epitopes provided a clearer cutoff for the effective gD2 mRNA dose than analyzing individual epitopes. Fourth, the antibody responses to all six epitopes matched the results of the HSV-2 challenge studies in that antibody titers were lowest in the 0.3-μg group and this was the only group with breakthrough infections, while the 1-μg dose was as protective as the 3- or 10-μg doses.

The study has certain limitations. First, the number of breakthrough infections was small, with only 3 animals developing infection. Immunizing mice with gD2 mRNA at doses lower than 0.3 μg may yield more breakthrough infections and improve our confidence in the value of epitope mapping to predict vaccine efficacy. Nevertheless, differences in breakthrough infections were statistically significant when comparing 0.3 μg with higher doses. Second, we evaluated sera for antibodies to gD2 epitopes at a single dilution of 1:50. Results may vary if sera were tested at multiple dilutions. We think this outcome is unlikely because almost all animals produced antibodies within the dynamic range of the assay, with few animals having no antibody response or producing antibody titers at the upper limit of detection.

Subsequent studies will evaluate the optimal dose of gC2 and gE2 mRNA-LNP to include in the trivalent vaccine based on the same principles explored here for gD2 mRNA-LNP. We conclude that epitope mapping adds a valuable new tool to more traditional immunology assays for deciding the dose of each mRNA immunogen to include in a multivalent vaccine during a phase 1 dose escalation study.

Author Contributions: Conceptualization, L.M.H. and H.M.F.; methodology, L.M.H., S.A., T.M.C., B.T.F., and K.P.E.; validation, L.M.H. and H.M.F.; formal analysis, L.M.H. and H.M.F.; investigation, L.M.H., S.A., T.M.C., B.T.F., and K.P.E.; resources, M.-G.A. and M.M.H.S.; data curation, L.M.H., B.T.F., K.P.E., and H.M.F.; writing—original draft preparation, L.M.H. and H.M.F.; writing—review and editing, L.M.H., G.H.C., and H.M.F.; visualization, L.M.H., K.P.E., and H.M.F.; supervision, D.W., G.H.C., and H.M.F.; project administration, D.W., G.H.C., and H.M.F.; funding acquisition, D.W., G.H.C., and H.M.F. All authors have read and agreed to the published version of the manuscript.

Funding: This research was funded by NIH NIAID grant AI139618, by the Penn Center for AIDS Research (CFAR) NIH grant P30 AI045008, and an unrestricted grant from BioNTech SE. The funders had no input or influence on the content of this manuscript.

Institutional Review Board Statement: The study was conducted according to the guidelines of the Declaration of Helsinki and approved by the Institutional Review Board of the University of Pennsylvania (protocol 805187 approved on 23 November 2021).

Data Availability Statement: All the data is available within the manuscript figures and text.

Acknowledgments: We thank Grace Choi and Alisa Stephens-Shields from the Department of Biostatistics, Epidemiology, and Informatics from the Perelman School of Medicine for their helpful discussions on biostatistical analyses.

Conflicts of Interest: In accordance with the University of Pennsylvania policies and procedures and our ethical obligations as researchers, we report that H.M.F., S.A., and G.H.C. are named on patents that describe the use of multiple subunit glycoprotein antigens for HSV vaccines. H.M.F., S.A., and D.W. are named on a patent claim that uses nucleoside-modified mRNA as a vaccine for HSV. D.W. is named on patents that describe the use of nucleoside-modified mRNA as a platform to deliver therapeutic proteins. D.W. is named on a patent describing the use of nucleoside-modified mRNA in LNP as a vaccine platform. We have disclosed those interests fully to the University of Pennsylvania, and we have in place an approved plan for managing any potential conflicts arising from licensing of our patents. M.M.H.S. is an employee of Acuitas Therapeutics, a company developing LNP for delivery of nucleic acid-based drugs. L.M.H., T.M.C., M-G.A., B.T.F., and K.P.E. declare no conflicts of interest. The funders had no role in the design of the study; in the collection, analyses, or interpretation of data; in the writing of the manuscript, or in the decision to publish the results.

References

1. Thompson, M.G.; Burgess, J.L.; Naleway, A.L.; Tyner, H.; Yoon, S.K.; Meece, J.; Olsho, L.E.W.; Caban-Martinez, A.J.; Fowlkes, A.L.; Lutrick, K.; et al. Prevention and Attenuation of Covid-19 with the BNT162b2 and mRNA-1273 Vaccines. *N. Engl. J. Med.* **2021**, *385*, 320–329. [CrossRef] [PubMed]
2. Feldman, R.A.; Fuhr, R.; Smolenov, I.; Ribeiro, A.; Panther, L.; Watson, M.; Senn, J.J.; Smith, M.; Almarsson, Ö.; Pujar, H.S.; et al. mRNA Vaccines against H10N8 and H7N9 Influenza Viruses of Pandemic Potential Are Immunogenic and Well Tolerated in Healthy Adults in Phase 1 Randomized Clinical Trials. *Vaccine* **2019**, *37*, 3326–3334. [CrossRef] [PubMed]
3. Alberer, M.; Gnad-Vogt, U.; Hong, H.S.; Mehr, K.T.; Backert, L.; Finak, G.; Gottardo, R.; Bica, M.A.; Garofano, A.; Koch, S.D.; et al. Safety Immunogenicity of a mRNA Rabies Vaccine in Healthy Adults: An Open-Label, Non-Randomised, Prospective, First-in-Human Phase 1 Clinical Trial. *Lancet* **2017**, *390*, 1511–1520. [CrossRef]
4. Awasthi, S.; Knox, J.J.; Desmond, A.; Alameh, M.G.; Gaudette, B.T.; Lubinski, J.M.; Naughton, A.; Hook, L.M.; Egan, K.P.; Tam, Y.K.; et al. Trivalent Nucleoside-Modified mRNA Vaccine Yields Durable Memory B Cell Protection against Genital Herpes in Preclinical Models. *J. Clin. Investig.* **2021**, *131*, e152310. [CrossRef] [PubMed]

5. Awasthi, S.; Hook, L.M.; Pardi, N.; Wang, F.; Myles, A.; Cancro, M.P.; Cohen, G.H.; Weissman, D.; Friedman, H.M. Nucleoside-Modified mRNA Encoding HSV-2 Glycoproteins C, D, and E Prevents Clinical and Subclinical Genital Herpes. *Sci. Immunol.* **2019**, *4*, eaaw7083. [CrossRef] [PubMed]
6. Egan, K.P.; Hook, L.M.; Naughton, A.; Pardi, N.; Awasthi, S.; Cohen, G.H.; Weissman, D.; Friedman, H.M. An HSV-2 Nucleoside-Modified mRNA Genital Herpes Vaccine Containing Glycoproteins gC, gD, and gE Protects Mice against HSV-1 Genital Lesions and Latent Infection. *PLoS Pathog.* **2020**, *16*, e1008795. [CrossRef] [PubMed]
7. LaTourette, P.C., 2nd; Awasthi, S.; Desmond, A.; Pardi, N.; Cohen, G.H.; Weissman, D.; Friedman, H.M. Protection against Herpes Simplex Virus Type 2 Infection in a Neonatal Murine Model Using a Trivalent Nucleoside-Modified mRNA in Lipid Nanoparticle Vaccine. *Vaccine* **2020**, *38*, 7409–7413. [CrossRef] [PubMed]
8. Jackson, L.A.; Anderson, E.J.; Rouphael, N.G.; Roberts, P.C.; Makhene, M.; Coler, R.N.; McCullough, M.P.; Chappell, J.D.; Denison, M.R.; Stevens, L.J.; et al. An mRNA Vaccine against SARS-CoV-2—Preliminary Report. *N. Engl. J. Med.* **2020**, *383*, 1920–1931. [CrossRef] [PubMed]
9. Mulligan, M.J.; Lyke, K.E.; Kitchin, N.; Absalon, J.; Gurtman, A.; Lockhart, S.; Neuzil, K.; Raabe, V.; Bailey, R.; Swanson, K.A.; et al. Phase I/II Study of COVID-19 RNA Vaccine BNT162b1 in Adults. *Nature* **2020**, *586*, 589–593. [CrossRef] [PubMed]
10. Ndeupen, S.; Qin, Z.; Jacobsen, S.; Estanbouli, H.; Bouteau, A.; Igyártó, B.Z. The mRNA-LNP Platform's Lipid Nanoparticle Component Used in Preclinical Vaccine Studies Is Highly Inflammatory. *Iscience* **2021**, *24*, 103479. [CrossRef] [PubMed]
11. Hook, L.M.; Cairns, T.M.; Awasthi, S.; Brooks, B.D.; Ditto, N.T.; Eisenberg, R.J.; Cohen, G.H.; Friedman, H.M. Vaccine-Induced Antibodies to Herpes Simplex Virus Glycoprotein D Epitopes Involved in Virus Entry and Cell-to-Cell Spread Correlate with Protection against Genital Disease in Guinea Pigs. *PLoS Pathog* **2018**, *14*, e1007095. [CrossRef] [PubMed]
12. Awasthi, S.; Hook, L.M.; Swaminathan, G.; Cairns, T.M.; Brooks, B.; Smith, J.S.; Ditto, N.T.; Gindy, M.E.; Bett, A.J.; Espeseth, A.S.; et al. Antibody Responses to Crucial Functional Epitopes as a Novel Approach to Assess Immunogenicity of Vaccine Adjuvants. *Vaccine* **2019**, *37*, 3770–3778. [CrossRef] [PubMed]
13. Whitbeck, J.C.; Huang, Z.Y.; Cairns, T.M.; Gallagher, J.R.; Lou, H.; Ponce-de-Leon, M.; Belshe, R.B.; Eisenberg, R.J.; Cohen, G.H. Repertoire of Epitopes Recognized by Serum IgG from Humans Vaccinated with Herpes Simplex Virus 2 Glycoprotein D. *J. Virol.* **2014**, *88*, 7786–7795. [CrossRef] [PubMed]
14. Awasthi, S.; Hook, L.M.; Shaw, C.E.; Friedman, H.M. A Trivalent Subunit Antigen Glycoprotein Vaccine as Immunotherapy for Genital Herpes in the Guinea Pig Genital Infection Model. *Hum. Vaccines Immunother.* **2017**, *13*, 2785–2793. [CrossRef] [PubMed]
15. Cairns, T.M.; Ditto, N.T.; Lou, H.; Brooks, B.D.; Atanasiu, D.; Eisenberg, R.J.; Cohen, G.H. Global Sensing of the Antigenic Structure of Herpes Simplex Virus gD Using High-Throughput Array-Based SPR Imaging. *PLoS Pathog* **2017**, *13*, e1006430. [CrossRef] [PubMed]
16. Kaushic, C.; Ashkar, A.A.; Reid, L.A.; Rosenthal, K.L. Progesterone Increases Susceptibility and Decreases Immune Responses to Genital Herpes Infection. *J. Virol.* **2003**, *77*, 4558–4565. [CrossRef] [PubMed]
17. Cairns, T.M.; Ditto, N.T.; Atanasiu, D.; Lou, H.; Brooks, B.D.; Saw, W.T.; Eisenberg, R.J.; Cohen, G.H. Surface Plasmon Resonance (SPR) Reveals Direct Binding of HSV Glycoproteins gH/gL to gD and Locates a gH/gL Binding Site on gD. *J. Virol.* **2019**, *93*, e00289-19. [CrossRef] [PubMed]
18. Atanasiu, D.; Saw, W.T.; Cairns, T.M.; Eisenberg, R.J.; Cohen, G.H. Using Split Luciferase Assay and Anti-HSV Glycoprotein Monoclonal Antibodies to Predict a Functional Binding Site between gD and gH/gL. *J. Virol.* **2021**, *95*, e00053-21. [CrossRef] [PubMed]
19. Lazear, E.; Whitbeck, J.C.; Ponce-de-Leon, M.; Cairns, T.M.; Willis, S.H.; Zuo, Y.; Krummenacher, C.; Cohen, G.H.; Eisenberg, R.J. Antibody-Induced Conformational Changes in Herpes Simplex Virus Glycoprotein gD Reveal New Targets for Virus Neutralization. *J. Virol.* **2012**, *86*, 1563–1576. [CrossRef] [PubMed]
20. Toh, Z.Q.; Kosasih, J.; Russell, F.M.; Garland, S.M.; Mulholland, E.K.; Licciardi, P.V. Recombinant Human Papillomavirus Nonavalent Vaccine in the Prevention of Cancers Caused by Human Papillomavirus. *Infect. Drug Resist.* **2019**, *12*, 1951–1967. [CrossRef] [PubMed]

viruses MDPI

Review

Rational Design of Live-Attenuated Vaccines against Herpes Simplex Viruses

Brent A. Stanfield [1], Konstantin G. Kousoulas [2,3,*], Agustin Fernandez [3] and Edward Gershburg [3,*]

1 Department of Pathobiological Sciences, School of Veterinary Medicine, Louisiana State University, Baton Rouge, LA 70803, USA; bstanf5@lsu.edu
2 Division of Biotechnology and Molecular Medicine, Louisiana State University, Baton Rouge, LA 70803, USA
3 Rational Vaccines Inc., Woburn, MA 01801, USA; af3@rationalvaccines.com
* Correspondence: vtgusk@lsu.edu (K.G.K.); ed.gershburg@rationalvaccines.com (E.G.)

Abstract: Diseases caused by human herpes simplex virus types 1 and 2 (HSV-1 and HSV-2) affect millions of people worldwide and range from fatal encephalitis in neonates and herpes keratitis to orofacial and genital herpes, among other manifestations. The viruses can be shed efficiently by asymptomatic carriers, causing increased rates of infection. Viral transmission occurs through direct contact of mucosal surfaces followed by initial replication of the incoming virus in skin tissues. Subsequently, the viruses infect sensory neurons in the trigeminal and lumbosacral dorsal root ganglia, where they are primarily maintained in a transcriptionally repressed state termed "latency", which persists for the lifetime of the host. HSV DNA has also been detected in other sympathetic ganglia. Periodically, latent viruses can reactivate, causing ulcerative and often painful lesions primarily at the site of primary infection and proximal sites. In the United States, recurrent genital herpes alone accounts for more than a billion dollars in direct medical costs per year, while there are much higher costs associated with the socio-economic aspects of diseased patients, such as loss of productivity due to mental anguish. Currently, there are no effective FDA-approved vaccines for either prophylactic or therapeutic treatment of human herpes simplex infections, while several recent clinical trials have failed to achieve their endpoint goals. Historically, live-attenuated vaccines have successfully combated viral diseases, including polio, influenza, measles, and smallpox. Vaccines aimed to protect against the devastation of smallpox led to the most significant achievement in medical history: the eradication of human disease by vaccination. Recently, novel approaches toward developing safe and effective live-attenuated vaccines have demonstrated high efficacy in various preclinical models of herpetic disease. This next generation of live-attenuated vaccines has been tailored to minimize vaccine-associated side effects and promote effective and long-lasting immune responses. The ultimate goal is to prevent or reduce primary infections (prophylactic vaccines) or reduce the frequency and severity of disease associated with reactivation events (therapeutic vaccines). These vaccines' "rational" design is based on our current understanding of the immunopathogenesis of herpesviral infections that guide the development of vaccines that generate robust and protective immune responses. This review covers recent advances in the development of herpes simplex vaccines and the current state of ongoing clinical trials in pursuit of an effective vaccine against herpes simplex virus infections and associated diseases.

Keywords: herpes simplex virus; herpesviruses; live-attenuated vaccines; vaccines

Citation: Stanfield, B.A.; Kousoulas, K.G.; Fernandez, A.; Gershburg, E. Rational Design of Live-Attenuated Vaccines against Herpes Simplex Viruses. *Viruses* **2021**, *13*, 1637. https://doi.org/10.3390/v13081637

Academic Editor: Barry J. Margulies

Received: 3 July 2021
Accepted: 13 August 2021
Published: 18 August 2021

1. Introduction

Human herpes simplex virus type 1 (HSV-1) and type 2 (HSV-2) are highly infectious and successful human pathogens. HSV-1 is estimated to infect 3.7 billion people worldwide, with transmission primarily occurring via the oral-to-oral route [1–3]. HSV-2 is estimated to infect half a billion people globally, and in the United States, these numbers are predicted to grow by >600,000 new infections per year until 2050 [1]. Infection with either HSV-1 or HSV-2 initially leads to an acute phase of infection in the host's mucosal epithelium. Productive replication of HSV-1 or HSV-2 in these tissues results in immunopathogenesis, observed as cold sores, blisters, and genital lesions. HSV-1 and HSV-2 infections are generally identified as oral/ocular (HSV-1) and genital (HSV-2) infections. However, HSV-1 causes an increasing proportion of new infections in genital tissues [4–6]. Changing sexual practices and the emergence of mutations affecting viral tropism may increase the prevalence of HSV-1 genital infections. A characteristic of all human alphaherpesviruses is their ability to infect and reside in the long-lived sensory neurons of the host's peripheral nervous system in a transcriptionally repressed state termed "latency" [7]. Epidemiological models predict that a prophylactic vaccine with a modest 50% efficacy can reduce the number of new infections by 58%, incidence by 60%, and seroprevalence by 21%, reducing the yearly rate of infection by 350,000 new cases per year by 2050 [8]. On a population scale, therapeutic vaccination is predicted to reduce new infections by 12%, incidence by 13%, and seroprevalence by 4%, and the number of new infections by 76,000 per year by 2050 [8]. Therapeutic vaccination to reduce or eliminate oral and genital herpes recurrence has long been a highly needed but elusive goal in herpes simplex vaccine development.

Recent advances in our understanding of effective anti-herpes immune responses have led to the development of many novel vaccine approaches [9]. Several academic laboratories and commercial entities are currently working toward developing a safe and effective herpes simplex vaccine in preclinical animal models (Table 1) and human trials (Table 2). In this section, we discuss recent developments in the preclinical pursuit of a safe and effective herpes simplex vaccine and review promising subunit/peptide, vectored/DNA/RNA, and live-attenuated vaccine technologies.

Table 1. Current herpes simplex vaccines under preclinical development.

Type of Vaccine	Description	Adjuvant	Type of Study	Animal Model	Route of Challenge	Results	Year	Refs.
Vectored/ DNA/RNA	Polyvalent HSV-2 glycoprotein DNA vaccine (gB2, gC2, gD2, gE2, gH2, gL2, and gI2)	DNA encoding IL-12	P	Mouse (Balb/c)	Genital HSV-2	DNA vaccines targeting optimal combinations of surface glycoproteins provide better protection than gD alone and similar survival benefits and disease symptom reductions compared with a potent live-attenuated HSV-2 0ΔNLS vaccine. However, mice vaccinated with HSV-2 0ΔNLS clear the virus much faster.	2017	[10]
Vectored/ DNA/RNA	Nucleoside-modified mRNA encoding HSV-2 gC2, gD2, and gE2	Lipid nanoparticle (LNP)	P	Mouse (Balb/c) and guinea pig (Hartley)	Genital HSV-2	The trivalent mRNA vaccine outperformed trivalent subunit-based vaccines, reducing latent viral load, shedding infectious virus, and PCR positive vaginal swabs.	2019	[11]
Vectored/ DNA/RNA	Modified vaccinia virus Ankara (MVA) expressing HSV-2 gD2	NA	Vector Stability	NA	NA	Serial passage of recombinant vaccinia vectors led to the loss of transgene expression	2020	[12]
Subunit	Asymptomatic CD8+ T cell peptide epitopes (UL44 aa400–408, UL9 aa196–204, and UL25 aa572–580)	CpG (Prime) followed by AAV8 vectored CXCL10 (Pull)	P	HLA transgenic rabbits	Ocular HSV-1	Prime/pull was effective at drawing HSV-1-specific CD8+ T cells to the cornea and trigeminal ganglia, reducing disease.	2018	[13]

Table 1. *Cont.*

Type of Vaccine	Description	Adjuvant	Type of Study	Animal Model	Route of Challenge	Results	Year	Refs.
Subunit	Bivalent HSV-2 Subunit (gD2 and gB2)	Nanoemulsion adjuvant NE01	P/T	Guinea pig (Hartley)	Genital HSV-2	Intranasal (IN) vaccination significantly reduced acute and recurrent disease scores and latent viral load compared to a placebo. Therapeutically, IN vaccination reduced recurrent lesion sores, days with the disease, animals shedding virus, and virus-positive vaginal swabs.	2019	[14]
Subunit	Trivalent HSV-2 subunit vaccine (gC2, gD2, and gE2)	CpG (5′-TCCATGAC GTTCCTG ACGTT-3′)/Alum	P	Neonatal Mouse (C57BL/6)	Intranasal (HSV-1/HSV-2)	Maternal vaccination protected offspring against neonatal disseminated disease and mortality from HSV-1 and HSV-2.	2020	[15]
Live-Attenuated	Replication-Competent Controlled HSV-1 Vectors (HSV-GS3 and HSV-GS7)	NA	P	Mouse (Swiss Webster)	Rear Footpad HSV-1	Inactivated HSV-1 vectors offered equivalent protection to inactivated vaccines. Activation of these controlled vaccines increased vaccine efficacy over inactivated vaccines.	2018	[16]
Live-Attenuated	Replication-defective HSV-2 dl5-29 (Lacking UL5 and UL29)	NA	P	Mouse (C57BL/6) and Neonatal Mouse (C57BL/6)	Adult Ocular (Corneal HSV-1 infection), Neonatal Mouse (Intranasal HSV-1 Infection)	Maternal vaccination led to the transfer of HSV-specific antibodies into neonatal circulation that protected against neonatal neurological disease and death.	2019	[17]
Live-Attenuated	HSV-1 0ΔNLS	NA	P	Mouse (C57BL/6)	Ocular HSV-1	Sterile immunity to ocular HSV-1 challenge with reduced infection of the nervous system. Vaccination preserved cornea free of pathology and complete preservation of visual acuity.	2019	[18]
Live-Attenuated	The non-neuroinvasive VC2 HSV-1 vaccine (Deletion of gK aa31-68 and UL20 aa4-22)	NA	P	Guinea pig (Hartley)	Genital HSV-2	The live-attenuated VC2 vaccine outperformed the gD2 subunit vaccine in the durability of vaccine-induced protection 6 months post-vaccination.	2019	[19]
Live-Attenuated	R2 non-neuroinvasive HSV-1 vaccine (HSV1-GS6264, 5 missense mutations in UL37)	NA	P	Guinea pig (Hartley)	Genital HSV-2	The live-attenuated prophylactic HSV vaccine, R2, was effective in the guinea pig model of genital HSV-2, especially when administered by the ID route.	2020	[20]
Live-Attenuated		NA	P	Mouse (Balb/c)	Ocular HSV-1	VC2 vaccination in mice produced superior protection and morbidity control compared to its parental strain HSV-1 (F).	2020	[21]

Abbreviations: P—Prophylactic, T—Therapeutic.

Table 2. Recent/current/pending clinical trials of herpes simplex vaccines.

Sponsor	Intervention	Summary	Status	ClinicalTrials.gov Identifier
Sanofi Pasteur	SP0148 (also known as ACAM 529 or HSV 529), a defective replication HSV-2 with deletions in UL5 and UL29	Estimated enrollment of 381 HSV-2 seropositive patients	Active, not recruiting; Phase 1/2	NCT04222985
Genocea Biosciences	GEN-003 is a subunit vaccine comprising HSV-2 glycoprotein D2 ($gD2\Delta TMR_{340-363}$) and infected cell polypeptide 4 ($ICP4_{383-766}$) adjuvanted with proprietary Matrix-M2	Genocea Biosciences, Inc. announced that they entered into a material transfer agreement and exclusive license option with Shionogi & Co., Ltd.	Terminated; Phase 2	NCT03146403
Vical	VCL-HB01 Plasmid-based vaccine encoding two HSV-2 proteins and VCL-HM01 Plasmid-based vaccine encoding one HSV-2 protein, both adjuvanted with Vaxfectin	VCL-HB01 was ineffective in reducing outbreaks in people who were infected with HSV-2	Completed; Phase 2	NCT02837575
Agenus	HerpV polyvalent peptide complex adjuvanted with QS-21	Stopped after Phase 2	Completed; Phase 2	NCT01687595
X-Vax Technology	HSV-2 ΔgD-2	Preparing for a Phase 1 clinical study	Preclinical	NA
UPenn in collaboration with BioNTech	HSV-2 mRNA vaccine coding gC2, gD2, and gE2	Preparing for a Phase 1 clinical study	Preclinical	NA
Rational Vaccines	RVx201 (derivative of HSV-2 0ΔNLS)	Preparing for a Phase 1 clinical study	Preclinical	NA
Rational Vaccines	RVx1001 (HSV-1 VC2)	Preparing for a Phase 1 clinical study	Preclinical	NA

1.1. Subunit/Peptide Vaccines

Subunit/peptide vaccines are desirable for vaccine development because they are reasonably stable, safe, and potentially effective. However, subunit-based vaccines against HSV-1 or HSV-2 have fallen short of meeting clinical endpoint criteria. Targeting the major entry mediators of the virus (gB/gD), which are major antigenic determinants, is a primary focus of subunit vaccine development as these immunogens stimulate highly effective neutralizing antibodies [22,23]. Additionally, gE has been utilized in subunit vaccines to target cell-to-cell spread and immune evasion to increase multivalent subunit vaccine efficacy [24,25]. Recently, the field of herpes vaccinology has expanded its focus by using subunit vaccines to include multiple herpes antigens and peptides. Khan et al. demonstrated the efficacy of vaccinating humanized rabbits with HSV-1-derived peptides identified in asymptomatic HSV-1^{+} individuals, followed by chemotactically pulling immune cells into the cornea. This immunization approach protected animals from an ocular challenge [13] (Table 1). The limited antigenic breadth of CD8^{+} T cell peptide epitopes (UL44 aa400–408, UL9 aa196–204, and UL25 aa572–580) reduced vaccine efficacy [13]. However, this "prime/pull" vaccination strategy is an innovative approach to vaccine administration and shows therapeutic efficacy in the most stringent animal models of the HSV-2 disease [26].

Antigenic breadth is of utmost importance when considering effective strategies for herpes vaccines. Previous estimates concluded that herpes simplex encodes 80 open reading frames (ORFs). More recently, with advances in multiomic technologies, it was discovered that HSV-1 encodes 284 ORFs, including 46 novel large ORFs, the functions of which are yet to be elucidated [27]. Considerable effort has been devoted to enhancing vaccine efficacy by increasing the number of antigens included in formulations. For instance, a bivalent HSV-2 subunit (gD2 and gB2) vaccine delivered by intranasal (IN) immunization elicited increased neutralizing antibody titers compared to a monovalent gD2 vaccine delivered IN. However, it was less effective than gD2-alone delivered intramuscularly. The bivalent gD2/gB2 vaccine reduced acute and recurrent disease scores and latent viral load compared to placebo. Therapeutically, IN vaccination reduced recurrent lesion sores, days with the disease, animals shedding virus, and virus-positive vaginal swabs [14].

Significant morbidity and mortality are associated with neonatal herpes simplex infections. Children that survive neonatal HSV infection may develop lifelong developmental and behavioral disorders. Vaccination of pregnant mice with a trivalent herpes simplex vaccine (gD2, gE2, and gC2) protected mice and offspring against lethal challenge with virulent HSV-1 and HSV-2 strains. Importantly, neonatal mice were protected from developing long-term behavioral morbidity [15]. These results suggest that an effective vaccination strategy can successfully combat neonatal infections.

1.2. Vectored/DNA/RNA Vaccines

Messenger RNA (mRNA)-based vaccines are promising technologies, which have been rapidly and successfully deployed against SARS-CoV-2, the causative agent of COVID-19. Moderna and Pfizer (in collaboration with BioNTech) have successfully launched two synthetic mRNA vaccines expressing the viral spike (S) glycoprotein. Both vaccines have been extensively used to vaccinate many people and proven to be safe and efficacious against SARS-CoV-2 infections, even conferring significant protection against variants that increase the rate of transmission [28,29]. With the demonstrated efficacy of mRNA vaccines under emergency use authorization, many novel mRNA-based vaccines are being pursued for other infectious disease pathogens, including herpesviruses. Specifically, Awashi et al. [11] demonstrated a trivalent, nucleoside-modified mRNA vaccine's efficacy in preventing clinical and subclinical genital HSV-2 disease in both mouse and guinea pig models of genital HSV-2 infection. Vaccination prevented the formation of genital lesions following guinea pigs and mice challenged with HSV-2. Additionally, two doses at 10 μg of the trivalent mRNA vaccine outperformed the three doses at 5 μg each of the trivalent subunit vaccine. The mRNA vaccination scheme stimulated superior systemic and vaginal HSV-2 specific IgG, neutralizing antibodies, and gD2 specific antibodies. This mRNA vaccine demonstrated superior immunogenicity, as evidenced by the stimulation of long-lived $CD4^+$ T cells, T follicular helper cells, and germinal center B cell responses. This trivalent mRNA vaccine is a promising candidate for future clinical trials in humans [11].

DNA has been proposed to be a valuable tool in the development of an effective HSV vaccine. It can be rapidly synthesized, purified, and is more stable than mRNA. Bagley et al. demonstrated that a DNA vaccine expressing a pool of HSV-2 glycoproteins (gB2, gC2, gD2, gE2, gH2, gL2, and gI2) adjuvanted with IL-12 outperformed the gD2 subunit vaccine but was not as effective in reducing virus shedding compared with the HSV-2 0ΔNLS live-attenuated vaccine. Thus, despite including seven prominent HSV-2 antigens, this DNA vaccine was not as effective as the live-attenuated vaccine. This work highlights the importance of antigenic breadth in vaccine efficacy against genital HSV-2 infection, which can only be reproduced effectively through an active infection with a live-attenuated virus [10]. To this end, live-attenuated vaccines have repeatedly demonstrated superior efficacy.

Vectored vaccines are becoming increasingly prevalent. Many of the vaccines deployed to combat the SARS-CoV-2 pandemic are replication-defective adenovirus vector vaccines expressing the SARS-CoV-2 spike (S) glycoprotein. These vaccines have demonstrated efficacy in preventing disease. Recently, safety concerns have stemmed from rare cardiac thrombotic and cardiomyopathy incidences of unexplained origin, which may be due to the vehicle carrier, and potential inflammatory properties of mRNA and the adenovirus vectors used to express the S glycoprotein. Vaccine stability is always a primary concern. Synthetic mRNA technology utilizes modified RNA nucleotides that may produce unwanted side effects and require very low temperatures to sustain vaccine stability. Adenovirus-based vaccines are much more stable than mRNA vaccines and do not require ultra-low temperatures for stability. Vaccinia (poxvirus)-based vaccines are extensively used due to their demonstrated efficacy in combating the smallpox epidemic. More recently, vaccinia vectors have been developed with improved safety profiles to be avirulent and induce high levels of transgene expression in the modified vaccinia virus Ankara (MVA) background. The MVA vector technology has demonstrated efficacy against HIV, influenza, parainfluenza, measles, flavivirus, and even malaria [30]. Atukorale et al. developed a vaccinia virus vectored HSV-2 vaccine expressing gD2 [12]. However, the transgene was lost following the vaccine's serial passage, pointing to potential vaccine stability issues. The authors also demonstrated that the transgene insertion site could dictate vector stability with a prolonged serial passage in cells, indicating that vaccinia vectors can be a viable platform for sound engineering.

1.3. Live-Attenuated Vaccines

Live-attenuated vaccines have been the most effective vaccines to combat human and animal viral infections in medical history. The repertoire of these successes includes the eradication of smallpox, poliomyelitis, measles, mumps, rubella, rotavirus, and others (reviewed in: [31]). A live-attenuated varicella-zoster virus (VZV) (human herpesvirus 3 (HHV-3) or chickenpox virus) vaccine is widely used worldwide and shown to be highly efficacious in controlling viral reactivation. Live varicella vaccine is generally safe and well-tolerated [32]. The success of the alphaherpesvirus VZV live-attenuated vaccines provides a primary example suggesting that a similar approach may be efficacious in combating herpes simplex infections which, like VZV, establish latency in neurons. In addition, the only FDA-approved oncolytic virotherapy on the market is a live-attenuated herpes simplex virus (TVEC or Imlygic) approved for the treatment of human melanoma. This virus was designed as an oncolytic and immunotherapeutic virus that augments anti-tumor immunological responses. Imlygic is a replication-competent HSV-1 mutant strain, with the deletion of both γ34.5 and ICP47 genes. These deletions limit virus replication in cancer cells and eliminate the inhibition of antigen presentation by the ICP47 gene. Additionally, the virus expresses human GM-CSF, which stimulates the recruitment of antigen presenting cells providing enhanced immunogenicity [33].

The generation of a safe and effective herpes simplex vaccine must focus on preparing attenuated viruses that can generate robust immune responses. HSV-1 and HSV-2 share ~83% of nucleotide identity, and cross-protective immunity may be achieved due to the extensive repertoire of cross-protective antigens [34]. To this end, novel live-attenuated vaccine strategies are being implemented to tame the virus in vivo. The replication-competent HSV-1 vectors (HSV-GS3 and HSV-GS7) demonstrated prophylactic efficacy in a mouse model of dermal HSV-1 infection. These vectors are controlled by placing one or two essential genes under the stringent control of a gene switch coactivated by heat and antiprogestin. In the absence of these activating factors, the controlled HSV-1 vectors do not replicate. In this study, the unactivated HSV-1 vectors offer equivalent protection to chemically inactivated vaccines. However, the activation of these controlled HSV-1 vectors increases vaccine efficacy over inactivated vaccines [16].

Recently the use of live-attenuated HSV-1 vaccines has demonstrated robust protection against ocular HSV-1 disease. More specifically, the HSV-1 0ΔNLS lacking a nuclear localization signal of the viral ubiquitin ligase ICP0, and the non-neurotrophic HSV-1 vaccine vector VC-2 with deletions in the amino terminus of both the gK and UL20 genes demonstrated effective protection against ocular HSV-1 challenge. Mice vaccinated with HSV-1 0ΔNLS showed superior protection against early viral replication, neuroinvasion, latency, and mortality than gD-2-vaccinated or naive mice following ocular challenge with a neurovirulent clinical isolate of HSV-1. Moreover, 0ΔNLS-vaccinated mice exhibited protection against ocular immunopathology and maintained corneal mechanosensory function. Vaccinated mice also showed suppressed T cell activation in the draining lymph nodes following the challenge. Vaccine efficacy correlated with serum neutralizing antibody titers.

Humoral immunity was identified as a significant correlate of protection against corneal neovascularization, HSV-1 shedding, and latency through passive immunization [35,36].

Interestingly, vaccination with the VC-2 vaccine protected mice from developing any appreciable ocular pathology, while vaccination with the attenuated parental HSV-1 (F) strain only offered partial protection. The corneas of VC-2 immunized mice demonstrated a significantly increased infiltration of T cells and limited infiltration of $Iba1^+$ macrophages compared to unvaccinated or parental HSV-1 (F) strain vaccinated groups. Animals vaccinated with VC-2 produced higher neutralizing antibody titers than the parental HSV-1 (F) strain post-challenge. Vaccination with VC-2 significantly increased the CD4 T central memory (TCM) subsets and CD8 T effector memory (TEM) T cell subsets in the draining lymph nodes following the ocular HSV-1 (McKrae) challenge, than unvaccinated mice or mice vaccinated with parental HSV-1 (F) strain, indicating that VC-2′s immunogenicity is superior to wild-type HSV-1 vaccination [21].

Neurotropism is the main hallmark of alphaherpesviruses and a major challenge in designing live-attenuated viruses that ideally should not establish latency in neurons. Recent attempts to inhibit virus entry into neuronal axons have yielded several novel live-attenuated HSV-1 vectors. The HSV-1 R2 live-attenuated vaccine has five missense mutations in the UL37 gene. UL37 has been shown to play a conserved role in alphaherpesvirus neurotropism by facilitating retrograde virion transport upon infection of neuronal axons [37]. The mutations in the R2 live-attenuated vaccine disrupt neuronal retrograde transport rendering the virus unable to establish latent infection in the nucleus of the neuronal cell body. In the guinea pig model of genital HSV-2 disease, intradermal (ID) vaccination with the R2 vaccine demonstrated superior performance to intramuscular (IM) vaccination with the gD2 monovalent subunit vaccine. Similarly, ID vaccination with R2 induced higher neutralizing antibody titers than IM vaccination with the gD2 subunit vaccine alone [20]. In comparison, the non-neuroinvasive HSV-1 VC2 vaccine demonstrated superior protection to the gD2 subunit vaccine while generating long-lasting efficacy up to 6 months post-vaccination in a guinea pig model of genital HSV-2 infection [19,38].

2. Rational Design of the VC-2 Vaccine

2.1. The Structure and Function of Glycoprotein K and the Membrane Protein UL20

Glycoprotein K (gK) is a highly hydrophobic glycoprotein having four transmembrane domains placing both amino and carboxy termini extracellularly. Glycoprotein K (gK) is required for efficient virus envelopment and functions as a heterodimer with the membrane protein UL20 [39,40]. The majority of mutations that cause enhanced virus-induced cell fusion are found within gK mediated primarily by interactions between gK and the amino terminus of gB [41–44]. Together gK and UL20 are highly conserved among neurotrophic alphaherpesviruses indicating highly conserved functions within this virus family [45–47]. Additionally, the amino terminus of gK is required for the interaction between gB and the cellular protein Akt. Upon binding to gB, Akt is phosphorylated and induces calcium release from the cell [48].

2.2. Herpes Simplex Virus Mechanism of Entry—Rational Design of the VC2 Live-Attenuated Vaccine

HSV is known to enter into cells by two mechanisms: fusion (between the viral envelope and the cellular plasma membrane) and endocytosis. Fusion requires the formation of a multiprotein complex including gB, gD, gH/gL, and their cellular receptors. This complex is known as the "core fusion machinery" and is essential for HSV entry into cells [49–52]. Membrane fusion is initiated upon gD binding to one of its cellular receptors (HVEM, Nectin-1, Nectin-2), which induces a conformational change in gD and activates gH/gL to act upon gB changing from its prefusion conformation to its postfusion conformation. These conformational changes induce fusion between the viral envelope and the host cell membrane by releasing the viral contents into the cell's cytoplasm [53].

In some cases, HSV will enter by endocytosis, resulting in a double-membraned virion in the cytoplasm. Escape from endocytic vesicles is pH-dependent; however, release from the endocytic vesicle ultimately requires fusion of the viral envelope with the membrane of the endocytic vesicle [54]. It has been proposed that the switch between endocytosis and direct fusion occurs upon gB binding to the cell surface receptor PILRα [55]. Specifically, this mechanistic switch is known to occur via interactions between gB and gK. HSV-1 lacking the amino terminus of gK (AA31-68) can no longer enter into PILRα cells, indicating gK mediates this phenotype [56]. However, entry into the axons of sensory neurons is strictly dependent on the direct fusion between the viral envelope and axonal cellular membranes [57]. Disruption of the ability of gK to induce gB-mediated membrane fusion restricts HSV-1 to replication in epithelial cells allowing for the presentation of all viral antigens. At the same time, the virus cannot establish latency in neurons. Interestingly, viral entry through endocytosis by the HSV-1 (VC-2) vaccine strain upregulated type I interferon responses and the induction of certain chemokines such as CXCL4 and TNF, which may result in the observed increased immunogenicity of VC2 compared to its parental wild-type virus HSV-1(F) (Clark and Kousoulas, unpublished).

3. Rational Design of the HSV-2 0ΔNLS Vaccine

3.1. The HSV ICP0 Protein

ICP0 is a ~775 amino acid polyfunctional protein, an E3 ubiquitin ligase bearing a RING-finger domain. The mature length of the ICP0 polypeptide may vary, depending on the HSV isolate. ICP0 is known to play a key role in activating HSV-1 gene expression, the disruption of ND10 structures, degrade cellular proteins via polyubiquitination, and evasion of the host cell's antiviral defenses [58]. Initially identified as a viral factor for viral replication in vitro, the ICP0-null virus demonstrated a significant growth defect, especially at low multiplicities of infection [59–63]. Subsequent in vivo experiments demonstrated the requirements of ICP0 for productive replication and reactivation from latent infection [64–67]. ICP0 is capable of transactivating promoters involved in all three phases of lytic transcriptional activation (α, β, and γ genes) [68–71]. Recent publications have identified ICP0 as a critical mediator of host cell chromatin architecture via the targeted degradation of the cellular epigenetic machinery. Specifically, ICP0 targets Schlafen 5 (SLFN5) for proteasomal degradation via ubiquitination of SLFN5. Infection with virus lacking ICP0 (HSV-1ΔICP0) SLFN5 binds to viral DNA to repress transcription via limiting RNA polymerase II access to immediate-early viral promoters [72]. Similarly, TRIM22 has been identified as an intrinsic host cell factor limiting HSV replication via the viral genome's heterochromatinization. ICP0 has been shown to disrupt this intrinsic defense in a mechanism independent of ICP0's ubiquitin ligase activity [73]. Additionally, ICP0 interacts with promyelocytic leukemia protein (PML) and facilitate its SUMO-independent degradation as a viral countermeasure to circumvent PML-mediated antiviral restrictions [74].

3.2. The Role of ICP0 Protein in Immune Evasion

Host cell recognition of cytosolic viral DNA is crucial for early antiviral defenses. Several cytosolic DNA sensors serve as pattern recognition receptors (PRRs) in the host cell defense against HSV infection. Interferon Gamma Inducible Protein 16 (IFI16) binds double-stranded DNA and is a member of the PYHIN family of proteins. IFI16 is primarily localized to the nucleus but shuttles between the nucleus and cytoplasm via acetylation by the histone acetyltransferase p300. Upon infection with HSV-1, IFI16 recognizes viral DNA in the nucleus and is rapidly acetylated for distribution to the cytoplasm, where it activates interferon production to restrict viral replication [75,76]. IFI16 is targeted by ICP0 for ubiquitination and degradation by the cellular proteasome [77–79]. Similarly, ICP0 has been shown to target IRF7 to limit antiviral interferon production [80].

The nuclear factor kappa-light-chain-enhancer of activated B cells (NF-κB) plays an essential role in regulating inflammation. ICP0 has been shown to suppress TNF-α mediated NF-κB activation via interaction with the p65 and p50 NF-κB subunits. ICP0 inhibits p65 nuclear translocation following TNF-α stimulation. ICP0 also actively targets the p50 NF-κB subunit for proteolytic degradation due to its E3 ubiquitin ligase activity. This ability to inhibit NF-kB activity is dependent on the RING-finger domain (RFD) of ICP0, and the RFD alone was sufficient to inhibit NF-κB activity in reporter assays [81].

HSV ICP0 is reported to alter the adaptive immune response to HSV infection significantly. A proposed mechanism for this property is ICP0's ability to inhibit CD83 expression in HSV-infected dendritic cells. This phenotype is mediated by the ICP0 RFD and is dependent on the proteolytic degradation of CD83 [82]. Also, ICP0 inhibits important components of the antigen presentation pathway in sentinel cells, which are responsible for activating the adaptive arm of the immune system. Virus lacking ICP0 is more immunogenic, increasing the breadth of antigen recognition by antibodies from immunized animals and generating superior protection compared with the gD2 subunit vaccine in mice and guinea pig models of genital HSV-2 disease [83–85].

Recently, it was reported that HSV-1 DNA activates the host cell DNA damage response (DDR) kinase pathways. Specifically, in cells infected with ICP0-null HSV-1, components of the host cell DDR facilitated viral replication (ATM and p53) or restricted viral replication (Mre11). However, ICP0 expression ablated these DDR effects, indicating ICP0 plays an important role in the viral evasion of host cell DDR [86]. Apparently, deletion of ICP0 unlocked the immune response to HSV infection, leading to greater antigen presentation and altering the inflammatory response to HSV infection. The polyfunctionality of the ICP0 protein establishes it an ideal target for vaccine and vector attenuation.

4. Clinical Trials of Herpes Simplex Vaccines

The only ongoing clinical trial evaluating the safety and efficacy of an HSV-2 vaccine is the Sanofi-Pasteur SP0148 vaccine (Table 2). The primary endpoints of this clinical trial include: (1) Evaluation of the safety profile of different investigational vaccine regimens against HSV-2; (2) evaluation of the relative efficacy of investigational vaccine regimens concerning the frequency of HSV shedding by PCR to detect viral DNA in the genital area (shedding rate) following the two-dose vaccine schedule; (3) determining the proportion of participants free of HSV genital recurrence at 6 months after the two-dose vaccine schedule. The secondary objectives of this study include: (1) Evaluating the impact of each investigational vaccine regimen in terms of the total number of days with genital lesions up to 6 months after the second vaccination, and number of recurrences 60 days after the second vaccination compared to the placebo group; (2) describing the efficacy of each investigational vaccine regimen concerning the frequency of HSV DNA detection in the genital area (shedding rate) 60 days following the first vaccination visit plus 60 days following the second vaccination visit compared to the placebo group; (3) describing the efficacy of the investigational vaccine regimens with respect to HSV DNA detection in the genital area (shedding rate) 60 days after the first vaccination visit compared to the placebo group.

Despite the historical failure to deliver an FDA-approved successful vaccine strategy by existing vaccine approaches, much knowledge has accumulated from past and ongoing studies regarding immunological features required for successfully confronting herpes simplex infections. Several novel vaccine approaches are in late-stage preclinical development, moving toward phase 1 trials in the coming years (Table 2). These approaches will likely demonstrate varied efficacy in clinical trials; although, they have demonstrated high efficacy in preclinical animal models. It is important to note that there were reports that an exacerbated CD8+T cell response through repeated reactivation may increase the rate of reactivation [87]. Therefore, an effective vaccine approach is required to protect without exacerbating the reactivation of the latent virus, suggesting that both inflammatory and immune-regulatory pathways and cellular milieus must be considered.

5. Conclusions

Live-attenuated, highly safe viruses generate a robust immune response, such as HSV-1 (VC2) and HSV-2 0ΔNLS, provide a promising approach as both prophylactic and therapeutic vaccines against HSV-1 and HSV-2 infections. Forthcoming phase I and II clinical trials are needed to provide necessary human data showing that these vaccines are well-tolerated while generating effective and broadly therapeutic immune responses. Mutating highly conserved genes within the herpes virus, used to circumvent the host's innate and adaptive immune responses, represents a novel strategy in the rational development of live-attenuated herpes vaccines. The HSV-2 0ΔNLS and VC2 vaccines represent two examples of this rational design approach. Importantly, these viruses can also be efficiently used as vectors for producing vaccines against other human pathogens due to their ability to express multiple genes as insertions into their genomes without appreciably affecting their viral infectivity.

Author Contributions: Conceptualization, B.A.S., K.G.K., E.G.; writing—original draft preparation, B.A.S., K.G.K.; writing—review and editing, K.G.K., A.F., E.G.; supervision—K.G.K., E.G.; funding acquisition—A.F. All authors have read and agreed to the published version of the manuscript.

Funding: This research received no external funding.

Institutional Review Board Statement: Not applicable.

Informed Consent Statement: Not applicable.

Data Availability Statement: Not applicable.

Conflicts of Interest: E.G. and K.G.K. are Rational Vaccines (RVx) employees and A.F. is a founder. RVx has licensed intellectual property rights to the VC2 and HSV-2 0ΔNLS vaccines and develops them for commercial use. B.A.S received consulting fees from RVx. These declared competing interests did not affect our adherence to MDPI policies.

References

1. James, C.; Harfouche, M.; Welton, N.; Turner, K.M.; Abu-Raddad, L.J.; Gottlieb, S.L.; Looker, K.J. Herpes simplex virus: Global infection prevalence and incidence estimates, 2016. *Bull. World Health Organ.* **2020**, *98*, 315–329. [CrossRef] [PubMed]
2. Looker, K.J.; Magaret, A.S.; May, M.T.; Turner, K.M.E.; Vickerman, P.; Gottlieb, S.L.; Newman, L.M. Global and Regional Estimates of Prevalent and Incident Herpes Simplex Virus Type 1 Infections in 2012. *PLoS ONE* **2015**, *10*, e0140765. [CrossRef]
3. Looker, K.J.; Magaret, A.S.; Turner, K.M.; Vickerman, P.; Gottlieb, S.L.; Newman, L.M. Global estimates of prevalent and incident herpes simplex virus type 2 infections in 2012. *PLoS ONE* **2015**, *10*, e114989. [CrossRef]
4. Durukan, D.; Fairley, C.K.; Bradshaw, C.S.; Read, T.R.H.; Druce, J.; Catton, M.; Caly, L.; Chow, E.P.F. Increasing proportion of herpes simplex virus type 1 among women and men diagnosed with first-episode anogenital herpes: A retrospective observational study over 14 years in Melbourne, Australia. *Sex. Transm. Infect.* **2018**, *95*, 307–313. [CrossRef]
5. Magdaleno-Tapial, J.; Hernández-Bel, P.; Valenzuela-Oñate, C.; Ortiz-Salvador, J.; García-Legaz-Martínez, M.; Martínez-Domenech, Á.; Pérez-Pastor, G.; Esteve-Martínez, A.; Zaragoza-Ninet, V.; Sánchez-Carazo, J.; et al. Genital Infection With Herpes Simplex Virus Type 1 and Type 2 in Valencia, Spain: A Retrospective Observational Study. *Actas Dermosifiliogr.* **2019**, *111*, 53–58. [CrossRef]
6. Spicknall, I.H.; Flagg, E.W.; Torrone, E.A. Estimates of the Prevalence and Incidence of Genital Herpes, United States, 2018. *Sex. Transm. Dis.* **2021**, *48*, 260–265. [CrossRef]
7. Stanfield, B.; Kousoulas, K.G. Herpes Simplex Vaccines: Prospects of Live-Attenuated HSV Vaccines to Combat Genital and Ocular Infections. *Curr. Clin. Microbiol. Rep.* **2015**, *2*, 125–136. [CrossRef]
8. Ayoub, H.H.; Chemaitelly, H.; Abu-Raddad, L.J. Epidemiological Impact of Novel Preventive and Therapeutic HSV-2 Vaccination in the United States: Mathematical Modeling Analyses. *Vaccines* **2020**, *8*, 366. [CrossRef] [PubMed]
9. Aschner, C.B.; Herold, B.C. Alphaherpesvirus Vaccines. *Curr. Issues Mol. Biol.* **2021**, *41*, 469–508. [CrossRef] [PubMed]
10. Bagley, K.C.; Schwartz, J.A.; Andersen, H.; Eldridge, J.H.; Xu, R.; Ota-Setlik, A.; Geltz, J.J.; Halford, W.P.; Fouts, T.R. An Interleukin 12 Adjuvanted Herpes Simplex Virus 2 DNA Vaccine Is More Protective Than a Glycoprotein D Subunit Vaccine in a High-Dose Murine Challenge Model. *Viral Immunol.* **2017**, *30*, 178–195. [CrossRef]
11. Awasthi, S.; Hook, L.M.; Pardi, N.; Wang, F.; Myles, A.; Cancro, M.P.; Cohen, G.H.; Weissman, D.; Friedman, H.M. Nucleoside-modified mRNA encoding HSV-2 glycoproteins C, D, and E prevents clinical and subclinical genital herpes. *Sci. Immunol.* **2019**, *4*, eaaw7083. [CrossRef]
12. Atukorale, V.N.; Weir, J.P.; Meseda, C.A. Stability of the HSV-2 US-6 Gene in the del II, del III, CP77, and I8R-G1L Sites in Modified Vaccinia Virus Ankara After Serial Passage of Recombinant Vectors in Cells. *Vaccines* **2020**, *8*, 137. [CrossRef] [PubMed]

13. Khan, A.A.; Srivastava, R.; Vahed, H.; Roy, S.; Walia, S.S.; Kim, G.J.; Fouladi, M.A.; Yamada, T.; Ly, V.T.; Lam, C.; et al. Human Asymptomatic Epitope Peptide/CXCL10-Based Prime/Pull Vaccine Induces Herpes Simplex Virus-Specific Gamma Interferon-Positive CD107 + CD8 + T Cells That Infiltrate the Corneas and Trigeminal Ganglia of Humanized HLA Transgenic Rabbits and Protect against Ocular Herpes Challenge. *J. Virol.* **2018**, *92*, e00535-18. [CrossRef] [PubMed]
14. Bernstein, D.I.; Cardin, R.D.; Bravo, F.J.; Hamouda, T.; Pullum, D.A.; Cohen, G.; Bitko, V.; Fattom, A. Intranasal nanoemulsion-adjuvanted HSV-2 subunit vaccine is effective as a prophylactic and therapeutic vaccine using the guinea pig model of genital herpes. *Vaccine* **2019**, *37*, 6470–6477. [CrossRef] [PubMed]
15. Patel, C.; Taylor, S.A.; Mehrbach, J.; Awasthi, S.; Friedman, H.M.; Leib, D.A. Trivalent Glycoprotein Subunit Vaccine Prevents Neonatal Herpes Simplex Virus Mortality and Morbidity. *J. Virol.* **2020**, *94*, e02163-19. [CrossRef] [PubMed]
16. Bloom, D.C.; Tran, R.K.; Feller, J.; Voellmy, R. Immunization by Replication-Competent Controlled Herpesvirus Vectors. *J. Virol.* **2018**, *92*, e00616-18. [CrossRef] [PubMed]
17. Patel, C.D.; Backes, I.M.; Taylor, S.A.; Jiang, Y.; Marchant, A.; Pesola, J.M.; Coen, D.M.; Knipe, D.M.; Ackerman, M.E.; Leib, D.A. Maternal immunization confers protection against neonatal herpes simplex mortality and behavioral morbidity. *Sci. Transl. Med.* **2019**, *11*, eaau6039. [CrossRef] [PubMed]
18. Royer, D.J.; Hendrix, J.F.; Larabee, C.M.; Reagan, A.M.; Sjoelund, V.H.; Robertson, D.M.; Carr, D.J.J. Vaccine-induced antibodies target sequestered viral antigens to prevent ocular HSV-1 pathogenesis, preserve vision, and preempt productive neuronal infection. *Mucosal Immunol.* **2019**, *12*, 827–839. [CrossRef]
19. Bernstein, D.I.; Cardin, R.D.; Pullum, D.A.; Bravo, F.J.; Kousoulas, K.G.; Dixon, D.A. Duration of protection from live attenuated vs. sub unit HSV-2 vaccines in the guinea pig model of genital herpes: Reassessing efficacy using endpoints from clinical trials. *PLoS ONE* **2019**, *14*, e0213401. [CrossRef]
20. Bernstein, D.I.; Cardin, R.D.; Smith, G.A.; Pickard, G.E.; Sollars, P.J.; Dixon, D.A.; Pasula, R.; Bravo, F.J. The R2 non-neuroinvasive HSV-1 vaccine affords protection from genital HSV-2 infections in a guinea pig model. *Npj Vaccines* **2020**, *5*, 104. [CrossRef]
21. Naidu, S.K.; Nabi, R.; Cheemarla, N.; Stanfield, B.; Rider, P.J.; Jambunathan, N.; Chouljenko, V.N.; Carter, R.; Del Piero, F.; Langohr, I.; et al. Intramuscular vaccination of mice with the human herpes simplex virus type-1(HSV-1) VC2 vaccine, but not its parental strain HSV-1(F) confers full protection against lethal ocular HSV-1 (McKrae) pathogenesis. *PLoS ONE* **2020**, *15*, e0228252. [CrossRef]
22. Straus, S.E.; Wald, A.; Kost, R.G.; McKenzie, R.; Langenberg, A.G.M.; Hohman, P.; Lekstrom, J.; Cox, E.; Nakamura, M.; Sekulovich, R.; et al. Immunotherapy of Recurrent Genital Herpes with Recombinant Herpes Simplex Virus Type 2 Glycoproteins D and B: Results of a Placebo-Controlled Vaccine Trial. *J. Infect. Dis.* **1997**, *176*, 1129–1134. [CrossRef]
23. Corey, L.; Langenberg, A.G.; Ashley, R.; Sekulovich, R.E.; Izu, A.E.; Douglas, J.M., Jr.; Handsfield, H.H.; Warren, T.; Marr, L.; Tyring, S.; et al. Recombinant glycoprotein vaccine for the prevention of genital HSV-2 infection: Two randomized controlled trials. Chiron HSV Vaccine Study Group. *JAMA* **1999**, *282*, 331–340. [CrossRef]
24. Polcicova, K.; Goldsmith, K.; Rainish, B.L.; Wisner, T.W.; Johnson, D.C. The Extracellular Domain of Herpes Simplex Virus gE Is Indispensable for Efficient Cell-to-Cell Spread: Evidence for gE/gI Receptors. *J. Virol.* **2005**, *79*, 11990–12001. [CrossRef] [PubMed]
25. Awasthi, S.; Huang, J.; Shaw, C.; Friedman, H.M. Blocking Herpes Simplex Virus 2 Glycoprotein E Immune Evasion as an Approach To Enhance Efficacy of a Trivalent Subunit Antigen Vaccine for Genital Herpes. *J. Virol.* **2014**, *88*, 8421–8432. [CrossRef] [PubMed]
26. Bernstein, D.I.; Cardin, R.D.; Bravo, F.J.; Awasthi, S.; Lu, P.; Pullum, D.A.; Dixon, D.A.; Iwasaki, A.; Friedman, H.M. Successful application of prime and pull strategy for a therapeutic HSV vaccine. *Npj Vaccines* **2019**, *4*, 33. [CrossRef] [PubMed]
27. Whisnant, A.W.; Jürges, C.S.; Hennig, T.; Wyler, E.; Prusty, B.; Rutkowski, A.J.; L'Hernault, A.; Djakovic, L.; Göbel, M.; Döring, K.; et al. Integrative functional genomics decodes herpes simplex virus 1. *Nat. Commun.* **2020**, *11*, 2038. [CrossRef] [PubMed]
28. Vitiello, A.; Ferrara, F. Brief review of the mRNA vaccines COVID-19. *Inflammopharmacology* **2021**, *29*, 645–649. [CrossRef]
29. Welsh, J. Coronavirus Variants-Will New mRNA Vaccines Meet the Challenge? *Engineering (Beijing)* **2021**, *7*, 712–714. [CrossRef] [PubMed]
30. Sutter, G.; Staib, C. Vaccinia vectors as candidate vaccines: The development of modified vaccinia virus Ankara for antigen delivery. *Curr. Drug Targets Infect Disord.* **2003**, *3*, 263–271. [CrossRef]
31. Minor, P.D. Live attenuated vaccines: Historical successes and current challenges. *Virology* **2015**, *479–480*, 379–392. [CrossRef] [PubMed]
32. Gabutti, G.; Bolognesi, N.; Sandri, F.; Florescu, C.; Stefanati, A. Varicella zoster virus vaccines: An update. *ImmunoTargets Ther.* **2019**, *8*, 15–28. [CrossRef] [PubMed]
33. Glorioso, J.C.; Cohen, J.B.; Goins, W.F.; Hall, B.; Jackson, J.W.; Kohanbash, G.; Amankulor, N.; Kaur, B.; Caligiuri, M.A.; Chiocca, E.A.; et al. *Oncolytic HSV Vectors and Anti-Tumor Immunity*; Caister Academic Press: Poole, UK, 2020. [CrossRef]
34. Dolan, A.; Jamieson, F.E.; Cunningham, C.; Barnett, B.C.; McGeoch, D.J. The genome sequence of herpes simplex virus type 2. *J. Virol.* **1998**, *72*, 2010–2021. [CrossRef] [PubMed]
35. Carr, D.J.J.; Berube, A.N.; Filiberti, A.; Gmyrek, G.B. Lack of neonatal Fc receptor does not diminish the efficacy of the HSV-1 0DeltaNLS vaccine against ocular HSV-1 challenge. *Vaccine* **2021**, *39*, 2526–2536. [CrossRef]
36. Carr, D.J.J.; Gmyrek, G.B.; Filiberti, A.; Berube, A.N.; Browne, W.P.; Gudgel, B.M.; Sjoelund, V.H. Distinguishing Features of High- and Low-Dose Vaccine against Ocular HSV-1 Infection Correlates with Recognition of Specific HSV-1–Encoded Proteins. *ImmunoHorizons* **2020**, *4*, 608–626. [CrossRef]

37. Richards, A.L.; Sollars, P.J.; Pitts, J.D.; Stults, A.M.; Heldwein, E.E.; Pickard, G.E.; Smith, G.A. The pUL37 tegument protein guides alpha-herpesvirus retrograde axonal transport to promote neuroinvasion. *PLOS Pathog.* **2017**, *13*, e1006741. [CrossRef]
38. Bernstein, D.I.; Pullum, D.A.; Cardin, R.D.; Bravo, F.J.; Dixon, D.A.; Kousoulas, K.G. The HSV-1 live attenuated VC2 vaccine provides protection against HSV-2 genital infection in the guinea pig model of genital herpes. *Vaccine* **2018**, *37*, 61–68. [CrossRef]
39. Foster, T.P.; Chouljenko, V.N.; Kousoulas, K.G. Functional and Physical Interactions of the Herpes Simplex Virus Type 1 UL20 Membrane Protein with Glycoprotein K. *J. Virol.* **2008**, *82*, 6310–6323. [CrossRef]
40. Foster, T.P.; Melancon, J.M.; Baines, J.D.; Kousoulas, K.G. The Herpes Simplex Virus Type 1 UL20 Protein Modulates Membrane Fusion Events during Cytoplasmic Virion Morphogenesis and Virus-Induced Cell Fusion. *J. Virol.* **2004**, *78*, 5347–5357. [CrossRef]
41. Chouljenko, V.N.; Iyer, A.V.; Chowdhury, S.; Chouljenko, D.V.; Kousoulas, K.G. The amino terminus of herpes simplex virus type 1 glycoprotein K (gK) modulates gB-mediated virus-induced cell fusion and virion egress. *J. Virol.* **2009**, *83*, 12301–12313. [CrossRef]
42. Chouljenko, V.N.; Iyer, A.V.; Chowdhury, S.; Kim, J.; Kousoulas, K.G. The Herpes Simplex Virus Type 1 UL20 Protein and the Amino Terminus of Glycoprotein K (gK) Physically Interact with gB. *J. Virol.* **2010**, *84*, 8596–8606. [CrossRef]
43. Hutchinson, L.; Goldsmith, K.; Snoddy, D.; Ghosh, H.; Graham, F.L.; Johnson, D.C. Identification and characterization of a novel herpes simplex virus glycoprotein, gK, involved in cell fusion. *J. Virol.* **1992**, *66*, 5603–5609. [CrossRef]
44. Melancon, J.M.; Luna, R.E.; Foster, T.P.; Kousoulas, K.G. Herpes Simplex Virus Type 1 gK Is Required for gB-Mediated Virus-Induced Cell Fusion, While neither gB and gK nor gB and UL20p Function Redundantly in Virion De-Envelopment. *J. Virol.* **2005**, *79*, 299–313. [CrossRef]
45. Jambunathan, N.; Charles, A.S.; Subramanian, R.; Saied, A.A.; Naderi, M.; Rider, P.; Brylinski, M.; Chouljenko, V.N.; Kousoulas, K.G. Deletion of a Predicted beta-Sheet Domain within the Amino Terminus of Herpes Simplex Virus Glycoprotein K Conserved among Alphaherpesviruses Prevents Virus Entry into Neuronal Axons. *J. Virol.* **2015**, *90*, 2230–2239. [CrossRef] [PubMed]
46. Rider, P.J.F.; Coghill, L.M.; Naderi, M.; Brown, J.M.; Brylinski, M.; Kousoulas, K.G. Identification and Visualization of Functionally Important Domains and Residues in Herpes Simplex Virus Glycoprotein K(gK) Using a Combination of Phylogenetics and Protein Modeling. *Sci. Rep.* **2019**, *9*, 14625. [CrossRef] [PubMed]
47. Rider, P.J.F.; Naderi, M.; Bergeron, S.; Chouljenko, V.N.; Brylinski, M.; Kousoulas, K.G. Cysteines and N-Glycosylation Sites Conserved among All Alphaherpesviruses Regulate Membrane Fusion in Herpes Simplex Virus 1 Infection. *J. Virol.* **2017**, *91*, e00873-17. [CrossRef] [PubMed]
48. Musarrat, F.; Jambunathan, N.; Rider, P.J.F.; Chouljenko, V.N.; Kousoulas, K.G. The Amino Terminus of Herpes Simplex Virus 1 Glycoprotein K (gK) Is Required for gB Binding to Akt, Release of Intracellular Calcium, and Fusion of the Viral Envelope with Plasma Membranes. *J. Virol.* **2018**, *92*, e01842-17. [CrossRef]
49. Eisenberg, R.J.; Atanasiu, D.; Cairns, T.M.; Gallagher, J.R.; Krummenacher, C.; Cohen, G.H. Herpes Virus Fusion and Entry: A Story with Many Characters. *Viruses* **2012**, *4*, 800–832. [CrossRef] [PubMed]
50. Fontana, J.; Atanasiu, D.; Saw, W.T.; Gallagher, J.R.; Cox, R.G.; Whitbeck, J.C.; Brown, L.M.; Eisenberg, R.J.; Cohen, G.H. The Fusion Loops of the Initial Prefusion Conformation of Herpes Simplex Virus 1 Fusion Protein Point Toward the Membrane. *mBio* **2017**, *8*, e01268-17. [CrossRef]
51. Sathiyamoorthy, K.; Chen, J.; Longnecker, R.; Jardetzky, T.S. The COMPLEXity in herpesvirus entry. *Curr. Opin. Virol.* **2017**, *24*, 97–104. [CrossRef]
52. Weed, D.; Nicola, A.V. Herpes simplex virus Membrane Fusion. *Adv. Anat. Embryol. Cell Biol.* **2017**, *223*, 29–47. [CrossRef]
53. Gianni, T.; Salvioli, S.; Chesnokova, L.S.; Hutt-Fletcher, L.M.; Campadelli-Fiume, G. alphavbeta6- and alphavbeta8-integrins serve as interchangeable receptors for HSV gH/gL to promote endocytosis and activation of membrane fusion. *PLoS Pathog.* **2013**, *9*, e1003806. [CrossRef]
54. Nicola, A.V. Herpesvirus Entry into Host Cells Mediated by Endosomal Low pH. *Traffic* **2016**, *17*, 965–975. [CrossRef]
55. Arii, J.; Kawaguchi, Y. The Role of HSV Glycoproteins in Mediating Cell Entry. *Adv. Exp. Med. Biol.* **2018**, *1045*, 3–21. [CrossRef] [PubMed]
56. Chowdhury, S.; Chouljenko, V.N.; Naderi, M.; Kousoulas, K.G. The Amino Terminus of Herpes Simplex Virus 1 Glycoprotein K Is Required for Virion Entry via the Paired Immunoglobulin-Like Type-2 Receptor Alpha. *J. Virol.* **2013**, *87*, 3305–3313. [CrossRef] [PubMed]
57. Madavaraju, K.; Koganti, R.; Volety, I.; Yadavalli, T.; Shukla, D. Herpes Simplex Virus Cell Entry Mechanisms: An Update. *Front. Cell. Infect. Microbiol.* **2021**, *10*, 852. [CrossRef]
58. Smith, M.; Boutell, C.; Davido, D.J. HSV-1 ICP0: Paving the way for viral replication. *Future Virol.* **2011**, *6*, 421–429. [CrossRef] [PubMed]
59. Cai, W.; Schaffer, P.A. Herpes simplex virus type 1 ICP0 regulates expression of immediate-early, early, and late genes in productively infected cells. *J. Virol.* **1992**, *66*, 2904–2915. [CrossRef] [PubMed]
60. Cai, W.Z.; Schaffer, P.A. Herpes simplex virus type 1 ICP0 plays a critical role in the de novo synthesis of infectious virus following transfection of viral DNA. *J. Virol.* **1989**, *63*, 4579–4589. [CrossRef]
61. Everett, R.D.; Rizzo, W.B.; Schulman, J.D.; Mukherjee, A.B. Construction and Characterization of Herpes Simplex Virus Type 1 Mutants with Defined Lesions in Immediate Early Gene 1. *J. Gen. Virol.* **1989**, *70*, 1185–1202. [CrossRef]
62. Sacks, W.R.; Schaffer, P.A. Deletion mutants in the gene encoding the herpes simplex virus type 1 immediate-early protein ICP0 exhibit impaired growth in cell culture. *J. Virol.* **1987**, *61*, 829–839. [CrossRef] [PubMed]

63. Stow, N.D.; Stow, E.C. Isolation and Characterization of a Herpes Simplex Virus Type 1 Mutant Containing a Deletion within the Gene Encoding the Immediate Early Polypeptide Vmw110. *J. Gen. Virol.* **1986**, *67*, 2571–2585. [CrossRef] [PubMed]
64. Cai, W.; Astor, T.L.; Liptak, L.M.; Cho, C.; Coen, D.M.; Schaffer, P.A. The herpes simplex virus type 1 regulatory protein ICP0 enhances virus replication during acute infection and reactivation from latency. *J Virol.* **1993**, *67*, 7501–7512. [CrossRef] [PubMed]
65. Halford, W.P.; Schaffer, P.A. Optimized Viral Dose and Transient Immunosuppression Enable Herpes Simplex Virus ICP0-Null Mutants To Establish Wild-Type Levels of Latency In Vivo. *J. Virol.* **2000**, *74*, 5957–5967. [CrossRef]
66. Halford, W.P.; Schaffer, P.A. ICP0 Is Required for Efficient Reactivation of Herpes Simplex Virus Type 1 from Neuronal Latency. *J. Virol.* **2001**, *75*, 3240–3249. [CrossRef]
67. Leib, D.A.; Coen, D.M.; Bogard, C.L.; Hicks, K.A.; Yager, D.R.; Knipe, D.M.; Tyler, K.L.; Schaffer, P.A. Immediate-early regulatory gene mutants define different stages in the establishment and reactivation of herpes simplex virus latency. *J. Virol.* **1989**, *63*, 759–768. [CrossRef]
68. Everett, R.D. Trans activation of transcription by herpes virus products: Requirement for two HSV-1 immediate-early polypeptides for maximum activity. *EMBO J.* **1984**, *3*, 3135–3141. [CrossRef] [PubMed]
69. Gelman, I.H.; Silverstein, S. Identification of immediate early genes from herpes simplex virus that transactivate the virus thymidine kinase gene. *Proc. Natl. Acad. Sci. USA* **1985**, *82*, 5265–5269. [CrossRef] [PubMed]
70. O'Hare, P.; Hayward, G.S. Three trans-acting regulatory proteins of herpes simplex virus modulate immediate-early gene expression in a pathway involving positive and negative feedback regulation. *J. Virol.* **1985**, *56*, 723–733. [CrossRef]
71. Perry, L.J.; Rixon, F.J.; Everett, R.D.; Frame, M.C.; McGeoch, D.J. Characterization of the IE110 Gene of Herpes Simplex Virus Type 1. *J. Gen. Virol.* **1986**, *67*, 2365–2380. [CrossRef]
72. Kim, E.T.; Dybas, J.M.; Kulej, K.; Reyes, E.D.; Price, A.M.; Akhtar, L.N.; Orr, A.; Garcia, B.A.; Boutell, C.; Weitzman, M.D. Comparative proteomics identifies Schlafen 5 (SLFN5) as a herpes simplex virus restriction factor that suppresses viral transcription. *Nat. Microbiol.* **2021**, *6*, 234–245. [CrossRef]
73. Reddi, T.S.; Merkl, P.E.; Lim, S.-Y.; Letvin, N.L.; Knipe, D.M. Tripartite Motif 22 (TRIM22) protein restricts herpes simplex virus 1 by epigenetic silencing of viral immediate-early genes. *PLoS Pathog.* **2021**, *17*, e1009281. [CrossRef]
74. Cuchet-Lourenço, D.; Vanni, E.; Glass, M.; Orr, A.; Everett, R.D. Herpes Simplex Virus 1 Ubiquitin Ligase ICP0 Interacts with PML Isoform I and Induces Its SUMO-Independent Degradation. *J. Virol.* **2012**, *86*, 11209–11222. [CrossRef] [PubMed]
75. Ansari, M.A.; Dutta, S.; Veettil, M.V.; Dutta, D.; Iqbal, J.; Kumar, B.; Roy, A.; Chikoti, L.; Singh, V.V.; Chandran, B. Herpesvirus Genome Recognition Induced Acetylation of Nuclear IFI16 Is Essential for Its Cytoplasmic Translocation, Inflammasome and IFN-beta Responses. *PLoS Pathog.* **2015**, *11*, e1005019. [CrossRef] [PubMed]
76. Li, T.; Diner, B.A.; Chen, J.; Cristea, I.M. Acetylation modulates cellular distribution and DNA sensing ability of interferon-inducible protein IFI16. *Proc. Natl. Acad. Sci. USA* **2012**, *109*, 10558–10563. [CrossRef] [PubMed]
77. Cuchet-Lourenco, D.; Anderson, G.; Sloan, E.; Orr, A.; Everett, R.D. The viral ubiquitin ligase ICP0 is neither sufficient nor necessary for degradation of the cellular DNA sensor IFI16 during herpes simplex virus 1 infection. *J. Virol.* **2013**, *87*, 13422–13432. [CrossRef] [PubMed]
78. Johnson, K.E.; Chikoti, L.; Chandran, B. Herpes simplex virus 1 infection induces activation and subsequent inhibition of the IFI16 and NLRP3 inflammasomes. *J. Virol.* **2013**, *87*, 5005–5018. [CrossRef] [PubMed]
79. Orzalli, M.H.; DeLuca, N.A.; Knipe, D.M. Nuclear IFI16 induction of IRF-3 signaling during herpesviral infection and degradation of IFI16 by the viral ICP0 protein. *Proc. Natl. Acad. Sci. USA* **2012**, *109*, E3008–E3017. [CrossRef] [PubMed]
80. Shahnazaryan, D.; Khalil, R.; Wynne, C.; Jefferies, C.A.; Gabhann-Dromgoole, J.N.; Murphy, C.C. Herpes simplex virus 1 targets IRF7 via ICP0 to limit type I IFN induction. *Sci. Rep.* **2020**, *10*, 22216. [CrossRef] [PubMed]
81. Zhang, J.; Wang, K.; Wang, S.; Zheng, C. Herpes simplex virus 1 E3 ubiquitin ligase ICP0 protein inhibits tumor necrosis factor alpha-induced NF-kappaB activation by interacting with p65/RelA and p50/NF-kappaB1. *J. Virol.* **2013**, *87*, 12935–12948. [CrossRef]
82. Kummer, M.; Turza, N.M.; Muhl-Zurbes, P.; Lechmann, M.; Boutell, C.; Coffin, R.S.; Everett, R.D.; Steinkasserer, A.; Prechtel, A.T. Herpes simplex virus type 1 induces CD83 degradation in mature dendritic cells with immediate-early kinetics via the cellular proteasome. *J. Virol.* **2007**, *81*, 6326–6338. [CrossRef]
83. Halford, W.P.; Puschel, R.; Gershburg, E.; Wilber, A.; Gershburg, S.; Rakowski, B. A live-attenuated HSV-2 ICP0 virus elicits 10 to 100 times greater protection against genital herpes than a glycoprotein D subunit vaccine. *PLoS ONE* **2011**, *6*, e17748. [CrossRef]
84. Halford, W.P.; Geltz, J.; Gershburg, E. Pan-HSV-2 IgG antibody in vaccinated mice and guinea pigs correlates with protection against herpes simplex virus 2. *PLoS ONE* **2013**, *8*, e65523. [CrossRef] [PubMed]
85. Geltz, J.J.; Gershburg, E.; Halford, W.P. Herpes simplex virus 2 (HSV-2) infected cell proteins are among the most dominant antigens of a live-attenuated HSV-2 vaccine. *PLoS ONE* **2015**, *10*, e0116091. [CrossRef] [PubMed]
86. Mertens, M.E.; Knipe, D.M. Herpes Simplex Virus 1 Manipulates Host Cell Antiviral and Proviral DNA Damage Responses. *mBio* **2021**, *12*, e03552-20. [CrossRef] [PubMed]
87. Holub, M.; Stranikova, A.; Chalupa, P.; Arientova, S.; Roubalova, K.; Beran, O. Frequent Recurrences of Genital Herpes Are Associated with Enhanced Systemic HSV-Specific T Cell Response. *Can. J. Infect. Dis. Med. Microbiol.* **2020**, *2020*, 5640960. [CrossRef]

viruses

Article

Antibodies Elicited in Response to a Single Cycle Glycoprotein D Deletion Viral Vaccine Candidate Bind C1q and Activate Complement Mediated Neutralization and Cytolysis

Maria Luisa Visciano [1], Aakash Mahant Mahant [1], Carl Pierce [1], Richard Hunte [1] and Betsy C. Herold [1,2,*]

1 Departments of Microbiology and Immunology, Albert Einstein College of Medicine, Bronx, NY 10461, USA; maria.visciano@einsteinmed.org (M.L.V.); aakash.mahant@einsteinmed.org (A.M.M.); Carl.Pierce@einsteinmed.org (C.P.); richard.hunte@einsteinmed.org (R.H.)
2 Department of Pediatrics, Albert Einstein College of Medicine, Bronx, NY 10461, USA
* Correspondence: betsy.herold@einsteinmed.org

Abstract: Herpes simplex virus (HSV) prevention is a global health priority but, despite decades of research, there is no effective vaccine. Prior efforts focused on generating glycoprotein D (gD) neutralizing antibodies, but clinical trial outcomes were disappointing. The deletion of gD yields a single-cycle candidate vaccine (ΔgD-2) that elicits high titer polyantigenic non-gD antibodies that exhibit little complement-independent neutralization but mediate antibody-dependent cellular cytotoxicity (ADCC) and phagocytosis (ADCP). Active or passive immunization with ΔgD-2 completely protects mice from lethal disease and latency following challenge with clinical isolates of either serotype. The current studies evaluated the role of complement in vaccine-elicited protection. The immune serum from the ΔgD-2 vaccinated mice exhibited significantly greater C1q binding compared to the serum from the gD protein vaccinated mice with infected cell lysates from either serotype as capture antigens. The C1q-binding antibodies recognized glycoprotein B. This resulted in significantly greater antibody-mediated complement-dependent cytolysis and neutralization. Notably, complete protection was preserved when the ΔgD-2 immune serum was passively transferred into C1q knockout mice, suggesting that ADCC and ADCP are sufficient in mice. We speculate that the polyfunctional responses elicited by ΔgD-2 may prove more effective in preventing HSV, compared to the more restrictive responses elicited by adjuvanted gD protein vaccines.

Keywords: herpes simplex viruses; vaccines; complement; C1q; glycoprotein D; glycoprotein B; complement-dependent cytolysis; complement-dependent neutralization

Citation: Visciano, M.L.; Mahant, A.M.; Pierce, C.; Hunte, R.; Herold, B.C. Antibodies Elicited in Response to a Single Cycle Glycoprotein D Deletion Viral Vaccine Candidate Bind C1q and Activate Complement Mediated Neutralization and Cytolysis. *Viruses* **2021**, *13*, 1284. https://doi.org/10.3390/v13071284

Academic Editor: Barry J. Margulies

Received: 25 May 2021
Accepted: 24 June 2021
Published: 30 June 2021

1. Introduction

Herpes simplex virus type 1 (HSV-1) and type 2 (HSV-2) are large DNA viruses that establish lifelong infection with periods of latency interspersed with episodes of asymptomatic or clinical reactivation. HSV-1 primarily causes oral mucocutaneous lesions, ocular disease and sporadic encephalitis, whereas both cause genital and neonatal infections. While HSV-2 dominates globally, HSV-1 is emerging as the more common cause of genital and neonatal disease in developed countries [1,2]. Immunocompromised hosts are at risk of more severe and prolonged symptoms with each of these syndromes and are at greater risk of viral dissemination. HSV-2, in particular, is a major cofactor fueling the HIV epidemic and is associated with an increased risk of HIV transmission and acquisition [3,4]. There are an estimated 3.7 billion people under the age of 50 years infected with HSV-1 and 491 million people between the ages of 15–49 years seropositive for HSV-2 [1,2], but despite the enormous health burden and the years of research in the field, there is no licensed HSV vaccine [5].

Various factors have contributed to the difficulty in designing an effective HSV vaccine, including the absence of defined correlates of immune protection and the ability of these viruses to evade innate and adaptive immune responses through diverse mechanisms [6]. All of the candidate vaccines that have been evaluated in clinical efficacy trials were predicated on the presumption that the neutralizing antibodies targeting the envelope glycoproteins D (gD) and/or B (gB) were correlates of immune protection [7–11]. However, results have been uniformly disappointing and highlight the need to consider other mechanisms of immune protection for vaccine development.

We recently engineered a single-cycle HSV-2 candidate vaccine strain deleted in gD (ΔgD-2), which provided complete protection against HSV-1 and HSV-2 and prevented the establishment of latency in murine models of vaginal, skin and ocular challenge [6,12–17]. The passive transfer of immune serum completely protected naïve mice from subsequent challenge, but surprisingly, there was little neutralization activity present. Rather, protection mapped to the ability of the Fc portion of the antibodies to engage Fc receptors and trigger antibody-dependent cellular cytotoxicity (ADCC), and to facilitate viral clearance by phagocytic cells [16,17]. The central role of the Fc receptor in mediating protection was confirmed by the observation that passive protection was lost when immune serum was transferred into FcγRIV knockout mice [18]. In contrast, adjuvanted recombinant gD protein vaccines elicited a predominant neutralizing response in the murine model, little ADCC and significantly less protection against disease following active or passive immunization when mice were challenged with clinical isolates. Moreover, the recombinant gD protein vaccine failed to prevent latency [15,18].

The Fc portion of antibodies may also protect through interactions with C1q. C1q binding may increase the potency of antibodies by modulating the stoichiometric requirements for neutralization [19], opsonization and phagocytosis, or activation of the complement cascade with the generation of membrane attack complexes on the infected cell surface, resulting in complement-dependent cytolysis (CDC). The prior neutralization studies were conducted after heat-inactivation of the ΔgD-2 immune serum and also did not evaluate C1q binding or CDC. Therefore, the current studies were designed to test the hypothesis that complement contributes to the immune protection mediated by ΔgD-2. We compared C1q binding, CDC and complement-dependent neutralization in vitro, using immune serum obtained from mice vaccinated with ΔgD-2 or an adjuvanted recombinant gD protein vaccine and then conducted passive transfer studies in C1q knockout mice.

2. Methods

2.1. Cells, Virus and Vaccines

Vero (African green monkey kidney, American Type Culture Collection (ATTC), Manassas, VA, USA), VD60 [20] and HaCat (human keratinocyte (ATCC PCS-200-011)) cells were grown in Dulbecco modified Eagle medium (DMEM) (Thermo-Fisher Scientific, Waltham, MA, USA) supplemented with 10% fetal bovine serum (FBS) (HyClone, Logan, UT) and 1% penicillin-streptomycin (Thermo-Fisher Scientific, Waltham, MA, USA). ΔgD-2 was propagated in VD60 cells and viral titers (PFU/mL) were quantified on complementing VD60 and non-complementing Vero cells [21]. HSV-1 (B^3x1.1) [15], HSV-2(G) [22], HSV-2(333)ZAG [23] (which expresses a green fluorescence protein under control of the cytomegalovirus promoter inserted at an intergenic site) and HSV-2(4674) [24] were propagated on Vero cells. HSV-2 gD protein (gD-2) was synthesized by the Einstein Protein Core Facility and combined with 150 μg of alum (Imject-Thermo Scientific, Thermo-Fisher Scientific, Waltham, MA, USA) and 12.5 μg of monophosphoryl lipid A (MPL) (Invivogen, San Diego, CA, USA) (rgD-2/Alum-MPL) [15].

2.2. Murine Vaccinations

Female Balb/c, C57BL/6 and C1qa knockout mice (C1qa$^{tmld(EUCOMM)Wtsi}$) were purchased from Jackson Laboratory (JAX, Bar Harbor, ME, USA). The use of mice for this study was approved by the Institutional Animal Care and Use Committee at the Albert Einstein College of Medicine, protocol 2018-0504. Balb/c or C57BL/6 mice (age 6 weeks) were vaccinated intramuscularly (prime) and then three weeks later (boost) with ΔgD-

2, rgD-2/Alum-MPL or a control VD60 lysate, as previously described [12]. Blood was obtained by retro-orbital sampling one week and three weeks post-boost.

2.3. C1q Binding ELISA

Overnight at 4 °C, 96-well plates (96 Well Flat Bottom Immuno Plate MaxiSorp (Thermo Fisher Scientific, Waltham, MA, USA) were coated with either 450 ng/mL of HSV infected (HSV-1 B^3x1.1 or HSV-2 G) or uninfected Vero cell lysates or with 250 ng/mL of HSV-1 recombinant gD-1 or gB-1 (produced in HEK293 cells by the Einstein Protein Core Facility), as described [18]. The plates were washed 4 times with PBS-0.5% Tween (washing buffer, WB) and then blocked with 5% Non-Fat Dry Milk (Bio-Rad, Hercules, CA, USA) in phosphate buffered-saline (PBS) with 0.1% Igepal-CA 630 (Millipore Sigma, St. Louis, MO, USA) (blocking buffer) for 1 h at room temperature (RT). The cells or proteins were then incubated (2 h RT) with serial two-fold dilutions of heat-inactivated immune sera followed by mouse C1q (1 µg/mL) (Complement Technology Inc., Tyler, TX, USA) and rat anti-mouse C1q-Biotin (0.5 µg/mL) (Cedarlane Labs, Burlington, NC, USA). Bound C1q was quantified using horse radish peroxidase conjugated streptavidin (Thermo Fisher Scientific, Waltham, MA, USA) (30 min, RT) followed by an addition of a substrate (OptEIA TMB Substrate Reagent Set, cat #555214, BD Bioscience, San Jose, CA, USA). The reaction was stopped by an addition of 2N H_2S0_4 and plates were read at 450 nm in a SpectraMax M5e Microplate Reader (Molecular Devices, San Jose, CA, USA). All dilutions were made in blocking buffer and plates were washed 4× with washing buffer after each step.

2.4. Viral Neutralization in the Absence or Presence of Complement

Neutralization was assessed using a plaque reduction assay with minor modifications [18]. Serial dilutions of heat-inactivated immune sera were incubated for 1 h at 37 °C with HSV-1 or HSV-2 (~100 PFU/well) in the absence or presence of 10% *v/v* rabbit complement (Cedarlane Labs, Burlington, NC, USA). Vero cells in 24-well cell culture plates (Costar-Corning, Kennebunk, ME, USA) were inoculated in duplicate with the virus–serum–complement mixture and plaques were counted after 48 h of incubation. The neutralization titer was defined as the highest dilution that yielded a 50% reduction in plaque numbers.

2.5. Complement Dependent Cytotoxicity

HaCat cells were infected with HSV-2(333)ZAG (0.1 PFU/cell) in 6-well cell culture plates (Costar-Corning, Kennebunk, ME, USA) for 1 h and then overlaid with media for 9 h. Cells were washed with PBS, and then heat-inactivated immune sera (1:50 dilution in incomplete DMEM) was added to cells. Plates were kept on ice for 30 min before adding 20% *v/v* rabbit complement. After a 4 h incubation at 37 °C in 5% CO_2, cells were detached with 500 µL/well Accutase (Thermo Fisher Scientific, Waltham, MA, USA), washed twice with PBS and stained with Zombie-NIR (BioLegend, San Diego, CA, USA) for 20 min at RT. Stained cells were then fixed with 2% paraformaldehyde and read with a Cytek Aurora 5 Laser System Flow cytometer (Cytek Bioscience, Freemont, CA, USA). Data were analyzed with FlowJo Software, version 10 (FlowJo-BD, Franklin Lakes, NJ, USA).

2.6. Passive Transfer Studies

Pooled serum containing 750 µg of total IgG (quantified by IgG ELISA, Invitrogen, Carlsbad, CA) harvested from intramuscularly ΔgD-2 or control (VD60) vaccinated C57Bl/6 mice was inoculated intraperitoneally into naïve WT or C1q-knockout BL/6 mice 24 h prior to skin challenge with HSV-2(4674) (5 × 10 PFU/mouse [13]), as previously described [18]. Mice were then monitored daily for epithelial and neurological disease and scored as follows: (1) erythema at inoculation site; (2) spread to distant site, zosteriform lesions, edema; (3) ulcerations, epidermal spread, limb paresis; (4) hind limb paralysis and (5) death. Mice were euthanized at a score of 4 and assigned a score of 5 the following day. At the time of euthanasia (when mice succumbed or day 14 post-challenge), sacral nerve tissue was collected and DNA isolated using the Qiagen Blood and Tissue DNA isolation kit (Qiagen, Hilden, Germany). A total of 10 ng of DNA per sample was loaded, and primers and probes specific for HSV polymerase were used to quantify HSV DNA (forward primer sequence, 5′-GGCCAGGCGCTTGTTGGTGTA-3′; reverse primer sequence, 5′-ATCACCGACCCGGAGAGGGA-3′; probe sequence, 5′-CCGCCGAACTGAGCAGACACCCGC-3′). Mouse β actin was used as a loading control (Applied Biosystems, Foster City, CA, USA), and qPCR was run in an Applied Biosystems QuantStudio 7 Flex.

2.7. Statistical Analysis

Analyses were performed using GraphPad Prism version 9 software (GraphPad Software, San Diego, CA, USA). The area under the curve (AUC) was calculated using trapezoid rule. A *p*-value of 0.05 was considered statistically significant. Survival curves were compared using the Gehan–Breslow–Wilcoxon test; other results were compared using *t*-tests or an ANOVA, as indicated.

3. Results

3.1. Immune Serum from ΔgD-2, but Not rgD-2Alum-MPL Vaccinated Mice Binds C1q

C1q binds to antibodies that are bound to viral particles or virally infected cells to promote activation of the complement cascade leading to CDC, opsonization and phagocytosis and/or complement-dependent neutralization. To determine if antibodies elicited in response to ΔgD-2 or rgD-2/Alum-MPL vaccination in mice exhibiting complement binding activity, a C1q sandwich binding ELISA was performed with immune serum ($n = 10$ mice per group). The immune serum from the ΔgD-2 prime-boost vaccinated mice exhibited significantly more C1q binding compared to rgD-2/Alum-MPL or compared to the VD60-control vaccinated mice when either HSV-1 (Figure 1A) or HSV-2 (Figure 1B) infected cell lysates were used as the capture antigen ($p < 0.001$ for both). In contrast, there was no significant increase in the C1q binding of the immune serum from rgD-2/Alum-MPL compared to the control mice. Notably, there was greater C1q binding of the ΔgD-2 immune serum when HSV-2, compared to HSV-1, infected cell lysates were used as the capture antigen (unpaired *t*-test comparing area under curve (AUC), 1079.0 ± 531.3 vs. 641.2 ± 134.3, $p = 0.02$).

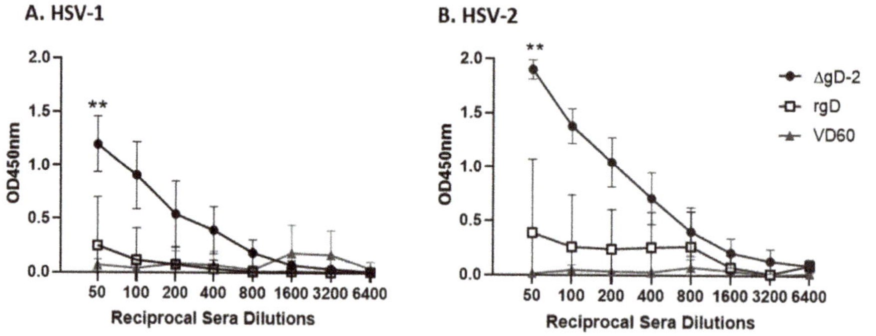

Figure 1. C1q binding of immune serum in mice vaccinated with ΔgD-2, adjuvanted recombinant gD or VD60 cell lysate. Serial 2-fold dilutions of heat-inactivated immune serum (1:50–1:6400) were assayed for ability to bind C1q using an ELISA with (**A**) HSV-1 B^{3}x1.1-infected Vero cells or (**B**) HSV-2(G) infected Vero cells. Results are shown as mean ± standard deviation (SD of the optical density units (OD450 nm) at each dilution (n = 9–10 mice per group) and the area under the curve was compared to VD60 controls using unpaired *t*-test with Welch's correction (** $p < 0.01$). There was no significant difference comparing C1q binding of adjuvanted rgD immune serum and VD60 controls.

The ΔgD-2 vaccine elicits a polyantigenic response including antibodies that bind gB, whereas rgD-2/Alum-MPL elicits only gD-directed responses [17,18]. Since the envelope glycoproteins, which are also expressed on the surface of infected cells, are likely targets of C1q activating antibodies, we compared the C1q binding of immune serum to gB or gD. The immune serum from the ΔgD-2 prime-boost vaccinated mice exhibited significant C1q binding to gB (but not gD) compared to the control or rgD-2/Alum-MPL mice ($p = 0.0003$ comparing AUC, $n = 10$ mice/group) (Figure 2A). In contrast, there was no significant C1q binding of the rgD-2/Alum-MPL immune serum to gD (Figure 2B), which is consistent with a lack of significant C1q capture by infected cell lysates (unpaired t-test comparing AUC 700.4 ± 235 (rgD-2) vs. 609.8 ± 76 (VD60), $p = 0.26$).

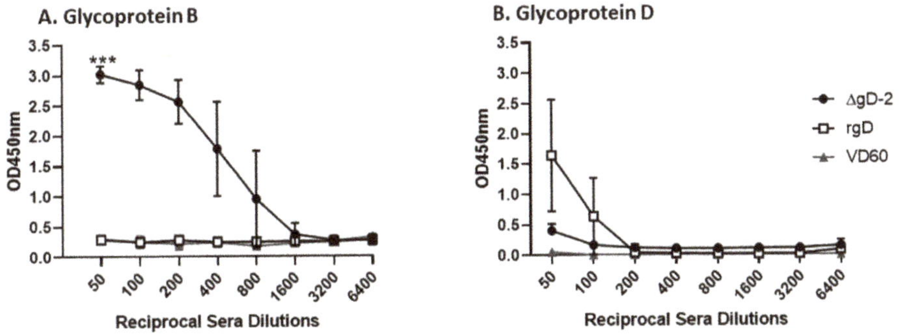

Figure 2. C1q binding of immune serum to glycoproteins gB or gD. Serial 2-fold dilutions of heat-inactivated immune sera (1:50–1:6400) were assayed for ability to bind C1q in ELISA with (**A**) recombinant gB or (**B**) recombinant gD protein. Results are shown as mean ± SD of the optical density units at each dilution ($n = 10$ mice per group) and the area under the curve was compared to VD60 controls by unpaired t-test with Welch's correction (*** $p < 0.001$).

3.2. gD-2 Immune Serum Mediates Complement Dependent Cytotoxicity

One of the major effects of C1q capture by antibody-bound infected cells is the assembly of the terminal components of complement to form a membrane attack complex leading to cell lysis. To determine if C1q binding translated into complement dependent cytolysis (CDC), HaCat cells were infected with HSV-2(333ZAG) for 9 h before adding immune serum and rabbit complement, and then analyzed using flow cytometry. In pilot studies, we confirmed that gB and gD are expressed on the infected cell surface by 6 h post-infection. The percentage of infected (GFP+) cells that were killed by the ΔgD-2 immune serum increased significantly from a mean of 11.77 to 76.09% when complement was added ($p < 0.001$, paired t-test) and compared to the serum from the VD60-immunized mice, with (11.29%) or without (8.21%) complement ($p < 0.0001$, two-way ANOVA) (Figure 3A,B). The addition of complement to the rgD-2/Alum-MPL immune serum had modest but significant effects on cytolysis (16.84 without vs. 29.57% with complement, $p = 0.04$, paired-t-test) and compared to the serum from the VD60 immunized mice when complement was added ($p < 0.05$, two-way ANOVA). The CDC activity of the ΔgD-2 immune serum was significantly greater than observed with the rgD-2 or VD60 immune serum ($p < 0.0001$, two-way ANOVA). Notably, there was a reduction in the GFP expression when infected cells were incubated with the ΔgD-2 immune serum and complement, likely reflecting a release of intracellular GFP as the cell was killed (Figure 3A, right panel).

3.3. Complement Enhances Neutralization Potency of ΔgD-2 Immune Serum

To investigate whether complement augments viral neutralization, plaque reduction assays were performed with serial dilutions of heat-inactivated sera obtained from the ΔgD-2, rgD-2/Alum-MPL or control VD60 immunized mice in the absence or presence of 10% rabbit complement. The addition of complement increased the neutralization titer (concentration of serum that inhibited 50% of viral plaques) from 26.75 ± 33.2 to 84.67 ± 40.4 for ΔgD-2 against HSV-1(B^3x1.1) ($p = 0.0024$, paired t-test) and from 52.3 ± 29.5 to 414.7 ± 107.1 for HSV-2(G) ($p = 0.0025$). The complement also increased the neutralization titer of the rgD-2 Alum/MPL immune serum against HSV-1 from 54.24 ± 25.08 to 63.75 ± 25/59 ($p = 0.0055$) but had no significant effect on the neutralization of HSV-2 (Figure 4). Notably, the complement-dependent neutralization titer of the ΔgD-2 immune serum was significantly higher than the complement-independent neutralization titer of the rgD-2/Alum-MPL2 immune serum for HSV-2 ($p = 0.004$, unpaired *t*-test).

3.4. C1q Is Not Required for Passive Protection

Previous studies demonstrated that the immune serum from the ΔgD-2 vaccinated (but not the adjuvanted rgD-2 protein vaccinated) mice passively protected the wild-type but not FcγRIV knockout mice from viral challenge, indicating that the activation of this FcR is critical for immune protection [15,18]. To determine if C1q binding is also required for passive protection, serum from the ΔgD-2 vaccinated mice was pooled and an equivalent amount of total IgG (750 μg/mouse) was administered intraperitoneally 1 day prior to challenging naïve C57Bl/6 or C1q knockout mice on the skin with an LD90 dose of HSV-2(4674). As a control, the wild-type mice received 750 μg/mouse of immune serum from the mice that had been immunized with VD60 cell lysate. Although the mice developed mild epithelial signs within the first few days following challenge, both the wild-type and C1q knockout mice that received the ΔgD-2 immune serum had significantly lower disease scores ($p < 0.0001$) and completely recovered, whereas all of the controls succumbed ($p < 0.01$) (Figure 5A,B). Moreover, the passive transfer of the ΔgD-2 immune serum reduced the amount of HSV-2 DNA detected in sacral ganglia tissue using a PCR at the time of euthanasia to below the limit of detection ($p < 0.0001$ compared to VD60 controls) (Figure 5C).

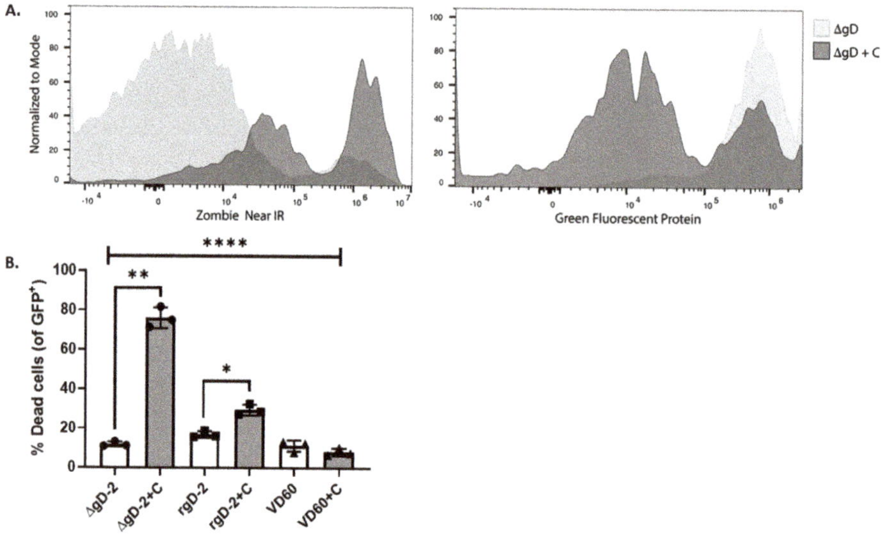

Figure 3. ΔgD-2 immune serum activates complement-dependent cytolysis. HaCAT cells were infected with HSV-2(333)ZAG, which expresses GFP, and then incubated for 4 h with heat-inactivated serum (1:50 dilution) obtained from mice prime-boost vaccinated with ΔgD-2, adjuvanted recombinant gD-2 (rgD-2), or VD60 control cell lysate with or without the addition of rabbit complement (+C). Cells were stained with Zombie NIR live-dead marker, fixed and then analyzed using flow cytometry to quantify the percentage of infected (GFP+) dead cells. (**A**) Representative histogram showing GFP staining (right) and Zombie NIR live/dead staining (left) when infected cells were incubated with ΔgD-2 immune serum obtained from a single mouse with or without complement. The *y*-axis is normalized to mode (e.g., the highest peak is set at 100% for each sample). (**B**) Bar graph showing percent of the GFP+ dead cells (mean ± SD) from a representative experiment (n =3 mice per group) (**** $p < 0.0001$, ** $p < 0.01$ and * $p < 0.05$, paired *t*-test comparing cytolysis with or without complement and two-way ANOVA with Tukey's corrections for multiple comparisons). Results are representative of 3 independent experiments.

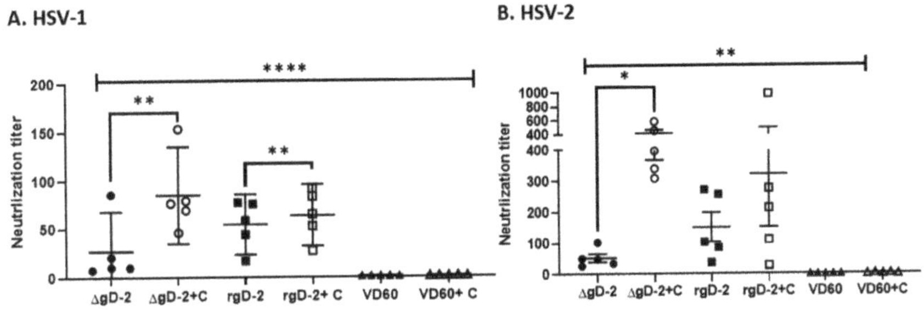

Figure 4. Complement enhances neutralization by ΔgD-2 immune serum. Neutralization of (**A**) HSV-1(B^{3}x1.1) or (**B**) HSV-2 (G) infection was determined using a plaque assay with serial dilutions of heat-inactivated immune serum from ΔgD-2, adjuvanted recombinant gD protein (gD-2) or VD60 lysate-vaccinated mice in the absence or presence of 10% rabbit complement (C) compared to plaques formed in the absence of serum. The serum dilution that inhibits 50% of plaque formation is shown as mean ± sd ($n = 5$ mice). **** $p < 0.0001$, ** $p < 0.01$ and * $p < 0.05$, paired t-test comparing neutralization titer with or without complement and two-way ANOVA with Tukey's corrections for multiple comparisons.

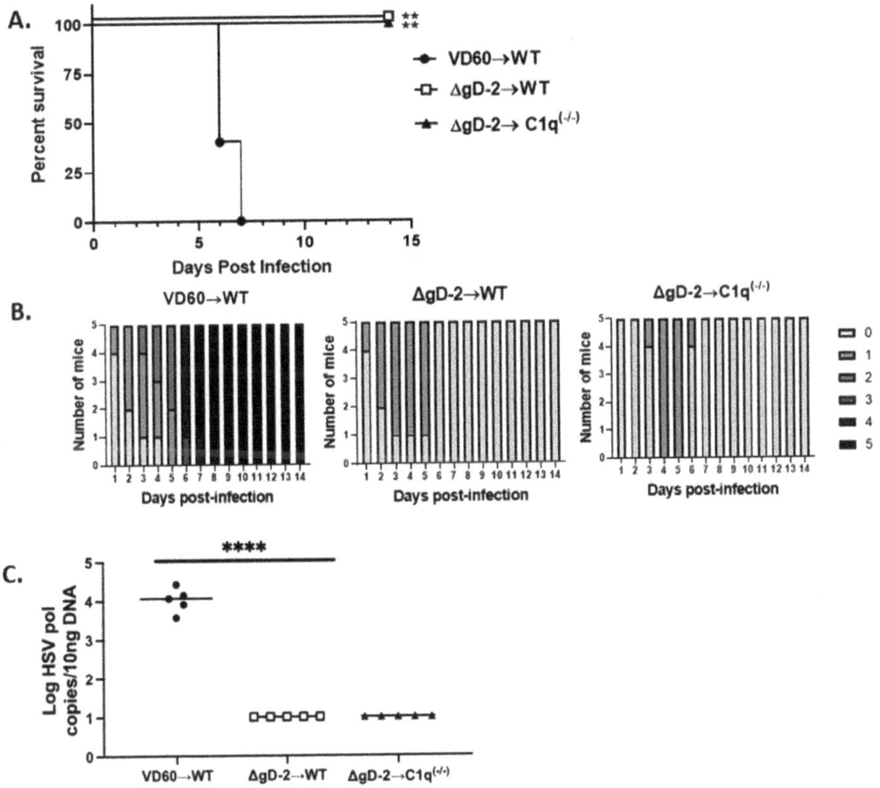

Figure 5. Passive transfer of immune serum from wild-type mice vaccinated with ΔgD-2 protects wild-type and *C1q-/-* mice. Pooled immune serum obtained from 5 ΔgD-2 vaccinated mice were assayed for IgG content and then administered intraperitoneally (750 μg total IgG/mouse) to wild-type or C1q-/- mice 1 day prior to challenging the mice by skin scarification with 5×10^4 PFU/mice of HSV-2 (4674). Survival curves (**A**) and disease scores (**B**) are shown, and the survival was compared using the Gehan-Breslow-Wilcoxon test ($n = 5$ mice per group ** $p < 0.01$). (**C**) Viral spread to sacral ganglia was determined using a quantitative PCR at time of euthanasia, **** $p < 0.0001$, ANOVA.

4. Discussion

The current studies extend our prior observations, highlighting differences in the immune response to the ΔgD-2 and rgD-2/Alum-MPL vaccinations. In addition to the previously documented more potent ADCC activity [12,15,18], the antibodies elicited by ΔgD-2 exhibit greater C1q binding compared to those elicited by the adjuvanted recombinant gD protein vaccine and these antibodies are associated with enhanced complement-dependent cytolysis and neutralization against both serotypes. C1q plays a pivotal role in initiating the lysis of virally infected cells by activating the classical complement cascade, which results in the assembly of the membrane attack complex on the cell surface and the formation of pores that disrupt the cell membrane. The mechanisms by which complement enhances antibody-dependent neutralization are not fully understood but may be mediated by C1q binding to the Fc component, thereby reducing the number of IgG molecules needed to neutralize viral particles, as was demonstrated for the West Nile virus [19]. Others have suggested that, in addition to C1q, the recruitment of other complement components (C4, C2 and C3) to the viral surface sterically blocks interactions between the virus and its receptors to prevent viral entry, as originally observed in studies with the Epstein–Barr virus [25].

Our prior findings, that antibodies elicited by the ΔgD-2 vaccine were only weakly neutralizing, were conducted with heat-inactivated serum (complement-independent) but were somewhat surprising, as the vaccine elicits polyantigenic responses that target glycoproteins B, C and E as well as other non-envelope viral proteins [17]. While gD is the dominant target of neutralizing responses, gB is also a major target [26]. However, preclinical rabbit studies of cytomegalovirus (CMV) gB vaccines found little neutralizing activity in the absence of complement. The addition of complement increased the neutralization titer, and a similar result was observed when complement was added to the human immune serum obtained from the participants in the CMV gB/MF59 clinical vaccine trials [27]. Monoclonal antibody (mAb) studies suggested that the epitope targeted, rather than the antibody avidity, determined the ability of the CMV gB mAbs to mediate complement-dependent neutralization. Our findings here suggest a similar phenomenon for ΔgD-2. Presumably, the stoichiometry of gB antibodies elicited by the ΔgD-2 vaccine and the epitopes targeted limit neutralization in the absence of complement.

The addition of complement to the neutralization assays had a greater effect for the ΔgD-2 immune serum, particularly against HSV-2, compared to the rgD-2 immune serum. The limited effect of complement on the rgD-2/Alum-MPL immune serum likely reflects the immune evasion properties of gE and gC. Specifically, gE binds to the Fc component of immunoglobulins to inhibit C1q binding, whereas gC binds C3b to inhibit complement-mediated neutralization and cytolysis. The deletion of gC from HSV-1 or HSV-2 results in an increased neutralization activity in the presence of human serum [28] and the neutralization titer of HSV gB mAbs was increased 2–16-fold when assayed against a gC null virus [28]. The importance of the antibodies that block the gE and gC immune evasion strategies is further supported by preclinical studies with a trivalent subunit protein or mRNA vaccine comprised of gD, gC and gE, which showed increased neutralizing titers and greater protection in small animal models compared to gD alone [29,30]. Presumably, ΔgD-2 overcomes these immune evasion strategies because it generates antibodies to gC and gE. This likely contributes to the observation that the neutralization titer of the ΔgD-2 immune serum in the presence of complement was at least as great as the neutralization titer of the rgD-2/Alum-MPL immune serum in the absence or presence of complement.

Although our in vitro studies demonstrated a role for complement in enhancing the neutralization and cytolytic activity of the ΔgD-2 immune serum, complete protection was preserved in passive transfer studies into C1q knockout mice, suggesting that the ADCC activity is sufficient to mediate protection in the murine model. This does not preclude the possibility that complement binding will contribute to protection in humans as the weaker activity of intrinsic mouse complement compared to humans may underestimate its role in mediating immune protection [31].

In summary, the current studies expand the characterization of the functionality of antibodies elicited in response to ΔgD-2 immunization, which includes not only the previously identified ADCC and antibody-dependent cellular phagocytosis (ADCP), but also antibody-mediated complement-dependent neutralization and cytolysis. This contrasts with recombinant gD protein vaccines, which elicit an almost exclusive complement-independent neutralization response. This more restrictive functional antibody response failed to protect in clinical trials [8]. Polyfunctional antibody responses are likely to be important for the prevention and control of other viral infections, including, for example, HIV, Ebolavirus and SARS-CoV-2 [32–35]. We speculate that prophylactic and therapeutic vaccines that elicit polyfunctional responses will prove more effective in preventing HSV and other viral infections.

Author Contributions: Conceptualization, M.L.V., A.M.M., R.H., C.P. and B.C.H.; methodology, M.L.V., A.M.M., R.H., C.P.; validation and formal analysis, A.M.M., C.P., B.C.H.; investigation; M.L.V., A.M.M., R.H., C.P.; writing and editing, M.L.V., A.M.M., R.H., C.P. and B.C.H., funding acquisition, B.C.H. All authors have read and agreed to the published version of the manuscript.

Funding: This research was funded by the National Institutes of Health, NIAID R01 AI17321, AI134367, P30 AI124414 and X-Vax Technologies. C.A.P. is supported by T32 AI007501 NIGMS MSTP training grant T32GM007288, R.H. is supported by T32 AI070117 and A.M.M. is supported by an Einstein-Montefiore CTSA training grant (TL1 TR002557).

Institutional Review Board Statement: The study was conducted according to the guidelines of the Declaration of Helsinki, use of mice for this study was approved by the Institutional Animal Care and Use Committee at the Albert Einstein College of Medicine, protocol 2018-0504 (approved 16.08.2018).

Informed Consent Statement: Not applicable.

Data Availability Statement: Data is available upon request.

Acknowledgments: The authors thank the Einstein Macromolecular Therapeutics Development Facility for producing recombinant glycoprotein D and glycoprotein B.

Conflicts of Interest: B.C.H. receives support for development of ΔgD-2 from X-Vax Technology, which holds the license for its development, and serves as a scientific advisor for the company. B.C.H. is an inventor on a patent for the ΔgD-2 vaccine.

References

1. Looker, K.J.; Magaret, A.S.; May, M.T.; Turner, K.M.E.; Vickerman, P.; Gottlieb, S.L.; Newman, L.M. Global and Regional Estimates of Prevalent and Incident Herpes Simplex Virus Type 1 Infections in 2012. *PLoS ONE.* **2015**, *10*, e0140765. [CrossRef]
2. Looker, K.J.; Magaret, A.S.; Turner, K.M.; Vickerman, P.; Gottlieb, S.L.; Newman, L.M. Global estimates of prevalent and incident herpes simplex virus type 2 infections in 2012. *PLoS ONE.* **2015**, *10*, e114989. [CrossRef] [PubMed]
3. Corey, L. Synergistic copathogens–HIV-1 and HSV-2. *N. Engl. J. Med.* **2007**, *356*, 854–856. [CrossRef]
4. Abu-Raddad, L.J.; Magaret, A.S.; Celum, C.; Wald, A.; Longini, I.M.; Self, S.G.; Corey, L. Genital herpes has played a more important role than any other sexually transmitted infection in driving HIV prevalence in Africa. *PLoS ONE* **2008**, *3*, e2230. [CrossRef] [PubMed]
5. Gottlieb, S.L.; Giersing, B.K.; Hickling, J.; Jones, R.; Deal, C.; Kaslow, D.C. Meeting report: Initial World Health Organization consultation on herpes simplex virus (HSV) vaccine preferred product characteristics, March 2017. *Vaccine* **2019**, *37*, 7408–7418. [CrossRef]
6. Aschner, C.B.; Herold, B.C. Alphaherpesvirus Vaccines. *Curr. Issues Mol. Biol.* **2021**, *41*, 469–508. [CrossRef]
7. Belshe, R.B.; Heineman, T.C.; Bernstein, D.I.; Bellamy, A.R.; Ewell, M.; Van Der Most, R.; Deal, C.D. Correlate of immune protection against HSV-1 genital disease in vaccinated women. *J. Infect. Dis.* **2014**, *209*, 828–836. [CrossRef]
8. Belshe, R.B.; Leone, P.A.; Bernstein, D.I.; Wald, A.; Levin, M.J.; Stapleton, J.T.; Gorfinkel, I.; Morrow, R.L.A.; Ewell, M.G.; Stokes-Riner, A.; et al. Efficacy results of a trial of a herpes simplex vaccine. *N. Engl. J. Med.* **2012**, *366*, 34–43. [CrossRef]
9. Bernstein, D.I.; Aoki, F.Y.; Tyring, S.K.; Stanberry, L.R.; Pierre, C.S.; Shafran, S.D.; Roels, G.L.; Van Herck, K.; Bollaerts, A.; Dubin, G.; et al. Safety and immunogenicity of glycoprotein D-adjuvant genital herpes vaccine. *Clin. Infect. Dis.* **2005**, *40*, 1271–1281. [CrossRef] [PubMed]

10. Stanberry, L.R.; Spruance, S.L.; Cunningham, A.L.; Bernstein, D.I.; Mindel, A.; Sacks, S.; Tyring, S.; Aoki, F.Y.; Slaoui, M.; Denis, M.; et al. Glycoprotein-D-adjuvant vaccine to prevent genital herpes. *N. Engl. J. Med.* **2002**, *347*, 1652–1661. [CrossRef]
11. Corey, L.; Langenberg, A.G.; Ashley, R.; Sekulovich, R.E.; Izu, A.E.; Douglas, J.M., Jr.; Handsfield, H.H.; Warren, T.; Marr, L.; Tyring, S.; et al. Recombinant glycoprotein vaccine for the prevention of genital HSV-2 infection: Two randomized controlled trials. Chiron HSV Vaccine Study Group. *JAMA* **1999**, *282*, 331–340. [CrossRef]
12. Aschner, C.B.; Pierce, C.; Knipe, D.M.; Herold, B.C. Vaccination Route as a Determinant of Protective Antibody Responses against Herpes Simplex Virus. *Vaccines* **2020**, *8*, 277. [CrossRef]
13. Ramsey, N.L.M.; Visciano, M.; Hunte, R.; Loh, L.N.; Aschner, C.B.; Jacobs, W.R.; Herold, B.C. A Single-Cycle Glycoprotein D Deletion Viral Vaccine Candidate, DeltagD-2, Elicits Polyfunctional Antibodies That Protect against Ocular Herpes Simplex Virus. *J. Virol.* **2020**, *94*, e00335-20. [CrossRef] [PubMed]
14. Kao, C.M.; Goymer, J.; Loh, L.N.; Mahant, A.; Burn Aschner, C.; Herold, B.C. Murine Model of Maternal Immunization Demonstrates Protective Role for Antibodies That Mediate Antibody-Dependent Cellular Cytotoxicity in Protecting Neonates From Herpes Simplex Virus Type 1 and Type 2. *J. Infect. Dis.* **2020**, *221*, 729–738. [CrossRef] [PubMed]
15. Burn, C.; Ramsey, N.; Garforth, S.J.; Almo, S.; Jacobs, W.R., Jr.; Herold, B.C. A Herpes Simplex Virus (HSV)-2 Single-Cycle Candidate Vaccine Deleted in Glycoprotein D Protects Male Mice from Lethal Skin Challenge with Clinical Isolates of HSV-1 and HSV-2. *J. Infect. Dis.* **2018**, *217*, 754–758.
16. Petro, C.D.; Weinrick, B.; Khajoueinejad, N.; Burn, C.; Sellers, R.; Jacobs, W.R., Jr.; Herold, B.C. HSV-2 DeltagD elicits FcgammaR-effector antibodies that protect against clinical isolates. *JCI Insight.* **2016**, *1*, e88529. [CrossRef]
17. Petro, C.; González, P.A.; Cheshenko, N.; Jandl, T.; Khajoueinejad, N.; Bénard, A.; Sengupta, M.; Herold, B.C.; Jacobs, W.R. Herpes simplex type 2 virus deleted in glycoprotein D protects against vaginal, skin and neural disease. *eLife* **2015**, *4*, e06054. [CrossRef] [PubMed]
18. Burn Aschner, C.; Loh, L.N.; Galen, B.; Delwel, I.; Jangra, R.K.; Garforth, S.J.; Chandran, K.; Almo, S.; Jacobs, W.R., Jr.; Ware, C.F.; et al. HVEM signaling promotes protective antibody-dependent cellular cytotoxicity (ADCC) vaccine responses to herpes simplex viruses. *Sci. Immunol.* **2020**, *5*. [CrossRef]
19. Mehlhop, E.; Nelson, S.; Jost, C.A.; Gorlatov, S.; Johnson, S.; Fremont, D.H.; Diamond, M.S.; Pierson, T.C. Complement protein C1q reduces the stoichiometric threshold for antibody-mediated neutralization of West Nile virus. *Cell Host Microbe* **2009**, *6*, 381–391. [CrossRef]
20. Ligas, M.W.; Johnson, D.C. A herpes simplex virus mutant in which glycoprotein D sequences are replaced by beta-galactosidase sequences binds to but is unable to penetrate into cells. *J. Virol.* **1988**, *62*, 1486–1494. [CrossRef]
21. Cheshenko, N.; Trepanier, J.B.; Stefanidou, M.; Buckley, N.; Gonzalez, P.; Jacobs, W.; Herold, B.C. HSV activates Akt to trigger calcium release and promote viral entry: Novel candidate target for treatment and suppression. *FASEB J.* **2013**, *27*, 2584–2599. [CrossRef] [PubMed]
22. Ejercito, P.M.; Kieff, E.D.; Roizman, B. Characterization of herpes simplex virus strains differing in their effects on social behaviour of infected cells. *J. Gen. Virol.* **1968**, *2*, 357–364. [CrossRef] [PubMed]
23. Nixon, B.; Stefanidou, M.; Mesquita, P.M.M.; Fakioglu, E.; Segarra, T.; Rohan, L.; Halford, W.; Palmer, K.; Herold, B.C. Griffithsin Protects Mice from Genital Herpes by Preventing Cell-to-Cell Spread. *J. Virol.* **2013**, *87*, 6257–6269. [CrossRef] [PubMed]
24. Segarra, T.J.; Fakioglu, E.; Cheshenko, N.; Wilson, S.S.; Mesquita, P.M.M.; Doncel, G.F.; Herold, B.C. Bridging the gap between preclinical and clinical microbicide trials: Blind evaluation of candidate gels in murine models of efficacy and safety. *PLoS ONE* **2011**, *6*, e27675. [CrossRef] [PubMed]
25. Nemerow, G.R.; Jensen, F.C.; Cooper, N.R. Neutralization of Epstein-Barr virus by nonimmune human serum. Role of cross-reacting antibody to herpes simplex virus and complement. *J. Clin. Investig.* **1982**, *70*, 1081–1091. [CrossRef]
26. Cairns, T.M.; Huang, Z.-Y.; Gallagher, J.R.; Lin, Y.; Lou, H.; Whitbeck, J.C.; Wald, A.; Cohen, G.H.; Eisenberg, R.J. Patient-Specific Neutralizing Antibody Responses to Herpes Simplex Virus Are Attributed to Epitopes on gD, gB, or Both and Can Be Type Specific. *J. Virol.* **2015**, *89*, 9213–9231. [CrossRef] [PubMed]
27. Li, F.; Freed, D.C.; Tang, A.; Rustandi, R.R.; Troutman, M.C.; Espeseth, A.S.; Zhang, N.; An, Z.; McVoy, M.; Zhu, H.; et al. Complement enhances in vitro neutralizing potency of antibodies to human cytomegalovirus glycoprotein B (gB) and immune sera induced by gB/MF59 vaccination. *NPJ Vaccines* **2017**, *2*, 1–8. [CrossRef]
28. Gerber, S.I.; Belval, B.J.; Herold, B.C. Differences in the role of glycoprotein C of HSV-1 and HSV-2 in viral binding may contribute to serotype differences in cell tropism. *Virology* **1995**, *214*, 29–39. [CrossRef]
29. Komala Sari, T.; Gianopulos, K.A.; Nicola, A.V. Glycoprotein C of Herpes Simplex Virus 1 Shields Glycoprotein B from Antibody Neutralization. *J. Virol.* **2020**, *94*, e01852-19. [CrossRef] [PubMed]
30. Awasthi, S.; Huang, J.; Shaw, C.; Friedman, H.M. Blocking herpes simplex virus 2 glycoprotein E immune evasion as an approach to enhance efficacy of a trivalent subunit antigen vaccine for genital herpes. *J. Virol.* **2014**, *88*, 8421–8432. [CrossRef] [PubMed]
31. Awasthi, S.; Hook, L.M.; Pardi, N.; Wang, F.; Myles, A.; Cancro, M.P.; Cohen, G.H.; Weissman, D.; Friedman, H.M. Nucleoside-modified mRNA encoding HSV-2 glycoproteins C, D, and E prevents clinical and subclinical genital herpes. *Sci. Immunol.* **2019**, *4*. [CrossRef] [PubMed]
32. Bergman, I.; Basse, P.H.; Barmada, M.A.; Griffin, J.A.; Cheung, N.K. Comparison of in vitro antibody-targeted cytotoxicity using mouse, rat and human effectors. *Cancer Immunol. Immunother.* **2000**, *49*, 259–266. [CrossRef] [PubMed]

33. Gunn, B.M.; Roy, V.; Karim, M.M.; Hartnett, J.N.; Suscovich, T.J.; Goba, A.; Momoh, M.; Sandi, J.D.; Kanneh, L.; Andersen, K.G.; et al. Survivors of Ebola Virus Disease Develop Polyfunctional Antibody Responses. *J. Infect. Dis.* **2020**, *221*, 156–161. [CrossRef] [PubMed]
34. Natarajan, H.; Crowley, A.R.; Butler, S.E.; Xu, S.; Weiner, J.A.; Bloch, E.M.; Littlefield, K.; Wendy Wieland-Alter, R.I.C.; Connor, R.I.; Wright, P.F.; et al. Markers of Polyfunctional SARS-CoV-2 Antibodies in Convalescent Plasma. *mBio* **2021**, *12*, e00765-21. [CrossRef]
35. Ackerman, M.E.; Mikhailova, A.; Brown, E.P.; Dowell, K.G.; Walker, B.D.; Bailey-Kellogg, C.; Suscovich, T.J.; Alter, G. Polyfunctional HIV-Specific Antibody Responses Are Associated with Spontaneous HIV Control. *PLoS Pathog.* **2016**, *12*, e1005315. [CrossRef] [PubMed]

viruses

MDPI

Article

Cross Strain Protection against Cytomegalovirus Reduces DISC Vaccine Efficacy against CMV in the Guinea Pig Model

K. Yeon Choi, Nadia S. El-Hamdi and Alistair McGregor *

Department Microbial Pathogenesis & Immunology, College of Medicine, Texas A&M University, Bryan, TX 77807, USA; yeonchoi@tamu.edu (K.Y.C.); nselhamdi@tamu.edu (N.S.E.-H.)
* Correspondence: mcgalistair2013@tamu.edu

Abstract: Congenital cytomegalovirus (CMV) is a leading cause of disease in newborns and a vaccine is a high priority. The guinea pig is the only small animal model for congenital CMV but requires guinea pig cytomegalovirus (GPCMV). Previously, a disabled infectious single cycle (DISC) vaccine strategy demonstrated complete protection against congenital GPCMV (22122 strain) and required neutralizing antibodies to various viral glycoprotein complexes. This included gB, essential for all cell types, and the pentamer complex (PC) for infection of non-fibroblast cells. All GPCMV research has utilized prototype strain 22122 limiting the translational impact, as numerous human CMV strains exist allowing re-infection and congenital CMV despite convalescent immunity. A novel GPCMV strain isolate (designated TAMYC) enabled vaccine cross strain protection studies. A GPCMV DISC (PC+) vaccine (22122 strain) induced a comprehensive immune response in animals, but vaccinated animals challenged with the TAMYC strain virus resulted in sustained viremia and the virus spread to target organs (liver, lung and spleen) with a significant viral load in the salivary glands. Protection was better than natural convalescent immunity, but the results fell short of previous DISC vaccine sterilizing immunity against the homologous 22122 virus challenge, despite a similarity in viral glycoprotein sequences between strains. The outcome suggests a limitation of the current DISC vaccine design against heterologous infection.

Keywords: guinea pig; cytomegalovirus; glycoproteins; neutralizing antibody; congenital CMV; pentamer complex; gB; epithelial cells; virus tropism; disabled infectious single cycle (DISC)

Citation: Choi, K.Y.; El-Hamdi, N.S.; McGregor, A. Cross Strain Protection against Cytomegalovirus Reduces DISC Vaccine Efficacy against CMV in the Guinea Pig Model. *Viruses* **2022**, *14*, 760. https://doi.org/10.3390/v14040760

Academic Editor: Barry J. Margulies

Received: 28 February 2022
Accepted: 30 March 2022
Published: 6 April 2022

1. Introduction

Human cytomegalovirus (HCMV), a betaherpesvirus, is a leading cause of congenital infection resulting in serious symptomatic diseases including cognitive and vision impairment as well as hearing loss in newborns [1,2]. Sensorineural hearing loss (SNHL) is the most common disease associated with congenital CMV and can continue to develop after birth [3]. Globally, congenital CMV occurs in approximately 1–5% of live births and this includes areas with high CMV seropositivity [4]. Primary CMV infection during pregnancy carries the greatest risk [4,5], but congenital CMV can also occur in women convalescent for the virus, and in these cases congenital infection may result from infection by a new strain [4]. Consequently, congenital infection can occur in mothers both seropositive and seronegative prior to pregnancy [6]. Ideally, a vaccine against congenital CMV should provide protection at the level higher than convalescent immunity to enable protection against infection by new strains of the virus.

Although the correlates of protection against congenital HCMV are poorly defined, it is generally thought that neutralizing antibodies to viral glycoprotein complexes significantly contributes to protection, but immune protection can also be enhanced by response to T cell target antigens (e.g., pp65) in convalescent immunity [7]. The evaluation of intervention strategies against CMV in a preclinical animal model is complicated by the species-specific nature of HCMV, making direct study of infection in animal models untenable. Species-specific animal CMV crosses the placenta in both the rhesus macaque (rhesus cytomegalovirus virus, RhCMV) and guinea pig (guinea pig cytomegalovirus, GPCMV) [8,9]. The guinea pig is the only small animal model for congenital CMV and the focus of this paper. Importantly, congenitally infected newborn pups have similar disease symptoms as humans, e.g., SNHL [10]. Various vaccine and intervention strategies have been evaluated against CMV in this model but studies have focused on the original prototype GPCMV strain 22122 (ATCC VR682) isolated in the 1950s [11]. Although this virus causes congenital infection, it is the only strain used in vaccine protection studies and was passed on fibroblast cells (>100) during the initial isolation which potentially attenuated the virus in contrast to clinical strains present in animal colonies. We recently isolated a new strain of GPCMV (designated TAMYC) from the salivary gland of an infected animal. This novel strain enabled the realistic evaluation of cross strain protection provided by promising CMV vaccine candidates against the 22122 strain in this translational animal model [12].

HCMV encodes multiple glycoprotein complexes (gB, gH/gL/gO, gM/gN and the pentamer complex (PC) gH/gL/UL128/UL130/UL131) important for cellular infection. The virus has two pathways of cell entry: direct entry which is independent of the pentamer complex (PC); and endocytic entry which requires PC in addition to other viral glycoproteins. The viral gB glycoprotein is essential for HCMV entry into all cell types, an immunodominant neutralizing antibody target, and remains a significant focus in various vaccine approaches, either as a standalone antigen, or in conjunction with other target viral antigens [13]. Although the gB protein generates neutralizing antibodies, these are less effective against virus neutralization on non-fibroblast cells including epithelial, endothelial and placental trophoblast cells where the viral pentamer complex (PC) is necessary for virus cell entry and the PC is an effective neutralizing antibody target [14,15]. In clinical trials, a subunit gB vaccine attains at best about 50% efficacy despite vaccine enhancement from non-neutralizing antibodies [16,17]. Consequently, the PC is also currently being evaluated in various CMV vaccine strategies as an important antigen target.

GPCMV encodes functional viral glycoprotein complexes to HCMV (gB, gH/gL/gO, gM/gN), which are important for virus cell entry [18–20]. Unlike murine cytomegalovirus, GPCMV also encodes a gH-based PC (gH/gLGP129/GP131/GP133) which is essential for GPCMV infection of all non-fibroblast cell types including epithelial and endothelial cells via an endocytic entry pathway similar to clinical strains of HCMV [19–21]. The PC is necessary for GPCMV dissemination and infection of placental trophoblasts and amniotic sac cells as well as congenital CMV [19,22,23]. As with HCMV, the GPCMV viral glycoprotein complexes are important neutralizing antibody targets [18,24–27]. GPCMV gB [25,28] is essential for virus infection of all cell types [18,19] and has been the most extensively studied vaccine antigen against congenital CMV in guinea pigs. However, in congenital protection studies, the various gB vaccine studies attained approximately 50% efficacy in the guinea pig model [28–31]. In HCMV, the endocytic pathway for cell entry is only partially defined and various candidate receptors have been identified [32–36]. Fibroblast cells that express the viral cell receptor platelet derived growth factor receptor alpha (PDGFRA) enable HCMV and GPCMV cell entry by direct cell fusion independent of the PC, but require gH/gL/gO triplex and gB [37–39]. Despite the essential nature of gB for infection of all cell types for HCMV and GPCMV, neutralizing antibodies directed to the PC might constitute a better vaccine target [40,41]. This is especially the case since antibodies directed to the PC are more effective at virus neutralization on placental trophoblasts and amniotic sac cell lines [14,23,27,38,42].

In addition to neutralizing antibodies, convalescent HCMV patients produce T cell responses to additional viral antigens including pp65 tegument protein and IE1 non-structural protein which are also thought to contribute to convalescent immunity [7,43]. Studies in animal models suggest that homologs of these antigens can also contribute to CMV vaccine-based protection. Consequently, the most effective CMV vaccine strategy might be one that evokes an immune response to various antibody and T cell target antigens. This potentially requires a complicated series of antigens to be present in candidate CMV vaccines to ensure a high level of efficacy. GPCMV encodes homolog T cell target antigens to HCMV such as pp65 (GP83), and a cell-mediated response to GP83 has been demonstrated to provide partial protection against congenital CMV [24,44,45], but has a limited impact as a standalone vaccine candidate [45,46]. Although various vaccine strategies have been evaluated in the guinea pig against congenital CMV, the most effective approach to date has been the use of a replication incompetent live viral strain or disabled infectious single cycle (DISC) vaccine [24]. The GPCMV DISC vaccine incorporates various antibody and T cell target antigens mimicking natural infection, but does not produce progeny virus in the host because of a lethal capsid gene mutation, and requires a complementing cell line for growth [24,38]. Protection against wild type virus (22122) challenge both horizontally and vertically was significantly increased with high efficacy and sterilizing immunity when this DISC vaccine strategy incorporated the unique PC components (GP129, GP131 and GP133) [38] compared to a GPCMV DISC (PC^-) vaccine that expressed only gH and gL but lacked the unique PC components [24]. A PC^+ DISC vaccine for HCMV based on a targeted viral protein destabilizing strategy is currently being evaluated in clinical trials [47].

In this current study, we hypothesized that a newly isolated strain of GPCMV (TAMYC strain) [12] may better resemble clinical strains present in guinea pig colonies. Consequently, this novel strain might provide a more significant test for CMV vaccine efficacy by evaluating heterologous cross strain vaccine protection in this model compared to previous homologous studies with the 22122 strain. Importantly, the TAMYC strain virus was highly cell associated similar to HCMV clinical strains and exhibited preferential tropism to various non-fibroblast cell types compared to the 22122 strain GPCMV [12]. An earlier cross strain protection study with a recombinant AdgB (22122 strain) vaccine failed to provide high level protection against the TAMYC virus challenge despite 99% identity in the gB sequence between strains [27,48]. This indicated a potential requirement for an immune response to multiple viral antigens for cross strain protection to be effective. Consequently, we evaluated the ability of the PC^+ 22122 strain based GPCMV DISC vaccine (designated DISCII) to cross protect against a challenge by the novel GPCMV strain (TAMYC) in vaccinated animals as this strategy had exhibited sterilizing immunity against the 22122 strain and induced a comprehensive immune response. Additionally, the ability of convalescent and hyperimmune animals (22122 strain) to protect against infection by the TAMYC strain GPCMV challenge was explored. Subsequently, antibody neutralization of both TAMYC and 22122 strains were separately evaluated with hyperimmune sera (TAMYC or 22122 strain infected animals) to ascertain differences between homologous and heterologous virus neutralization on fibroblast and epithelial cells. Overall, the results suggest a minimum threshold expectation for an effective vaccine strategy that exhibits cross strain protection against CMV in this model.

2. Materials and Methods

2.1. Virus, Cells, Synthetic Genes and Oligonucleotides

Wild type GPCMV (strain 22122, ATCC VR682 or new strain isolate, designated TAMYC) were propagated on guinea pig fibroblast lung cells (GPL; ATCC CCL 158) and renal epithelial (REPI) cell lines as previously described [19,22]. Both 22122 and TAMYC strain viruses were PC positive. Virus stocks for antibody neutralization assays were generated on renal epithelial cells. Virus titers were determined by GPCMV titration on renal epithelial and fibroblast cells [19]. Recombinant defective adenovirus (Ad5) vectors encoding GPCMV glycoproteins (gB, gH, gL, GP129, GP131 and GP133) were previously described [18,19,27]. Oligonucleotides were synthesized by Sigma-Genosys (The Woodlands, TX, USA).

2.2. Animal Studies

Guinea pig (Hartley) animal studies were performed under IACUC (Texas A&M University, College Station, TX, USA) permit 2017-0227. All study procedures were carried out in strict accordance with the recommendations in the "Guide for the Care and Use of Laboratory Animals of the National Institutes of Health". Animals were observed daily by trained animal care staff, and animals that required care were referred to the attending veterinarian for immediate care or euthanasia. Terminal euthanasia was carried out by lethal CO_2 overdose followed by cervical dislocation in accordance with IACUC protocol and NIH guidelines. Animals purchased from Charles River Laboratories were verified as seronegative for GPCMV by anti-GPCMV ELISA of sera collected by toenail clip bleed as previously described [18]. Animal studies were performed to evaluate: (a) immune response to GPCMV infection; (b) virus dissemination in seropositive and seronegative animals; (c) vaccine protection against GPCMV infection. Animals were made immune to GPCMV by single injection (SQ, 1×10^5 pfu) or hyperimmune by 3 sequential injections of the same strain of GPCMV with each injection separated by 3–4-week intervals. Infected animals were bled by toenail clip and serum from individual animals evaluated for anti-GPCMV titer by ELISA to verify seroconversion. Anti-glycoprotein complex ELISA titers (gB, gH/gL, gM/gN, PC) were also evaluated at approximately 2 months post final virus injection/vaccination. Sera of animals within each group with similar anti-GPCMV ELISA titers were pooled for further study. Hyperimmune pooled anti-GPCMV sera was previously described [24]. The antibody immune response to specific glycoprotein complexes (gB, gH/gL, gM/gN and PC) was evaluated by ELISAs for pooled sera for each group following the previously described assays [38]. Neutralization assays were evaluated on fibroblast and renal epithelial cells as previously described [38] for pooled sera from each group or seronegative control sera. Animals were vaccinated with DISCII (strain 22122) GPCMV (SQ 1×10^3 pfu) followed by two sequential DISCII vaccine booster shots as described for hyperimmune animals. DISCI (PC negative) vaccine sera was historical pooled sera as previously described [38].

2.3. GPCMV Glycoprotein ELISAs

Specific glycoprotein complex ELISAs were carried out as previously described using positive coating antigen derived from renal epithelial cell monolayers transduced with recombinant replication defective adenovirus (Ad) vectors expressing specific glycoprotein complexes, or control recombinant Ad vectors expressing GFP for negative coating antigen [18,19,24,27]. This was except for the case of gM/gN ELISA which utilized transient expression plasmid with synthetic codon optimized expression plasmids for transfection onto guinea pig cells [18]. Harvested cells were washed with PBS and cell pellets fixed prior to processing as coating antigen. Protein concentration was normalized by a Bradford assay. MaxiSorp ELISA plates (NUNC) were coated with 0.5 µg of either Ag+ or Ag- preparations diluted in carbonate coating buffer overnight at 4 °C, washed in 1X PBST then blocked with 2% nonfat dry milk. Test sera were diluted in blocking buffer from 1:80 to 1:20,480 in doubling dilutions, incubated for 2 h at 37 °C and then reacted with anti-Guinea Pig IgG peroxidase antibody (Sigma-Aldrich, St. Louis, MO, USA) diluted (1:2000) in blocking buffer for an additional 1 h at 37 °C before reacting with TMB membrane peroxidase substrate (KPL). Net OD (absorbance 450 nm) was attained by subtracting the OD of Ag- from the OD of Ag+. All ELISAs described in this report were carried out with the same batch of coating antigen. The described approach is based on similar strategies for glycoprotein complex expression for HCMV and RhCMV and ELISAs [49,50]. All ELISAs were run a minimum of three times in duplicates. ELISA reactivity was considered positive if the net OD was greater than, or equal to, 0.2, as determined by GPCMV negative serum.

2.4. GPCMV Neutralization Assays

GPCMV neutralization assays (NA_{50}) were performed on GPL fibroblasts and renal epithelial (REPI) cells with PC^+ GPCMV (22122 strain or TAMYC strain) virus stocks generated on renal epithelial cells [18,19] using pooled sera from a specific group of GPCMV convalescent or DISC vaccinated animals as previously described [24]. Serially diluted sera were incubated with approximately 1×10^5 pfu PC^+ GPCMV in media containing 1% rabbit complement (Equitech Bio, Kerrville, TX, USA) for 90 min at 37 °C before infecting

REPI cells for 1 h. For neutralization on GPL cells, 1×10^3 pfu PC+ GPCMV was used. Infected cells and supernatant were collected on day 4 then titrated on GPLs. The final neutralizing antibody titer was the inverse of the highest dilution, producing 50% or greater reduction in plaques compared to the virus only control. NA_{50} were performed from each sample three times concurrently with the same virus stocks between groups.

2.5. Real Time PCR

Blood and tissues (lung, liver, spleen, salivary gland) were collected from euthanized guinea pigs to determine the viral load as previously described [18,24]. Briefly, for tissue DNA extraction, FastPrep 24 (MP Biomedicals, Solon, OH, USA) was used to homogenize tissues as a 10% weight/volume homogenate in Lysing Matrix D (MP Biomedicals). To obtain DNA from whole blood, blood was collected into tubes containing ACD anticoagulant and 200 μL of blood was subsequently used per extraction. DNA was extracted using the QIAcube (Qiagen Inc., Germantown, MD, USA) according to the manufacturer's liquid (blood) or tissue protocol instructions. Viral load was determined by real time PCR on LightCycler 480 (Roche Life Science, Indianapolis, IN, USA) using primers and a hydrolysis probe to amplify a product from the GPCMV GP44 gene. The PCR master mix contained LightCycler ProbesMaster (Roche Life Science, Indianapolis, IN, USA), 0.4 μM primers and 0.1 μM probe, and 0.4U uracil N-glycosylase (UNG) in 25 μL of the total reaction volume including 10 μL of DNA per reaction. Standard controls and no template controls (NTC) were run with each assay for quantification. LightCycler 480 amplification parameters were: UNG step for 10 min at 40 °C followed by activation at 95 °C for 10 min, then 45 cycles of denaturation at 95 °C for 15 s, annealing at 56 °C for 15 s, and elongation at 72 °C for 10 s. Data were collected by 'single' acquisition during the extension step. The standard curve was generated using the GPCMV GP44 plasmid [51] for quantification and assay sensitivity. The sensitivity of the assay was determined to be 5 copies/reaction. The viral load was expressed as genome copies/mL of blood or genome copies/mg tissue. Results calculated were a mean value of triplicate PCR runs per sample.

2.6. Statistical Analysis

All statistical analyses were conducted with GraphPad Prism (version 7) software. Replicate means were analyzed using Student's *t* test (unpaired), with significance taken as a p value of <0.05 or as specified in the figure legends.

3. Results

3.1. Comparative Ability of GPCMV DISC Vaccine (PC^+ or PC^-) to Neutralize TAMYC Strain

Previously, we demonstrated that inclusion of the PC in a GPCMV DISC vaccine strategy improved virus neutralization as well as vaccine efficacy against prototype strain 22122, providing sterilizing immunity against dissemination and congenital infection [38]. The ability of a DISC vaccine strategy to provide cross strain GPCMV protection was unknown and a limitation of the current model. A new strain of GPCMV (TAMYC) was isolated from the salivary gland of an infected commercial colony animal. A comparison of encoded GPCMV glycoprotein indicated that apart from the gO glycoprotein there was relatively high similarity between the respective strain glycoproteins at the predicted amino acid level and percentage homology [12]: gB (99%); gN (92%); gO (75%); gH (84%); gM (99%); gL (98%); GP129 (88%); GP131 (89%); GP133 (91%). Consequently, cross strain protection against the TAMYC strain was potentially possible with the current PC+ GPCMV DISC (22122) vaccine strategy, DISCII [38].

A group of GPCMV seronegative female animals (n = 12) were vaccinated with a sequential three-dose vaccine regime of the DISCII vaccine (1×10^3 pfu/shot, SQ). The first vaccine was given at day 0, followed by a booster at days 26 and 49-post original shot. Animals were bled at 24 and 48 days after original day 0 to determine anti-GPCMV antibody titer. On day 70, a final bleed was used to evaluate immune response to specific glycoprotein complexes (gB, gH/gL, gM/gN and PC) [18,24]. Historical pooled sera from

22122 strain DISCI (PC$^-$) vaccinated animals [38] generated under the same vaccine regime to DISCII were compared with DISCII vaccine sera for immune responses to GPCMV glycoprotein complexes, and additionally evaluated for virus neutralization (TAMYC strain). Sera antibody immune response comparisons between the DISCI and DISCII vaccine strategies are shown in Figure 1: anti-GPCMV ELISA (Figure 1A); anti-glycoprotein complex ELISAs (Figure 1B,C).

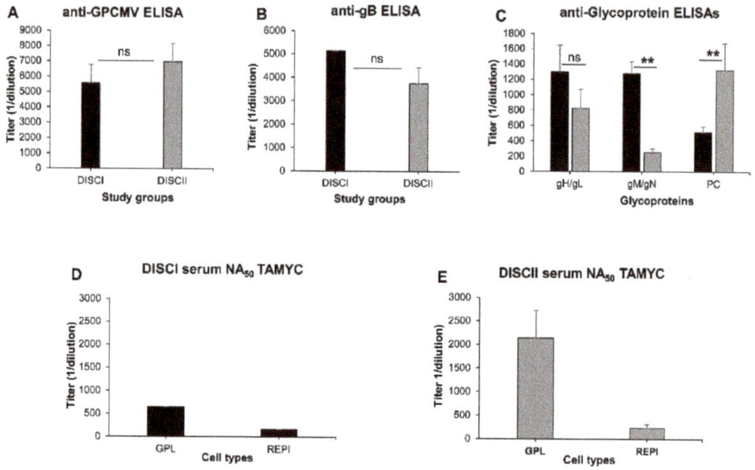

Figure 1. Comparative immune responses to DISC vaccine (DISCI vs. DISCII) and GPCMV (TAMYC strain) neutralization on fibroblast and epithelial cells. (**A–C**) Immune response of DISCII animal sera was compared to that of previous historical DISCI pooled sera from animals vaccinated with identical protocol [38]. (**A**) Anti-GPCMV ELISA titer; (**B**) anti-gB glycoprotein ELISA titer; (**C**) anti-glycoprotein complex ELISA titers (gH/gL, gM/gN, PC) from sera of DISCI (black) or DISCII (gray) vaccinated animals. Neutralizing antibody titers (NA_{50}) against TAMYC strain virus on GPL (fibroblast) or REPI (epithelial) cells of pooled sera from either DISCI animals (**D**) or DISCII-vaccinated animals (**E**). Mean ELISA and neutralization values are a result of assay triplicates with each sample run a minimum of three independent times. Statistical analysis was determined by unpaired Student's *t* test; ** $p < 0.005$; ns = non-significant.

DISCII vaccine results were similar to that previously observed in DISCII vaccinated animals [38] and included a specific response to PC. DISCII induced a higher anti-GPCMV ELISA titer compared to historical DISCI sera (5947 vs. 6950) but was not significant (Figure 1A). DISCI vaccine sera induced slightly higher anti-gB antibody titers compared to DISCII (5120 vs. 3750) but was not statistically significant (Figure 1B). However, DISCI vaccine sera induced approximately five-fold higher anti-gM/gN titer compared to DISCII, but anti-gH/gL titers were more similar between DISC vaccines (Figure 1C). Next, DISC vaccine sera were evaluated for their ability to neutralize the TAMYC strain GPCMV on both fibroblast (GPL) and epithelial (REPI) cells. Both DISCI and DISCII sera were more effective at neutralizing the virus on GPL cells (Figure 1D,E), with DISCII having a higher NA_{50} than DISCI (2133 vs. 640). This was despite the essential nature of gB, higher anti-gB titer in DISCI sera and 99% identity in gB sequence between TAMYC and 22122 strains. Both DISCI and DISCII sera had reduced neutralizing titers on epithelial cells with approximately four and nine-fold reductions, respectively, compared to on GPL cells (Figure 1D,E). Previous studies with 22122 neutralization and DISC vaccine sera indicated that inclusion of the PC improved virus neutralization on both fibroblast and non-fibroblast cells, and this would appear to be a similar outcome against the TAMYC virus (Figure 1D,E) [38]. Previously, depletion of antibodies to specific viral glycoprotein complexes from DISCII sera and 22122 hyperimmune GPCMV (PC$^+$/PC$^-$) sera [38] demonstrated that improved virus neutralization on non-fibroblast cells was attributed to anti-PC antibodies. The presence of anti-PC improved the DISCII virus NA_{50} titer against the TAMYC virus, but this was only two-fold greater than that of DISCI sera (Figure 1D,E) and suggests a more limited impact of anti-PC against the TAMYC strain. This might relate to similar levels of anti-gH/gL antibodies generated in both DISC vaccine strategies. Possibly gH/gL might be present on the virion surface of TAMYC in a greater level than PC compared to the 22122 strain, despite both virus stocks being generated on epithelial virus. The levels of specific viral glycoprotein complexes related to gH/gL have been reported to differ between HCMV strain types related to gO strain type, and this might impact on specific neutralizing antibodies titer directed to PC [52–54].

3.2. *DISC Vaccine Cross Protection against GPCMV (TAMYC Strain) Virus Challenge*

DISCII vaccinated animals from the previous section were subsequently challenged with wild type (strain TAMYC) GPCMV (1×10^5 pfu, SQ), and a matching control group of unvaccinated animals (pre-screened GPCMV negative) were similarly challenged with TAMYC strain GPCMV. At subsequent time points (4, 8, 12 and 27 days post-infection, dpi), three animals per group were randomly selected for the evaluation of viral load (liver, lung, spleen and blood). The outcome (Figure 2) demonstrated that the DISCII vaccine did not provide sterilizing immunity to the TAMYC strain challenge.

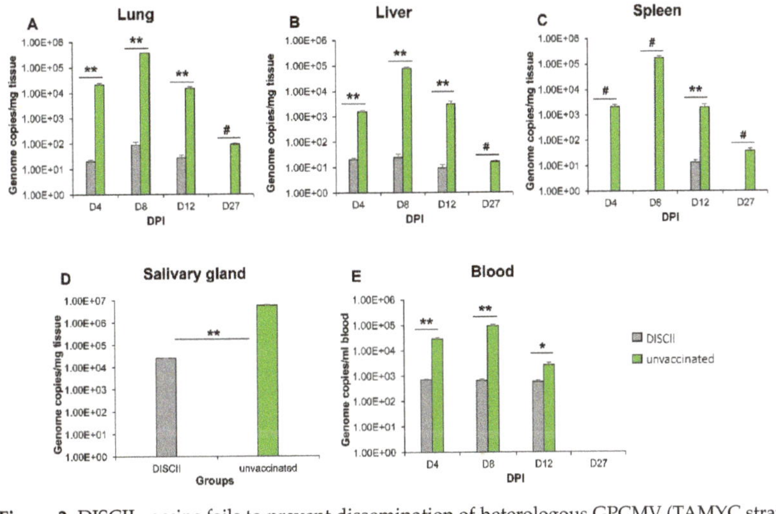

Figure 2. DISCII vaccine fails to prevent dissemination of heterologous GPCMV (TAMYC strain) to target organs in vaccinated animals. Seronegative animals (n = 12) were vaccinated with 3 sequential shots of DISCII vaccine. Animals were evaluated for immune response (Figure 1) and at 3 weeks post-last vaccination animals were challenged with GPCMV (TAMYC strain, 1×10^5 pfu, SQ). A control group (n = 12) of seronegative (unvaccinated, green) animals were similarly challenged with virus. At 4, 8, 12 and 27 dpi, 3 animals per group were evaluated for viral load in target organs. Target organs: lung (**A**); liver (**B**); spleen (**C**) plotted as genome copies/mg tissue over 4, 8, 12 and 27 dpi. Salivary gland (**D**) was only evaluated at 27 dpi and plotted as genome copies/mg tissue. (**E**) Viremia at 4, 8, 12 and 27 dpi was plotted as genome copies/mL blood. Statistical analysis determined by unpaired Student's t test; * $p < 0.05$; ** $p < 0.005$; ns = non-significant; # = DISCII vaccinated group value below the level of detection.

Consequently, the DISCII vaccine had a more limited impact on virus dissemination in the vaccinated group. GPCMV (TAMYC strain) disseminated to all target organs in the vaccine group, but the viral load was reduced compared to the unvaccinated groups at all time points (Figure 2). The reduction in virus load was most effective in the spleen with the virus detected only at 12 dpi in the vaccine group, but present at all time points in the control group. The virus was detected in the blood at a constant level (approximately 10^3 genome copies/mL blood) at 4, 8 and 12 dpi in the vaccine group, but peaked at earlier time points in the unvaccinated group at 4 and 8 dpi and was slightly above the vaccine group load at 12 dpi (Figure 2E). The virus continued to be detected in the salivary gland tissue at 27 dpi in vaccinated animals with a reduction of 2 logs compared to the unvaccinated group (Figure 2D). Results indicated a limitation of the current DISC vaccine strategy against cross strain heterologous virus protection compared to previous homologous protection studies against the 22122 strain challenge [38].

It was concluded that the DISCII vaccine strategy provided a limited ability to cross protect against the new strain virus challenge, and potentially would fail to completely prevent congenital infection, especially since there was a sustained viral load in the blood which would potentially enable significant placental infection in pregnant animals.

3.3. *Limitation of Cross Strain Protection in Animals Convalescent for 22122 Strain*

Next, we investigated if the DISCII vaccine provided higher level of protection compared to natural convalescent immunity against the 22122 strain, or animals hyperimmune to the 22122 strain. Animals that have been naturally infected with GPCMV or received a single dose of GPCMV to mimic natural infection induced a lower antibody response to viral glycoprotein complexes compared to animals given multiple injections of PC^+ wild type virus to render them hyperimmune [12,38]. GPCMV seronegative animals (n = 12/group) were initially infected with either a single dose, to mimic natural infection, or animals received three sequential doses of the 22122 strain (1×10^5 pfu, SQ) to render animals hyperimmune to GPCMV. Animals were evaluated for immune response at 2 months post-viral infection, and antibody titers are compared in Figure 3 between groups (22122-X1 and 22122-HI): Anti-GPCMV ELISA (Figure 3A); Anti-glycoprotein complexes (gB, gH/gL, gM/gN and PC) ELISAs (Figure 3B). Although anti-GPCMV titers were similar between groups (Figure 3A), the hyperimmune group had significantly higher antibody ELISA titers to all viral glycoprotein complexes (Figure 3B).

Subsequently, cross strain protection was evaluated in convalescent groups of animals (22122-X1 or 22122-HI) by challenging animals with TAMYC strain virus (1×10^5 pfu, SQ). At subsequent time points post-infection (4, 8, 12 and 27 days post infection, dpi), three animals per group were randomly selected for evaluation of viral load (liver, lung, spleen and blood). The results demonstrated that the 22122-X1 group of animals (Figure 3C,D) had reduced the viral load in target organs compared to a control group of seronegative animals (Figure 3G,H). In the 22122-X1 group of animals, no virus was present in the blood by 12 dpi, and the virus was only detectable in the spleen and salivary gland by 27 dpi. However, the viral load in the salivary gland was still relatively high compared to control seronegative animals but with a 2 log reduction (Figure 3C,G). In hyperimmune animals (22122-HI), the viral load was substantially more reduced or non-detectable at different time points in target tissues (Figure 3E) and was below detection limits in the blood (Figure 3F). However, the virus continued to be shed in all tissues at 27 dpi with the viral load in salivary gland very similar to the viral load observed in the 22122-X1 convalescent group of animals. Overall, results indicated that the 22122 hyperimmune animals were better protected against the heterologous TAMYC virus challenge compared to the 22122-X1 convalescent animals or the DISCII vaccinated animals (Figure 2). However, the results indicate a limitation of cross strain protection by convalescent immunity from 22122 against re-infection by strain TAMYC, with the ability to prevent detectable viremia, but not virus dissemination to target organs.

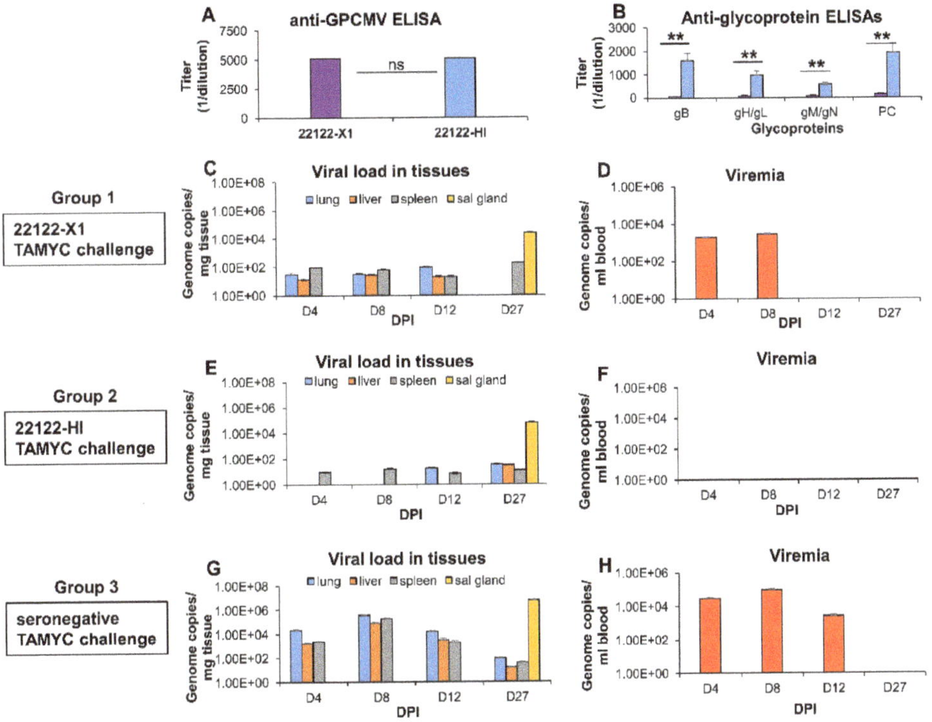

Figure 3. Comparative heterologous GPCMV (TAMYC strain) dissemination in convalescent (22122 strain) or control seronegative animals. Animals were infected with GPCMV (22122 strain) by single injection to establish convalescent natural immunity (22122-X1) or 3 sequential injections to establish hyperimmune status (22122-HI) prior to challenge (1×10^5 pfu, SQ) with GPCMV (TAMYC strain). Convalescent animals were evaluated for anti-GPCMV ELISA titer and specific anti-glycoprotein ELISA titers. (**A**) Mean anti-GPCMV ELISA titer comparison of sera from animals in 22122-X1 group (purple) or 22122-HI group (blue). (**B**) Comparative mean anti-glycoprotein complex ELISA titers (gB, gH/gL, gM/gN, PC) from sera of animals in 22122-X1 (purple) or 22122-HI group (blue). Statistical analysis determined by unpaired Student's *t* test; ** $p < 0.005$; ns = non-significant. (**C–H**) Comparative GPCMV (TAMYC strain) dissemination in convalescent animals: (**C**,**D**) group 1 (22122-X1); (**E**,**F**) group 2 hyperimmune (22122-HI); or (**G**,**H**) group 3 control seronegative animals. Animals ($n = 12$/group) were injected with 1×10^5 pfu, SQ of GPCMV (TAMYC strain). On days 4, 8, 12 and 27 post infection (dpi), 3 animals from each group were evaluated for viral load in target organs (lung, liver and spleen), by real-time PCR of DNA extracted from tissue. Viral load plotted as viral genome copies/mg tissue. Salivary gland (sal gland) tissue was only evaluated at 27 dpi (**C**,**E**,**G**). Viremia detected at 4, 8, 12 and 27 dpi was plotted as genome copies/mL blood (**D**,**F**,**H**).

3.4. Comparative Antibody Neutralization of 22122 and TAMYC GPCMV Strains by Hyperimmune Convalescent Sera from Animals (22122 or TAMYC Strain)

Since the 22122 strain-based immune response had a more limited impact against the heterologous TAMYC strain, we compared the antibody ELISA and neutralizing titers from the 22122 hyperimmune animals with the TAMYC hyperimmune animals. Specifically, we evaluated the ability of sera from hyperimmune animals (22122 or TAMYC) to neutralize homologous and heterologous virus infection on fibroblast and epithelial cells in an effort to determine if there was the potential for improvement of cross strain protection by a DISC vaccine strategy based on neutralizing antibodies. Pooled hyperimmune sera were derived from this current study (TAMYC strain hyperimmune sera) or from historical pooled sera (22122 strain hyperimmune sera) [38]. Figure 4 compares the pooled sera antibody ELISA titers from convalescent hyperimmune (22122 or TAMYC strain) animals: anti-GPCMV (Figure 4A), and specific glycoprotein complexes gB, gH/gL, gM/gM, and PC (Figure 4B,C).

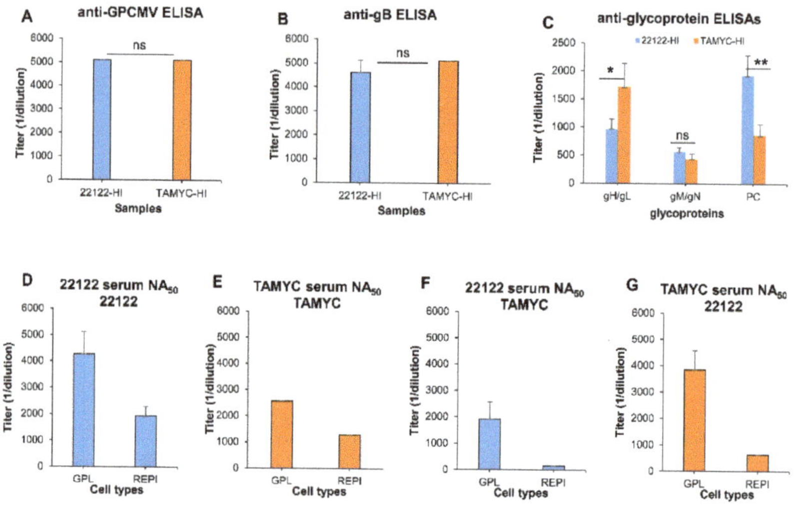

Figure 4. GPCMV hyperimmune convalescent sera antibody responses and virus neutralization on fibroblast and epithelial cells. (**A–C**) Comparative ELISAs of 22122-HI (blue) or TAMYC-HI (orange) sera. (**A**) Mean anti-GPCMV ELISA titers; (**B**) mean anti-gB glycoprotein ELISA titers; (**C**) mean anti-glycoprotein complex ELISA titers (gH/gL, gM/gN, PC) of sera from animals infected with GPCMV 22122 strain (22122-HI, blue) or TAMYC strain (TAMYC-HI, orange). (**D–G**) Comparative GPCMV neutralization (NA_{50}) on GPL (fibroblast) or REPI (epithelial) cells by hyperimmune sera. (**D**) 22122-HI sera (blue) neutralization (NA_{50}) of 22122 strain virus. (**E**) TAMYC-HI sera (orange) NA_{50} of TAMYC strain virus. (**F**) 22122-HI sera (blue) neutralization (NA_{50}) of TAMYC strain virus. (**G**) TAMYC-HI sera (orange) NA_{50} of 22122 strain virus. Mean ELISA and neutralization values are a result of assay triplicates with each sample run a minimum of three independent times. Statistical analysis determined by unpaired Student's *t* test; * $p < 0.05$; ** $p < 0.005$; ns = non-significant.

ELISAs were based on the 22122 strain GPCMV coating antigen and specific glycoprotein complexes. Results demonstrate that regardless of the strain, the anti-GPCMV ELISA titer was similar between groups (5120), as were anti-gB (approximately 5000). However, there was more of a contrast with the anti-gH/gL titer, which was higher for the TAMYC strain (1707 vs. 960). The anti-PC was two-fold higher for 22122 compared to TAMYC (1920 vs. 853). The response to gM/gN was relatively low for both TAMYC and 22122 sera.

The ability of antibodies in convalescent hyperimmune (22122 or TAMYC strain) sera to neutralize (NA_{50}) GPCMV (either 22122 or TAMYC strain) on fibroblast and epithelial cells were evaluated. Homologous neutralization of 22122 pooled sera against 22122 strain virus was most effective on GPL fibroblasts (titer = 4267) but had >two-fold lower NA_{50} titers on REPI epithelial cells (titer = 1920) (Figure 4D). The TAMYC sera of homologous TAMYC strain virus neutralization (Figure 1E) were also more effective on GPL fibroblasts (titer = 2560) compared to on epithelial cells (titer = 1280), with two-fold lower NA_{50} on REPI than on GPL cells. However, compared to 22122 sera homologous 22122 strain virus neutralization, titers on both fibroblast and epithelial cells were lower. In cross protective neutralization assays, the effectiveness of 22122 sera neutralization against heterologous TAMYC strain virus was evaluated (Figure 4F). Cross neutralization on both fibroblast (titer = 1920) and epithelial cells (titer = 160) was lower (Figure 4F) compared to homologous neutralization assays (Figure 4D). On GPL cells, the NA_{50} titer was >two-fold lower, while the titer on REPI cells decreased by 12-fold. The reverse comparative evaluation of TAMYC sera of the heterologous 22122 strain was evaluated (Figure 4G). TAMYC sera were more effective against the 22122 strain on GPL (titer = 3840) compared to REPI cells (titer = 640), Figure 4G. TAMYC sera had three-fold lower NA_{50} titers against the 22122 strain on epithelial cells, compared to the 22122 sera of the 22122 strain (Figure 4D,G). Overall, it was concluded that convalescent hyperimmune sera had the ability to neutralize virus infection but worked best on fibroblast cells compared to epithelial cells. Additionally, virus neutralizations of the 22122 strain by homologous sera (22122) and TAMYC sera (heterologous) were highly effective especially on fibroblast cells where NA_{50} titers were similar. In contrast, homologous and heterologous sera were less effective against the TAMYC virus, with 22122 sera particularly limited in NA_{50} titers against TAMYC epithelial infection (Figure 4F), compared to homologous NA_{50} titers (Figure 4G) against TAMYC on REPI cells. This potentially indicated that a DISC vaccine strategy based on strain 22122 is likely to be less effective against the GPCMV TAMYC strain virus challenge or similar clinical strain which is supported by vaccine protection outcome findings (Figure 2). Overall, a DISC vaccine based on a clinical strain (TAMYC) might have better efficacy against GPCMV homologous and heterologous infections. Potentially, this indicates a limitation of the current HCMV DISC vaccine strategy, which is based on a lab-adapted AD169 HCMV strain [47].

4. Discussion

An important requirement of an effective CMV vaccine is an ability to provide protection greater than that of convalescent natural immunity because the risk of congenital CMV is not only by primary infection during pregnancy but also from re-infection by new strains of the virus. Indeed, it is the ability to attain significant cross strain protection that likely increases the challenge for a successful vaccine against congenital CMV. Although preclinical animal models are available for the evaluation of CMV vaccine efficacy, they potentially suffer from various factors that reduce the translational impact. Firstly, HCMV cannot be directly studied in an animal model because of species specificity, which precludes direct evaluation of HCMV that might be available for other viral pathogens in animals models (e.g., influenza virus) [55]. Consequently, animal species-specific CMV studies are necessary. Although mouse models of murine cytomegalovirus have the advantage of powerful immunological tools, and gene knockout animals, there is a lack of strain variation in MCMV at the amino acid protein coding sequence level which limits the ability to evaluate the impact of viral strain infection on vaccine protection. The most commonly studied strains (K181 and Smith) are identical at the protein level [56]. Furthermore, MCMV does not cause congenital CMV, nor does it encode a PC. MCMV encodes a second gH-based trimer more similar to Epstein-Barr virus [57], which affects the translational impact of MCMV vaccine studies.

Although a NHP congenital CMV model with RhCMV has recently been developed for congenital CMV [58], no vaccine protection studies against vertical transmission have been evaluated. Importantly, RhCMV encodes a homolog PC that is required for virus tropism to non-fibroblast cells and pathogenicity in the NHP model [59]. Interestingly, a hyperimmune globulin (HIG) therapy strategy in the NHP applied to pregnant CD4+ T cell-depleted animals resulted in protection against congenital RhCMV, which implied that neutralizing antibodies were sufficient to protect against congenital CMV, but protection required inclusion of potent antibodies to PC [60]. In contrast, HIG therapy against congenital CMV in a human clinical trial did not reach statistical significance [61,62]. Potentially, protection against congenital RhCMV may have requirements different from those for protection against congenital HCMV. However, in the congenital RhCMV studies, the virus was introduced by intravenous route, rendering it cell free and potentially easier to rapidly neutralize, which likely weakens the study. The major focus of RhCMV vaccine research with the NHP model has been on horizontal transmission with varying levels of success, but no specific approach has attained sterilizing immunity [63]. Although a DISC vaccine strategy has been developed for RhCMV, it is based on the knockout of the gL glycoprotein gene which forms the basis of two important gH-based glycoprotein complexes (gH/gL/gO and PC) that impact the immune response to these entry complexes [64]. The availability of various RhCMV strains enables the potential for evaluation of cross strain protection to a level more similar to that of the HCMV infection of humans. However, a significant limitation to this NHP model is the small number of available CMV negative animals, as well as the prohibitive cost involved that precludes high throughput vaccine studies against congenital CMV.

Consequently, the guinea pig remains an important model for the development of intervention strategies against congenital CMV. This animal model suffers from limitations associated with available reagents which impact various human disease models based on this animal. However, the recent in-depth sequencing of the guinea pig genome has enabled the application of the CRISPR/Cas9 gene knockout strategy, as well as the ability to generate synthetic genes for cellular innate immune studies [38,39,46,65]. Furthermore, our laboratory and other investigators have established novel non-fibroblast guinea pig cell lines for virus tropism studies. However, an additional limitation of this model has been the use of a single strain of GPCMV (22122), which was isolated more than 50 years ago and passaged multiple times on fibroblasts, increasing the likelihood of adaptation that potentially limits the pathogenicity of this virus, despite the ability to cause congenital infection. The lack of additional GPCMV strains available prevented an ability to evaluate cross strain protection by candidate CMV vaccine strategies. We consider the latter an important benchmark for advancement of any CMV candidate vaccine, and this was compounded by the recent milestone achievement of complete protection against congenital GPCMV (22122 strain) by the use of two different candidate vaccine approaches: DISC vaccine [38]; and interferon sensitive attenuated live vaccine strain [66]. The recent isolation of a new strain of GPCMV (TAMYC) [12] without passage on fibroblast cells has enabled the bar to be raised for vaccine efficacy studies in this model by the evaluation of cross strain protection by utilizing the TAMYC strain virus. As with clinical HCMV strains, the greatest range of sequence variation between 22122 and TAMYC strains is the gO protein with 25% difference at the predicted amino acid level [12]. Other viral glycoproteins additionally differ between strains but the difference is not as profound and similar to that seen between HCMV strains [12]. Importantly, the TAMYC strain virus encodes a PC similar to the 22122 strain virus [12].

The correlates of protection against congenital CMV are poorly understood, but it is thought that antibody response is a significant driver for protection. The gB protein is essential for both HCMV and GPCMV infection of all cell types and an immunodominant antibody target. Consequently, gB has been a central focus or corner stone of many vaccine strategies against CMV both in preclinical and clinical studies. However, a standalone gB vaccine fails to achieve better than 50% efficacy in the guinea pig or in clinical trials. A limitation of gB vaccine efficacy in the guinea pig model was, until recently, the use of various truncated gB constructs. These strategies lacked the ability to form a trimeric complex found on the virion, and therefore limited the vaccine neutralizing titer because of the absence of higher order antigens. We recently evaluated recombinant Ad vector vaccines encoding either GPCMV gB lacking a transmembrane domain or a full length gB. Although both vaccines produced similar high antibody titers, the full length gB vaccine (AdgBWT), capable of forming a trimeric complex, produced higher neutralizing titers on both fibroblast and non-fibroblast cell types [27]. The current DISC vaccine is capable of both monomeric and trimeric gB complex formation; the antibody titer is lower than that of the AdgB vaccine, but is considered to have similar anti-gB neutralizing titers to that of hyperimmune convalescent animals based on anti-gB sera absorption studies [38]. In HCMV, non-neutralizing gB antibodies also contribute to gB vaccine efficacy, and it is likely that the DISC vaccine also produces non-neutralizing antibodies not only to gB but to other viral antigens. The impact of non-neutralizing gB antibodies for GPCMV would appear to have a minimal impact on vaccine protection [27], but remains to be more fully evaluated in future studies. However, it is clear that the gB immune response is limited in efficacy as a vaccine candidate failing to fully protect against GPCMV (22122 strain), despite improvements in neutralizing titers. Additionally, the limitation of a gB-only based vaccine strategy is further compounded when evaluated for cross strain protection against the TAMYC strain virus, despite 99% similarity in amino acid sequence [48]. Importantly, the TAMYC strain virus is more similar to clinical HCMV strains, highly cell associated and preferentially is tropic for non-fibroblast cells, in contrast to 22122 strain GPCMV [12]. The failure of the gB vaccine to cross protect between strains has also been demonstrated in the RhCMV NHP horizontal transmission model [67], which further indicates the limitation of gB as a standalone CMV vaccine candidate.

In HCMV, the PC is a potent neutralizing target antigen in convalescent-phase patients and in vaccine studies [40,41,68]. In GPCMV, the PC is necessary for virus tropism to non-fibroblast cells (including epithelial, endothelial and trophoblasts) and congenital infection. Furthermore, inclusion of the PC in a GPCMV DISC vaccine strategy improved virus neutralization on non-fibroblast cells by generation of PC-specific neutralizing antibodies [38]. This resulted in complete protection against congenital CMV (22122 strain) in this animal model, as well as sterilizing immunity compared to a previous DISC vaccine lacking PC [24,38]. Additionally, the inclusion of the PC in a live attenuated GPCMV vaccine strategy also resulted in complete protection against congenital CMV [66]. These recent vaccine studies demonstrated the importance of the PC to improve vaccine efficacy in this animal model. Both approaches induce an immune response to all glycoprotein complexes, but the inclusion of the PC in the vaccine design dramatically improved the protective immune response [24,38,66,69]. However, the DISCII vaccine sera did not reach the level of virus neutralization on both fibroblast and epithelial cells against the 22122 strain observed for hyperimmune sera from animals convalescent for GPCMV (22122 strain). This suggests room for improvement of the vaccine neutralizing titer, more especially since the DISCII vaccine was less effective at neutralizing the heterologous TAMYC strain virus on both fibroblast and epithelial cells compared to the 22122 strain NA_{50} titers. Likely, there is a limitation of virus neutralization evoked by cross strain protection from the 22122 strain background, since the 22122 strain hyperimmune sera are less effective against the TAMYC virus. In contrast, TAMYC hyperimmune sera are more effective against the TAMYC virus, especially on epithelial cells with higher neutralizing titers, than against the 22122 strain. Potentially, this indicates that a DISC vaccine built in the backdrop of the clinical TAMYC strain may have better efficacy and cross strain protection, but awaits future study since no recombinant virus has been generated based on the TAMYC strain. This might also indicate a potential failing of an HCMV DISC vaccine strategy based on the backdrop of the AD169 strain; a fibroblast adapted HCMV strain with restored ability to express the PC [70]. Strain-specific neutralizing target antigens have been identified in HCMV, and most recently in gH [71], which are likely to impact vaccine efficacy.

As with an RhCMV gB-based vaccine strategy, an RhCMV PC-based vaccine failed to provide complete protection against horizontal viral transmission [72]. Potentially, this indicates a general failing of a gB or a PC-based standalone vaccine strategy which does re-enforce the advantage of a DISC vaccine approach. Recently, a potent therapeutic antibody was identified that targets both gB and PC in HCMV, which indicates the likely interdependent importance of both of these antigens as neutralizing targets and the value of including both antigens in CMV vaccine design [73]. Potentially, CMV DISC vaccine efficacy could be enhanced by the inclusion of gB or gH, and unique PC ORFs from various important divergent viral strains to improve cross strain protection. This is a possible avenue for study in future HCMV or animal CMV DISC vaccine design. It is important to note that the TAMYC strain mainly infects by cell-cell spread with limited levels of cell release virus, similar to HCMV clinical strains. Potentially, cell-cell spread limits the effect of neutralizing antibodies and may serve as an effective escape mechanism from the host antibody response.

In convalescent CMV immunity, the T cell response is considered to be important and likely contributes to protection against congenital CMV. Indeed, the evasion of CD8 T cell response is critical for CMV superinfection [74]. In addition to antibody response, the GPCMV DISC vaccine strategy has previously been shown to evoke a cell-mediated response against pp65 tegument protein (GP83) in both PC^+ and PC^- DISC vaccines [24,38]. In HCMV, pp65 is thought to be the immunodominant T cell target, but this may not equate with the most effective target antigen for a protective T cell response. The non-structural IE1 protein in HCMV induces a T cell response and has been demonstrated to be partially protective in RhCMV studies [75]. Potentially, other viral antigens also induce a cell-mediated immune response in GPCMV such as GPCMV IE1 [65], and this is currently under evaluation. In both HCMV and GPCMV, the pp65 tegument protein is an innate immune evasion factor targeting cGAS and IFI16 [46,76]. The GP83 cell-mediated response has been demonstrated to be partially protective in various vaccine strategies against GPCMV [30,45,46]. However, the protective effect of the GP83 antigen T cell response is further limited in the context of cross strain GPCMV protection. In a recent Ad vector vaccine study encoding GPCMV GP83 (AdGP83), we demonstrated AdGP83 induced a cell-mediated immune response similar to GPCMV convalescent and DISC vaccinated animals; however, cross strain protection against the TAMYC challenge virus in AdGP83 vaccinated animals was relatively poor compared to protection in the 22122 challenged animals [46]. This was despite a 100% identity in the predicted GP83 amino acid sequence between the GPCMV 22122 and TAMYC strains. Thus, although the DISC vaccine has been demonstrated to generate a cell mediated response to GP83, it is unlikely to be an effective cross protective antigen based on the AdGP83 based vaccine studies [46]. An ability to comprehensively evaluate the T cell response against GPCMV in the guinea pig is currently lacking, and is a limitation of studies in this model, and should be a focus for future development.

5. Conclusions

In conclusion, the current GPCMV DISC vaccine strategy, although highly successful against the homologous strain (22122 strain) virus challenge dissemination and congenital infection in the animal, fails to provide high level protection against the heterologous virus (TAMYC strain) challenge. Consequently, the current version of the DISC vaccine would be unlikely to provide a high level of protection against congenital infection, more especially given the sustained viral load in the blood in the TAMYC virus challenged vaccinated animals. The ability for a CMV vaccine to cross protect against infection by a new strain of virus is an important additional stage of evaluation for any pre-clinical CMV vaccine. Studies in GPCMV hyperimmune immune convalescent animals suggest that the efficacy of the current DISC vaccine can be improved, but this is likely to require modifications to the DISC vaccine to enhance both the antibody and cell-mediated immune response. Since the DISC vaccine virus is cloned as an infectious BAC plasmid, additional modifications are easily attained via modifications of the viral genome in bacteria. Overall, the current results suggest that an HCMV DISC vaccine strategy will also likely require additional modifications to maximize cross strain protection, which becomes a significant factor in areas or groups endemic for HCMV and the potential exposure to multiple strains of the virus.

Author Contributions: Conceptualization, A.M. and K.Y.C.; Methodology, A.M., K.Y.C. and N.S.E.-H.; Validation, A.M., K.Y.C. and N.S.E.-H.; Formal Analysis, A.M., K.Y.C. and N.S.E.-H.; Investigation, A.M., K.Y.C. and N.S.E.-H.; Resources, A.M. and K.Y.C.; Data Curation, A.M. and K.Y.C.; Writing—Original Draft Preparation, A.M., K.Y.C. and N.S.E.-H.; Writing—Review and Editing, A.M., K.Y.C. and N.S.E.-H.; Visualization, A.M., K.Y.C. and N.S.E.-H.; Supervision, A.M. and K.Y.C.; Project Administration, A.M. and K.Y.C.; Funding Acquisition, A.M. All authors have read and agreed to the published version of the manuscript.

Funding: Research was supported by funding from NIH. NIAID (R01AI098984; R01AI100933; R01AI155561) and NICHD (R01HD090065).

Institutional Review Board Statement: Animal studies. Guinea pig animal studies were performed under IACUC (Texas A&M University) permit 2017-0227. All study procedures were carried out in strict accordance with the recommendations in the "Guide for the Care and Use of Laboratory Animals of the National Institutes of Health".

Informed Consent Statement: Not applicable.

Data Availability Statement: Not applicable.

Acknowledgments: We would like to thank Michael A. McVoy (VCU) for the gift of the second-generation GPCMV BAC.

Conflicts of Interest: The authors declare no conflict of interest. The funders had no role in the design of the study; in the collection, analyses, or interpretation of data; in the writing of the manuscript, or in the decision to publish the results.

References

1. Ross, S.A.; Boppana, S.B. Congenital cytomegalovirus infection: Outcome and diagnosis. *Semin. Pediatr. Infect. Dis.* **2005**, *16*, 44–49. [CrossRef] [PubMed]
2. Griffiths, P.D.; Walter, S. Cytomegalovirus. *Curr. Opin. Infect. Dis.* **2005**, *18*, 241–245. [CrossRef] [PubMed]
3. Fowler, K.B.; Dahle, A.J.; Boppana, S.B.; Pass, R.F. Newborn hearing screening: Will children with hearing loss caused by congenital cytomegalovirus infection be missed? *J. Pediatr.* **1999**, *135*, 60–64. [CrossRef]
4. Manicklal, S.; Emery, V.C.; Lazzarotto, T.; Boppana, S.B.; Gupta, R.K. The "silent" global burden of congenital cytomegalovirus. *Clin. Microbiol. Rev.* **2013**, *26*, 86–102. [CrossRef]
5. Enders, G.; Daiminger, A.; Bader, U.; Exler, S.; Enders, M. Intrauterine transmission and clinical outcome of 248 pregnancies with primary cytomegalovirus infection in relation to gestational age. *J. Clin. Virol.* **2011**, *52*, 244–246. [CrossRef]
6. Fowler, K.B.; Stagno, S.; Pass, R.F. Maternal immunity and prevention of congenital cytomegalovirus infection. *JAMA* **2003**, *289*, 1008–1011. [CrossRef]
7. Sylwester, A.W.; Mitchell, B.L.; Edgar, J.B.; Taormina, C.; Pelte, C.; Ruchti, F.; Sleath, P.R.; Grabstein, K.H.; Hosken, N.A.; Kern, F.; et al. Broadly targeted human cytomegalovirus-specific CD4+ and CD8+ T cells dominate the memory compartments of exposed subjects. *J. Exp. Med.* **2005**, *202*, 673–685. [CrossRef]
8. Yue, Y.; Barry, P.A. Rhesus cytomegalovirus a nonhuman primate model for the study of human cytomegalovirus. *Adv. Virus Res.* **2008**, *72*, 207–226. [CrossRef]
9. Griffith, B.P.; McCormick, S.R.; Fong, C.K.; Lavallee, J.T.; Lucia, H.L.; Goff, E. The placenta as a site of cytomegalovirus infection in guinea pigs. *J. Virol.* **1985**, *55*, 402–409. [CrossRef]
10. Woolf, N.K.; Koehrn, F.J.; Harris, J.P.; Richman, D.D. Congenital cytomegalovirus labyrinthitis and sensorineural hearing loss in guinea pigs. *J. Infect. Dis.* **1989**, *160*, 929–937. [CrossRef]
11. Hartley, J.W.; Rowe, W.P.; Huebner, R.J. Serial propagation of the guinea pig salivary gland virus in tissue culture. *Proc. Soc. Exp. Biol. Med.* **1957**, *96*, 281–285. [CrossRef] [PubMed]
12. Choi, K.Y.; El-Hamdi, N.S.; McGregor, A. Convalescent Immunity to Guinea Pig Cytomegalovirus Induces Limited Cross Strain Protection against Re-Infection but High-Level Protection against Congenital Disease. *Int. J. Mol. Sci.* **2020**, *21*, 5997. [CrossRef] [PubMed]
13. Schleiss, M.R.; Permar, S.R.; Plotkin, S.A. Progress toward Development of a Vaccine against Congenital Cytomegalovirus Infection. *Clin. Vaccine Immunol.* **2017**, *24*, e00268-17. [CrossRef] [PubMed]
14. Tabata, T.; Petitt, M.; Fang-Hoover, J.; Freed, D.C.; Li, F.; An, Z.; Wang, D.; Fu, T.M.; Pereira, L. Neutralizing Monoclonal Antibodies Reduce Human Cytomegalovirus Infection and Spread in Developing Placentas. *Vaccines* **2019**, *7*, 135. [CrossRef] [PubMed]
15. Sandonis, V.; Garcia-Rios, E.; McConnell, M.J.; Perez-Romero, P. Role of Neutralizing Antibodies in CMV Infection: Implications for New Therapeutic Approaches. *Trends Microbiol.* **2020**, *28*, 900–912. [CrossRef] [PubMed]
16. Nelson, C.S.; Huffman, T.; Jenks, J.A.; Cisneros de la Rosa, E.; Xie, G.; Vandergrift, N.; Pass, R.F.; Pollara, J.; Permar, S.R. HCMV glycoprotein B subunit vaccine efficacy mediated by nonneutralizing antibody effector functions. *Proc. Natl. Acad. Sci. USA* **2018**, *115*, 6267–6272. [CrossRef]
17. Pass, R.F.; Zhang, C.; Evans, A.; Simpson, T.; Andrews, W.; Huang, M.L.; Corey, L.; Hill, J.; Davis, E.; Flanigan, C.; et al. Vaccine prevention of maternal cytomegalovirus infection. *N. Engl. J. Med.* **2009**, *360*, 1191–1199. [CrossRef]
18. Coleman, S.; Hornig, J.; Maddux, S.; Choi, K.Y.; McGregor, A. Viral Glycoprotein Complex Formation, Essential Function and Immunogenicity in the Guinea Pig Model for Cytomegalovirus. *PLoS ONE* **2015**, *10*, e0135567. [CrossRef]
19. Coleman, S.; Choi, K.Y.; Root, M.; McGregor, A. A Homolog Pentameric Complex Dictates Viral Epithelial Tropism, Pathogenicity and Congenital Infection Rate in Guinea Pig Cytomegalovirus. *PLoS Pathog.* **2016**, *12*, e1005755. [CrossRef]

20. Auerbach, M.; Yan, D.; Fouts, A.; Xu, M.; Estevez, A.; Austin, C.D.; Bazan, F.; Feierbach, B. Characterization of the guinea pig CMV gH/gL/GP129/GP131/GP133 complex in infection and spread. *Virology* **2013**, *441*, 75–84. [CrossRef]
21. Choi, K.Y.; El-Hamdi, N.; McGregor, A. Endothelial cell infection by guinea pig cytomegalovirus is a lytic or persistent infection dependent upon tissue origin but requires viral pentamer complex and pp65 tegument protein. *J. Virol.* **2021**.
22. Coleman, S.; Choi, K.Y.; McGregor, A. Cytomegalovirus UL128 homolog mutants that form a pentameric complex produce virus with impaired epithelial and trophoblast cell tropism and altered pathogenicity in the guinea pig. *Virology* **2017**, *509*, 205–221. [CrossRef]
23. Choi, K.Y.; El-Hamdi, N.S.; McGregor, A. Requirements for guinea pig cytomegalovirus tropism and antibody neutralization on placental amniotic sac cells. *J. Gen. Virol.* **2020**, *101*, 426–439. [CrossRef] [PubMed]
24. Choi, K.Y.; Root, M.; McGregor, A. A Novel Non-Replication-Competent Cytomegalovirus Capsid Mutant Vaccine Strategy Is Effective in Reducing Congenital Infection. *J. Virol.* **2016**, *90*, 7902–7919. [CrossRef] [PubMed]
25. Britt, W.J.; Harrison, C. Identification of an abundant disulfide-linked complex of glycoproteins in the envelope of guinea pig cytomegalovirus. *Virology* **1994**, *201*, 294–302. [CrossRef]
26. Schleiss, M.R.; Jensen, N.J. Cloning and expression of the guinea pig cytomegalovirus glycoprotein B (gB) in a recombinant baculovirus: Utility for vaccine studies for the prevention of experimental infection. *J. Virol. Methods* **2003**, *108*, 59–65. [CrossRef]
27. Choi, K.Y.; El-Hamdi, N.S.; McGregor, A. Neutralizing antibodies to gB based CMV vaccine requires full length antigen but reduced virus neutralization on non-fibroblast cells limits vaccine efficacy in the guinea pig model. *Vaccine* **2020**, *38*, 2340–2349. [CrossRef]
28. Schleiss, M.R.; Bourne, N.; Stroup, G.; Bravo, F.J.; Jensen, N.J.; Bernstein, D.I. Protection against congenital cytomegalovirus infection and disease in guinea pigs, conferred by a purified recombinant glycoprotein B vaccine. *J. Infect. Dis.* **2004**, *189*, 1374–1381. [CrossRef]
29. Hashimoto, K.; Yamada, S.; Katano, H.; Fukuchi, S.; Sato, Y.; Kato, M.; Yamaguchi, T.; Moriishi, K.; Inoue, N. Effects of immunization of pregnant guinea pigs with guinea pig cytomegalovirus glycoprotein B on viral spread in the placenta. *Vaccine* **2013**, *31*, 3199–3205. [CrossRef]
30. Cardin, R.D.; Bravo, F.J.; Pullum, D.A.; Orlinger, K.; Watson, E.M.; Aspoeck, A.; Fuhrmann, G.; Guirakhoo, F.; Monath, T.; Bernstein, D.I. Replication-defective lymphocytic choriomeningitis virus vectors expressing guinea pig cytomegalovirus gB and pp65 homologs are protective against congenital guinea pig cytomegalovirus infection. *Vaccine* **2016**, *34*, 1993–1999. [CrossRef]
31. Swanson, E.C.; Gillis, P.; Hernandez-Alvarado, N.; Fernandez-Alarcon, C.; Schmit, M.; Zabeli, J.C.; Wussow, F.; Diamond, D.J.; Schleiss, M.R. Comparison of monovalent glycoprotein B with bivalent gB/pp65 (GP83) vaccine for congenital cytomegalovirus infection in a guinea pig model: Inclusion of GP83 reduces gB antibody response but both vaccine approaches provide equivalent protection against pup mortality. *Vaccine* **2015**, *33*, 4013–4018. [CrossRef] [PubMed]
32. Martinez-Martin, N.; Marcandalli, J.; Huang, C.S.; Arthur, C.P.; Perotti, M.; Foglierini, M.; Ho, H.; Dosey, A.M.; Shriver, S.; Payandeh, J.; et al. An Unbiased Screen for Human Cytomegalovirus Identifies Neuropilin-2 as a Central Viral Receptor. *Cell* **2018**, *174*, 1158–1171.e1119. [CrossRef] [PubMed]
33. Xiaofei, E.; Meraner, P.; Lu, P.; Perreira, J.M.; Aker, A.M.; McDougall, W.M.; Zhuge, R.; Chan, G.C.; Gerstein, R.M.; Caposio, P.; et al. OR14I1 is a receptor for the human cytomegalovirus pentameric complex and defines viral epithelial cell tropism. *Proc. Natl. Acad. Sci. USA* **2019**, *116*, 7043–7052. [CrossRef]
34. Vanarsdall, A.L.; Pritchard, S.R.; Wisner, T.W.; Liu, J.; Jardetzky, T.S.; Johnson, D.C. CD147 Promotes Entry of Pentamer-Expressing Human Cytomegalovirus into Epithelial and Endothelial Cells. *mBio* **2018**, *9*, e00781-18. [CrossRef]
35. Stein, K.R.; Gardner, T.J.; Hernandez, R.E.; Kraus, T.A.; Duty, J.A.; Ubarretxena-Belandia, I.; Moran, T.M.; Tortorella, D. CD46 facilitates entry and dissemination of human cytomegalovirus. *Nat. Commun.* **2019**, *10*, 2699. [CrossRef]
36. Feire, A.L.; Koss, H.; Compton, T. Cellular integrins function as entry receptors for human cytomegalovirus via a highly conserved disintegrin-like domain. *Proc. Natl. Acad. Sci. USA* **2004**, *101*, 15470–15475. [CrossRef]
37. Wu, Y.; Prager, A.; Boos, S.; Resch, M.; Brizic, I.; Mach, M.; Wildner, S.; Scrivano, L.; Adler, B. Human cytomegalovirus glycoprotein complex gH/gL/gO uses PDGFR-alpha as a key for entry. *PLoS Pathog.* **2017**, *13*, e1006281. [CrossRef]
38. Choi, K.Y.; El-Hamdi, N.S.; McGregor, A. Inclusion of the Viral Pentamer Complex in a Vaccine Design Greatly Improves Protection against Congenital Cytomegalovirus in the Guinea Pig Model. *J. Virol.* **2019**, *93*, e01442-19. [CrossRef]
39. El-Hamdi, N.S.; Choi, K.Y.; McGregor, A. Guinea pig cytomegalovirus trimer complex gH/gL/gO uses PDGFRA as universal receptor for cell fusion and entry. *Virology* **2020**, *548*, 236–249. [CrossRef]
40. Freed, D.C.; Tang, Q.; Tang, A.; Li, F.; He, X.; Huang, Z.; Meng, W.; Xia, L.; Finnefrock, A.C.; Durr, E.; et al. Pentameric complex of viral glycoprotein H is the primary target for potent neutralization by a human cytomegalovirus vaccine. *Proc. Natl. Acad. Sci. USA* **2013**, *110*, E4997–E5005. [CrossRef]
41. Ha, S.; Li, F.; Troutman, M.C.; Freed, D.C.; Tang, A.; Loughney, J.W.; Wang, D.; Wang, I.M.; Vlasak, J.; Nickle, D.C.; et al. Neutralization of Diverse Human Cytomegalovirus Strains Conferred by Antibodies Targeting Viral gH/gL/pUL128-131 Pentameric Complex. *J. Virol.* **2017**, *91*, e02033-16. [CrossRef] [PubMed]
42. Chiuppesi, F.; Wussow, F.; Johnson, E.; Bian, C.; Zhuo, M.; Rajakumar, A.; Barry, P.A.; Britt, W.J.; Chakraborty, R.; Diamond, D.J. Vaccine-Derived Neutralizing Antibodies to the Human Cytomegalovirus gH/gL Pentamer Potently Block Primary Cytotrophoblast Infection. *J. Virol.* **2015**, *89*, 11884–11898. [CrossRef] [PubMed]

43. Wills, M.R.; Mason, G.M.; Sissons, J.G.P. Adaptive Cellular Immunity to Human Cytomegalovirus. In *Cytomegaloviruses: From Molecular Pathogenesis to Intervention*; Reddehase, M.J., Ed.; Caister Academic Press: Norfolk, UK, 2013; Volume II, pp. 142–172.
44. McGregor, A.; Liu, F.; Schleiss, M.R. Molecular, biological, and in vivo characterization of the guinea pig cytomegalovirus (CMV) homologs of the human CMV matrix proteins pp71 (UL82) and pp65 (UL83). *J. Virol.* **2004**, *78*, 9872–9889. [CrossRef]
45. Schleiss, M.; Lacayo, J.; Belkaid, Y.; McGregor, A.; Stroup, G.; Rayner, J.; Alterson, K.; Chulay, J.; Smith, J. Preconceptual administration of an alphavirus replicon UL83 (pp65 homolog) vaccine induces humoral and cellular immunity and improves pregnancy outcome in the guinea pig model of congenital cytomegalovirus infection. *J. Infect. Dis.* **2007**, *195*, 789–798. [CrossRef] [PubMed]
46. Choi, K.Y.; El-Hamdi, N.; Hornig, J.; McGregor, A. Guinea pig cytomegalovirus protective T cell antigen GP83 is a functional pp65 homolog for innate immune evasion and pentamer dependent virus tropism. *J. Virol.* **2021**, *95*, e00324-21. [CrossRef] [PubMed]
47. Wang, D.; Freed, D.C.; He, X.; Li, F.; Tang, A.; Cox, K.S.; Dubey, S.A.; Cole, S.; Medi, M.B.; Liu, Y.; et al. A replication-defective human cytomegalovirus vaccine for prevention of congenital infection. *Sci. Transl. Med.* **2016**, *8*, 362ra145. [CrossRef] [PubMed]
48. Choi, K.Y.; El-Hamdi, N.S.; McGregor, A. A trimeric capable gB CMV vaccine provides limited protection against a highly cell associated and epithelial tropic strain of cytomegalovirus in guinea pigs. *J. Gen. Virol.* **2021**, *102*, 001579. [CrossRef]
49. Yue, Y.; Zhou, S.S.; Barry, P.A. Antibody responses to rhesus cytomegalovirus glycoprotein B in naturally infected rhesus macaques. *J. Gen. Virol.* **2003**, *84*, 3371–3379. [CrossRef]
50. Ryckman, B.J.; Chase, M.C.; Johnson, D.C. HCMV gH/gL/UL128-131 interferes with virus entry into epithelial cells: Evidence for cell type-specific receptors. *Proc. Natl. Acad. Sci. USA* **2008**, *105*, 14118–14123. [CrossRef]
51. McGregor, A.; Choi, K.Y.; Schleiss, M.R. Guinea pig cytomegalovirus GP84 is a functional homolog of the human cytomegalovirus (HCMV) UL84 gene that can complement for the loss of UL84 in a chimeric HCMV. *Virology* **2011**, *410*, 76–87. [CrossRef]
52. Zhou, M.; Yu, Q.; Wechsler, A.; Ryckman, B.J. Comparative analysis of gO isoforms reveals that strains of human cytomegalovirus differ in the ratio of gH/gL/gO and gH/gL/UL128-131 in the virion envelope. *J. Virol.* **2013**, *87*, 9680–9690. [CrossRef]
53. Zhang, L.; Zhou, M.; Stanton, R.; Kamil, J.; Ryckman, B.J. Expression Levels of Glycoprotein O (gO) Vary between Strains of Human Cytomegalovirus, Influencing the Assembly of gH/gL Complexes and Virion Infectivity. *J. Virol.* **2018**, *92*, e00606-18. [CrossRef] [PubMed]
54. Day, L.Z.; Stegmann, C.; Schultz, E.P.; Lanchy, J.M.; Yu, Q.; Ryckman, B.J. Polymorphisms in Human Cytomegalovirus Glycoprotein O (gO) Exert Epistatic Influences on Cell-Free and Cell-to-Cell Spread and Antibody Neutralization on gH Epitopes. *J. Virol.* **2020**, *94*, e02051-19. [CrossRef] [PubMed]
55. Lowen, A.C.; Mubareka, S.; Tumpey, T.M.; Garcia-Sastre, A.; Palese, P. The guinea pig as a transmission model for human influenza viruses. *Proc. Natl. Acad. Sci. USA* **2006**, *103*, 9988–9992. [CrossRef] [PubMed]
56. Smith, L.M.; McWhorter, A.R.; Masters, L.L.; Shellam, G.R.; Redwood, A.J. Laboratory strains of murine cytomegalovirus are genetically similar to but phenotypically distinct from wild strains of virus. *J. Virol.* **2008**, *82*, 6689–6696. [CrossRef]
57. Wagner, F.M.; Brizic, I.; Prager, A.; Trsan, T.; Arapovic, M.; Lemmermann, N.A.; Podlech, J.; Reddehase, M.J.; Lemnitzer, F.; Bosse, J.B.; et al. The viral chemokine MCK-2 of murine cytomegalovirus promotes infection as part of a gH/gL/MCK-2 complex. *PLoS Pathog.* **2013**, *9*, e1003493. [CrossRef] [PubMed]
58. Roark, H.K.; Jenks, J.A.; Permar, S.R.; Schleiss, M.R. Animal Models of Congenital Cytomegalovirus Transmission: Implications for Vaccine Development. *J. Infect. Dis.* **2020**, *221*, S60–S73. [CrossRef] [PubMed]
59. Taher, H.; Mahyari, E.; Kreklywich, C.; Uebelhoer, L.S.; McArdle, M.R.; Mostrom, M.J.; Bhusari, A.; Nekorchuk, M.; E, X.; Whitmer, T.; et al. In vitro and in vivo characterization of a recombinant rhesus cytomegalovirus containing a complete genome. *PLoS Pathog.* **2020**, *16*, e1008666. [CrossRef]
60. Nelson, C.S.; Cruz, D.V.; Tran, D.; Bialas, K.M.; Stamper, L.; Wu, H.; Gilbert, M.; Blair, R.; Alvarez, X.; Itell, H.; et al. Preexisting antibodies can protect against congenital cytomegalovirus infection in monkeys. *JCI Insight* **2017**, *2*, e94002. [CrossRef]
61. Revello, M.G.; Lazzarotto, T.; Guerra, B.; Spinillo, A.; Ferrazzi, E.; Kustermann, A.; Guaschino, S.; Vergani, P.; Todros, T.; Frusca, T.; et al. A randomized trial of hyperimmune globulin to prevent congenital cytomegalovirus. *N. Engl. J. Med.* **2014**, *370*, 1316–1326. [CrossRef]
62. Hughes, B.L.; Clifton, R.G.; Rouse, D.J.; Saade, G.R.; Dinsmoor, M.J.; Reddy, U.M.; Pass, R.; Allard, D.; Mallett, G.; Fette, L.M.; et al. A Trial of Hyperimmune Globulin to Prevent Congenital Cytomegalovirus Infection. *N. Engl. J. Med.* **2021**, *385*, 436–444. [CrossRef] [PubMed]
63. Itell, H.L.; Kaur, A.; Deere, J.D.; Barry, P.A.; Permar, S.R. Rhesus monkeys for a nonhuman primate model of cytomegalovirus infections. *Curr. Opin. Virol.* **2017**, *25*, 126–133. [CrossRef] [PubMed]
64. Valencia, S.; Gill, R.B.; Dowdell, K.C.; Wang, Y.; Hornung, R.; Bowman, J.J.; Lacayo, J.C.; Cohen, J.I. Comparison of vaccination with rhesus CMV (RhCMV) soluble gB with a RhCMV replication-defective virus deleted for MHC class I immune evasion genes in a RhCMV challenge model. *Vaccine* **2019**, *37*, 333–342. [CrossRef]
65. Hornig, J.; Choi, K.Y.; McGregor, A. The essential role of guinea pig cytomegalovirus (GPCMV) IE1 and IE2 homologs in viral replication and IE1-mediated ND10 targeting. *Virology* **2017**, *504*, 122–140. [CrossRef] [PubMed]
66. Choi, K.Y.; McGregor, A. A Fully Protective Congenital CMV Vaccine Requires Neutralizing Antibodies to Viral Pentamer and gB Glycoprotein Complexes but a pp65 T-Cell Response Is Not Necessary. *Viruses* **2021**, *13*, 1467. [CrossRef] [PubMed]
67. Abel, K.; Strelow, L.; Yue, Y.; Eberhardt, M.K.; Schmidt, K.A.; Barry, P.A. A heterologous DNA prime/protein boost immunization strategy for rhesus cytomegalovirus. *Vaccine* **2008**, *26*, 6013–6025. [CrossRef]

68. Gerna, G.; Revello, M.G.; Baldanti, F.; Percivalle, E.; Lilleri, D. The pentameric complex of human Cytomegalovirus: Cell tropism, virus dissemination, immune response and vaccine development. *J. Gen. Virol.* **2017**, *98*, 2215–2234. [CrossRef]
69. Schleiss, M.R.; Buus, R.; Choi, K.Y.; McGregor, A. An Attenuated CMV Vaccine with a Deletion in Tegument Protein GP83 (pp65 Homolog) Protects against Placental Infection and Improves Pregnancy Outcome in a Guinea Pig Challenge Model. *Future Virol.* **2013**, *8*, 1151–1160. [CrossRef]
70. Liu, Y.; Freed, D.C.; Li, L.; Tang, A.; Li, F.; Murray, E.M.; Adler, S.P.; McVoy, M.A.; Rupp, R.E.; Barrett, D.; et al. A Replication-Defective Human Cytomegalovirus Vaccine Elicits Humoral Immune Responses Analogous to Those with Natural Infection. *J. Virol.* **2019**, *93*, e00747-19. [CrossRef]
71. Thomas, M.; Kropff, B.; Schneider, A.; Winkler, T.H.; Gorzer, I.; Sticht, H.; Britt, W.J.; Mach, M.; Reuter, N. A Novel Strain-Specific Neutralizing Epitope on Glycoprotein H of Human Cytomegalovirus. *J. Virol.* **2021**, *95*, e0065721. [CrossRef]
72. Wussow, F.; Yue, Y.; Martinez, J.; Deere, J.; Longmate, J.; Herrmann, A.; Barry, P.; Diamond, D. A vaccine based on the rhesus cytomegalovirus UL128 complex induces broadly neutralizing antibodies in rhesus macaques. *J. Virol.* **2013**, *87*, 1322–1332. [CrossRef] [PubMed]
73. Su, H.; Ye, X.; Freed, D.C.; Li, L.; Ku, Z.; Xiong, W.; Gao, P.; Liu, X.; Montgomery, D.; Xu, W.; et al. Potent Bispecific Neutralizing Antibody Targeting Glycoprotein B and the gH/gL/pUL128/130/131 Complex of Human Cytomegalovirus. *Antimicrob. Agents Chemother.* **2021**, *65*, e02422-20. [CrossRef] [PubMed]
74. Hansen, S.G.; Powers, C.J.; Richards, R.; Ventura, A.B.; Ford, J.C.; Siess, D.; Axthelm, M.K.; Nelson, J.A.; Jarvis, M.A.; Picker, L.J.; et al. Evasion of CD8+ T cells is critical for superinfection by cytomegalovirus. *Science* **2010**, *328*, 102–106. [CrossRef] [PubMed]
75. Abel, K.; Martinez, J.; Yue, Y.; Lacey, S.F.; Wang, Z.; Strelow, L.; Dasgupta, A.; Li, Z.; Schmidt, K.A.; Oxford, K.L.; et al. Vaccine-induced control of viral shedding following rhesus cytomegalovirus challenge in rhesus macaques. *J. Virol.* **2011**, *85*, 2878–2890. [CrossRef]
76. Biolatti, M.; Dell'Oste, V.; Pautasso, S.; Gugliesi, F.; von Einem, J.; Krapp, C.; Jakobsen, M.R.; Borgogna, C.; Gariglio, M.; De Andrea, M.; et al. Human Cytomegalovirus Tegument Protein pp65 (pUL83) Dampens Type I Interferon Production by Inactivating the DNA Sensor cGAS without Affecting STING. *J. Virol.* **2018**, *92*, e01774-17. [CrossRef] [PubMed]

viruses

Review

Antiviral Active Compounds Derived from Natural Sources against Herpes Simplex Viruses

Lukas van de Sand [1,†], Maren Bormann [1,†], Yasmin Schmitz [2], Christiane Silke Heilingloh [1], Oliver Witzke [1] and Adalbert Krawczyk [1,2,*]

1 West German Centre of Infectious Diseases, Department of Infectious Diseases, University Hospital Essen, University of Duisburg-Essen, 45147 Essen, Germany; lukas.vandesand@uk-essen.de (L.v.d.S.); maren.bormann@uk-essen.de (M.B.); christiane.heilingloh@uk-essen.de (C.S.H.); oliver.witzke@uk-essen.de (O.W.)
2 Institute of Virology, University Hospital Essen, University of Duisburg-Essen, 45147 Essen, Germany; yasmin.schmitz@stud.uni-due.de
* Correspondence: adalbert.krawczyk@uni-due.de
† These authors contributed equally to this work.

Abstract: Herpes simplex viruses (HSV) are ubiquitously distributed with a seroprevalence ranging up to 95% in the adult population. Refractory viral infections with herpes simplex virus type 1 (HSV-1) and type 2 (HSV-2) represent a major global health issue. In particular, the increasing occurrence of resistance to conventional antiviral drugs make the therapy of such infections even more challenging. For instance, the frequent and long-term use of acyclovir and other nucleoside analogues targeting the viral DNA-polymerase enhance the development of resistant viruses. Particularly, the incidental increase of those strains in immunocompromised patients is alarming and represent a major health concern. Alternative treatment concepts are clearly needed. Natural products such as herbal medicines showed antiherpetic activity in vitro and in vivo and proved to be an excellent source for the discovery and isolation of novel antivirals. By this means, numerous plant-derived compounds with antiviral or antimicrobial activity could be isolated. Natural medicines and their ingredients are well-tolerated and could be a good alternative for treating herpes simplex virus infections. This review provides an overview of the recent status of natural sources such as plants, bacteria, fungi, and their ingredients with antiviral activity against herpes simplex viruses. Furthermore, we highlight the most potent herbal medicines and ingredients as promising candidates for clinical investigation and give an overview about the most important drug classes along with their potential antiviral mechanisms. The content of this review is based on articles that were published between 1996 and 2021.

Keywords: herpes simplex viruses; natural products; antiherpetic drugs; resistance

Citation: van de Sand, L.; Bormann, M.; Schmitz, Y.; Heilingloh, C.S.; Witzke, O.; Krawczyk, A. Antiviral Active Compounds Derived from Natural Sources against Herpes Simplex Viruses. *Viruses* **2021**, *13*, 1386. https://doi.org/10.3390/v13071386

Academic Editor: Barry J. Margulies

Received: 12 June 2021
Accepted: 14 July 2021
Published: 16 July 2021

1. Introduction

Herpes simplex virus infections are considered a major public health issue worldwide. These human pathogen DNA viruses belong to the family of *Alphaherpesvirinae*. Upon primary infection, the herpes simplex viruses type 1 and 2 (HSV-1 and HSV-2) persist lifelong in the autonomic and sensory ganglia of its host. Especially HSV-1 infections are ubiquitously distributed with a seroprevalence ranging up to 95% in the adult population [1]. After reactivation, HSV may cause symptoms ranging from painful, but self-limited infections of the oral or genital mucosa to severe infections of the eye or life-threatening infections in immunocompromised hosts or newborns [2,3]. Active HSV-1 infections are usually associated with oral or facial herpes, while HSV-2 predominately causes genital infections. Reactivated HSV-2 infections often exhibit painful genital lesions providing a higher risk for other sexually transmitted diseases and invasive cervical carcinoma [4].

Although numerous vaccine candidates have been investigated in clinical trials, there is no licensed vaccine available for the prevention of HSV infections. Over the last decades, many different antiviral drugs targeting the viral DNA-polymerase were approved for the treatment of acute HSV infections. The most widely used antiviral agents against HSV are acyclovir (ACV), valacyclovir, famciclovir, cidofovir, and foscarnet. ACV and the related nucleoside analogues can successfully inhibit viral replication and thereby mediate cure from HSV-related symptoms, but the emergence of drug resistance to ACV has created a barrier for the treatment of HSV infections [5]. Moreover, it has been demonstrated that ACV therapy in HIV/HSV-co-infected patients reduces HIV serum levels and may protract the necessity of an antiretroviral therapy [6–8]. However, ACV may interact directly with the HIV reverse transcriptase in HIV-infected cells, which may increase the occurrence of the reverse transcriptase mutants that are associated with a reduced sensitivity of the virus to antiretroviral therapy [9,10]. Furthermore, corneal morbidity and blindness are common issues of ACV-refractory HSV infections of the cornea in industrial nations [11]. ACV-resistant infections are frequently observed in immunocompromised patients. Due to a long-term prophylactic or pre-emptive antiviral treatment in these patients, the occurrence of ACV resistance is particularly high in this group [12]. In the average adult population, the frequency of ACV-resistant HSV was determined with 0.27% (n = 368) [12]. In contrast, the frequency of ACV-resistant HSV was assessed with 7.03% in immunocompromised patients [12]. The highest rates of ACV resistance were reported in patients undergoing hematopoietic stem cell transplantation (14.3%), followed by HIV-infected patients (3.92%) or patients suffering from various tumor diseases (3.85%) [12]. Cross-resistance to other nucleoside analogs targeting the viral HSV thymidine kinase (TK) are frequent, since a reduced sensitivity of HSV to ACV is mostly caused by mutations in the TK gene [5,13]. However, resistance not only emerges against drugs such as famciclovir or penciclovir that target HSV-TK but also against the viral DNA-polymerase inhibitors foscarnet and cidofovir [14], the latter severely in patients undergoing stem cell transplantation [12]. DNA-polymerase inhibitors can be used for the treatment of ACV-resistant HSV infections. However, their use is limited due to possible serious side effects, especially in patients with comorbidities [5].

Clearly, there is an urgent need to explore new effective and well-tolerated approaches for the treatment of HSV infections and reactivations. Traditional herbal medicines are an abundant source of antimicrobial or antiviral active substances. Plant extracts and other natural products have been used for hundreds of years for the treatment of infectious diseases. We screened the PubMed database to find relevant articles by using the keywords natural products, medicinal plants, medicinal herbs, herbal medicine, plant oils, herpes simplex virus, herpes labialis, and herpes genitalis. Articles included in our analysis were published from 1996 to 2021. We searched for studies that described compounds that were isolated from natural sources such as plants, fungi, and other sources. We focused on well-characterized compounds with already uncovered mechanisms of how these compounds interfere with the viral replication. This strategy allows for conclusions about the potential antiviral activity of these compounds against ACV-resistant viruses. The review gives an overview of the distinct compounds isolated from plants and other natural sources and summarizes the results from in vitro and in vivo studies conducted thus far.

2. Antiviral Active Ingredients from Natural Sources

Herbal medicines have been used for centuries to treat infectious diseases. Within the last decades, numerous compounds with antiviral activity against HSV and other viruses could be isolated from distinct natural sources such as plants or fungi. The antiviral active ingredients include alkaloids, terpenes, polysaccharides, flavonoids, phenolic acids, and steroids (Figure 1). The compounds inhibit the viral replication by using different mechanisms, which are summarized in Figure 2 and Table 1 and described below in more detail.

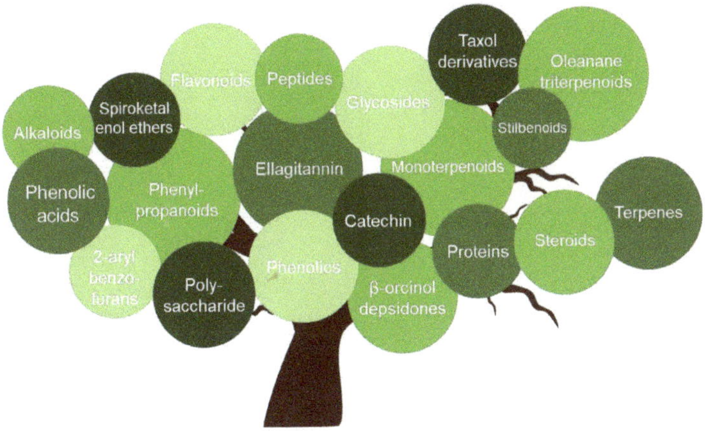

Figure 1. Classification of antiherpetic agents derived from natural sources. Natural sources such as plants or fungi are rich in different groups of bioactive compounds. Several of these groups (e.g., alkaloids, terpenes, polysaccharides, flavonoids, phenolic acids, and steroids) were identified as antiviral active agents against HSV-1 and HSV-2.

Table 1. Chemical compounds and their anti-HSV activity. CC_{50} = 50% cytotoxic concentration, EC_{50} = 50% effective concentration, IC_{50} = 50% inhibitory concentration, SI = selectivity index, HSV = herpes simplex virus, CPE = cytopathogenic effect, XTT = 2,3-bis[2-methoxy-4-nitro-5-sulphophenyl]-5-[(phenylamino)carbonyl-2H-tetrazolium hydroxide], ELISA = enzyme-linked immunosorbent assay, MAPK = mitogen-activated protein kinase, CCECs = cerebral capillary vessel endothelial cells, PMNs = polymorphonuclear leukocytes, TK = thymidine kinase.

No.	Group	Compound	Plant/Other	Assay Employed; Cell Line	CC_{50}	HSV-1 EC_{50}/IC_{50}; SI	HSV-2 EC_{50}/IC_{50}; SI	Virus	Mechanism of Action/Target Structure	Refs.
1	Alkaloid	Harmine	*Peganum harmala*	CPE; Hec-1-A cells	>300 µM	4.56 µM	1.47 µM	HSV-1 F; HSV-2 G	Tyrosine phosphorylation-regulated kinase inhibitor; downregulation of cellular NF-κB and MAPK pathways.	[15,16]
2	Anthraquinone	Emodin	*Rheum tanguticum*	CPE; HEp-2 cells	>1000 µg/mL (>3.7 mM)	n/A	n/A	HSV-1 F; HSV-2 (333)	Inhibition of viral replication.	[17]
3	Catechin	Epigallocatechin (EGC)	*Thea sinensis* L.	CPE; Vero cells	500 µM	4 µM; 125	63 µM; 7.9	HSV-1 KOS; HSV-2 G	Glycoproteins B and D.	[18,19]
4		Palmitoyl-EGCG (*p*-EGCG)		Plaque assay; Vero cells	>75 µM	<50 µM	n/A	HSV-1 UL46	Glycoprotein D expression is reduced.	[20]
5		Samarangenin B (Sam B)	*Limonium sinense* L.		>100 µM	11.4 µM	n/A	HSV-1 KOS	Suppresses expression of ICP0 and ICP4 genes and viral DNA-polymerase (ß transcripts).	[21,22]
6	Ellagitannin	Casuarinin	*Terminalia arjuna Linn*	Plaque assay; Vero cells	89 ± 1 µM	n/A	1.5 µM; 59	HSV-2 (196)	Inhibition of viral attachment and penetration.	[23]
7	Flavonoid	Baicalein	*Scutellaria baicalensis*	Plaque assay; Vero cells	>200 µM	n/A	12.4 µM; >16.1	HSV-1 F	Inactivation of free viral particles and downregulating cellular NF-κB.	[24]
				HaCat cells	>200 µM	n/A	20.1 µM; >9.95			
8		(−)-epigallocatechin 3-O-gallate (EGCG)	*Camellia sinensis*	Titer reduction; Vero cells	n/A	$10^{2.0}/10^{4.4}$ reduction at 100 µM	$10^{4.0-5.0}/10^{4.0}$ reduction at 100 µM	HSV-1 F; HSV-2 (333)	Glycoproteins B and D.	[25]
9		Galangin	*Helichrysum aureonitens*	CPE; Vero cells	1000 µM	2.5 µM; 400	n/A	HSV-1 KOS	Inhibition of of viral adsorption.	[18]
10		Houttuynoid A	*Houttuynia cordata*	Plaque assay; Vero cells	166.36 ± 9.27 µM	23.50 ± 1.82 µM		HSV-1 F	Blocking viral attachment.	[26]
11		Isoquercitrin	*Houttuynia cordata*		>100 µg/mL (215.34 µM)	0.42 µg/mL (0.9 µM); >512.8			Downregulation of cellular NF-κB.	[27]
12		Quercetin	*Caesalpinia pulcherrima*	XTT; BCC-1/KMC cells	496.9 µg/mL (16.44 mM)	22.6 ± 4.2 µg/mL (74.78 ± 13.89 µM); 22.0	86.7 ± 7.4 µg/mL (286.86 ± 24.48); 5.7	HSV-1 KOS; HSV-2 (196)	Downregulation of cellular NF-κB and blocks viral entry (gD cellular binding site).	[27,28]
13	Glycosides	Pterocarnin A	*Pterocarya stenoptera*	XTT; Vero cells	31.7 ± 1.6 µM	n/A	5.4 ± 0.3 µM; 5.9	HSV-2 (196)	Inhibition of of viral attachment.	[29]

Table 1. *Cont.*

No.	Group	Compound	Plant/Other	Assay Employed; Cell Line	CC_{50}	HSV-1 EC_{50}/IC_{50}; SI	HSV-2 EC_{50}/IC_{50}; SI	Virus	Mechanism of Action/Target Structure	Refs.
14	Harmaline	7-methoxy-1-methyl-4,9-dihydro-3H-pyrido[3,4-b]indole (HM)	*Ophiorrhiza nicobarica Balkr*	Plague assay; Vero cells	30 μg/mL (120.14 μM)	1.1 ± 0.1 μg/mL (4.41 ± 0.4 μM); 27.27	1.5 ± 0.1 μg/mL (6.01 ± 0.4 μM); 20	HSV-1 F; HSV-2 G	Suppression of viral immediate early gene expression.	[30,31]
15	Monoterpenoid	Geraniol	*Thymus bovei*	Titer reduction; Vero cells	>210 μg/mL (1361.42 μM)	n/A	1.92 ± 0.84 μg/mL (12.45 ± 5.45 μM); >109.38	HSV-2	In silico: Interacts with HSV-2 protease.	[32]
16	Oleanane triterpenoid	Glycyrrhetinic acid methylester	*Glycyrrhiza glabra*	Plaque assay; Vero cells	>207 μM	8.1 ± 0.2 μM/mL; >26	n/A	HSV-1 KOS	Inhibition of HSV-1 replication.	[33]
17		Glycyrrhetinic acid			84.0 ± 2.8 μM	21.7 ± 0.6 μM; 3.9			Induces the autophagy activator Beclin 1 → blocks HSV replication.	[33]
18		Glycyrrhizin			>608 μM	225 ± 24.1 μM/mL; >2.7			Reduces adhesion force between CCECs and PMNs.	[33,34]
19	Phenolic acid	Chebulinic acid	*Terminalia chebula*	Plaque assay; Vero cells	>200 μg/mL	17.02 ± 2.82 μM; 18.62	0.06 ± 0.002 μg/mL	HSV-1 KOS; HSV-2 G	Prevention of HSV-1 glycoprotein-mediated cell fusion events and attachment of HSV-2.	[35,36]
20		Gallic acid	*Galla*	Plaque assay; Vero cells and GMK AH1	668.7 ± 54.5 μM	57.1 ± 2.3 μM; 11.72	33.56; 64.35 μM (during; after infection)	HSV-1 KOS; HSV-2 (333)	Inhibition of ICP2, gC, gD, and VP5 expression (effects on viral attachment).	[37,38]
21	Phenolic	Curcumin	*The curry spice turmeric*	CPE; Vero cells	49.8 ± 0.4 μg/mL (135.18 ± 1.09 μM)	n/A	n/A	HSV-1 (17)	P300/CBP histone acetyltransferase.	[39,40]
22	Phenylpropanoid	Verbascoside	*Lepechinia speciosa*	Plaque assay; Vero cells	>200 μg/mL (320.21 μM)	58 μg/mL (92.86 μM); >3.4	8.9 μg/mL (14.25 μM); >22.4	HSV-1; HSV-2 (clinical isolates)	HSV-1: prevention of viral adsorption, intracellular viral inhibition; HSV-2: inhibition of attachment and penetration.	[41]
23	Polysaccharide	MI-S	*Agaricus brasiliensis*	Plaque assay; Vero cells	2415.29 ± 389.21 μg/mL (134.18 ± 21.61 μM)	1.24 ± 0.05 μg/mL (0.07 μM), 1948; 5.50 ± 0.58 μg/mL (0.31 ± 0.03 μM), 439 (during; after infection)	0.39 ± 0.17 μg/mL (0.02 ± 0.01 μM), 6193; 4.30 ± 0.36 μg/mL (0.24 ± 0.02 μM), 562 (during; after infection)	HSV-1 KOS; HSV-2 333	Inhibition of attachment, penetration and cell-to-cell spread.	[42]

Table 1. *Cont.*

No.	Group	Compound	Plant/Other	Assay Employed; Cell Line	CC_{50}	HSV-1 EC_{50}/IC_{50}; SI	HSV-2 EC_{50}/IC_{50}; SI	Virus	Mechanism of Action/Target Structure	Refs.
24		Scleroglucan	*Scierotium glucanicum*	CPE; Vero cells	400 μg/mL (559.83 μM)	5 μg/mL (7 μM); 80	*n*/A	HSV-1 F	Glycoproteins of HSV-1 (inhibits adsorption step).	[43]
25	Spiroketal-enol ether derivative	(E)-2-(2,4-hexa-diynyliden)-1,6dioxaspiro[4.5] dec-3-ene	*Tanacetum vulgare*	Time-of-addition assay; Vero cells	>30 μg/mL (>149.83 μM)	0.146 ± 0.013 μg/mL (0.73 ± 0.06 μM); >205	0.127 ± 0.009 μg/mL (0.63 ± 0.04 μM); >236	HSV-1 (AY240815.1); HSV-2 (HM011430.1)	Suppression of viral RNA synthesis.	[44]
26	Steroid	Halistanol sulfate	*Petromica citrina*	Plaque assay; Vero cells	13.83 ± 3.75 μg/mL (20.08 ± 5.44 μM)	5.63 ± 1.3 μg/mL (8.17 ± 1.89 μM); 2.46	*n*/A	HSV-1 KOS	Inhibition of attachment and penetration. Impairs HSV-1 gD and ICP27 levels.	[45]
27	Stilbenoid and 2-arylbenzofuran	Kuwanon X	*Moru salba* L.	Plaque assay; Vero cells	80.3 ± 3.2 μg/mL (128.15 ± 5.12 μM)	2.2 ± 0.1 μg/mL (3.5 ± 0.16 μM); 37	2.5 ± 0.3 μg/mL (3.99 ± 0.48 μM); 32	HSV-1 (15577); HSV-2 (333)	Downregulation of cellular NF-κB and viral RNA/DNA synthesis.	[46]
28		Oxyresveratrol	*Artocarpus lakoocha*		>100 μM	63.5 μM	55.3 μM	HSV-1; HSV-2	Inhibition of early and late replication.	[47,48]
29	Taxol derivative	*n*-benzoyl-(2′R,3′S)-3′phenylisoserine	*Lactarius*	CPE; Vero cells	>500 μg/mL	21.7 μg/mL (76.06 μM); >23	*n*/A	HSV-1 (McIntyre)	Inhibition of HSV-1 replication (possibly related to mitotic division).	[49]
30	Terpene	28-Deacetylsendanin (28-DAS)	*Melia azedarach*	ELISA; Vero cells	>400 μg/mL (696.11 μM)	1.46 μg/mL (2.54 μM)	*n*/A	HSV-1 (McIntyre)	Reduces activity of TK.	[50]
31		Isoborneol	*Salvia fruticosa*	Plaque assay; Vero cells	*n*/A	*n*/A		HSV-1 F	Affected TK-independent glycosylation process of viral glycoproteins B and D.	[51]
32		1-cinnamoyl-3,11-dihydroxymeliacarpin (CDM)	*Melia azedarach*	Plaque assay; HCLE cells	>100 μM	0.78 μM		HSV-1 KOS	Inhibition of glycoproteins B, gC, gD intracellular trafficking and downregulates cellular NF-κB.	[52–54]
33		Triptofordin C-2	*Tripterygium wilfordii*	Plaque assay; HeLa cells	89 ± 9.5 μg/mL (145.76 ± 15.56 μM)	3.7 ± 0.90 μg/mL (6.06 ± 1.47 μM); 24 ± 3.2		HSV-1 HF	Suppression of viral immediate early gene expression.	[55]

Table 1. *Cont.*

No.	Group	Compound	Plant/Other	Assay Employed; Cell Line	CC_{50}	HSV-1 EC_{50}/IC_{50}; SI	HSV-2 EC_{50}/IC_{50}; SI	Virus	Mechanism of Action/Target Structure	Refs.
34	β-orcinol depsidone	Psoromic acid	*Usnea*	Plaque assay; Vero cells	>310 µM	1.9 ± 0.42 µM; >163.2	2.7 ± 0.43 µM; 114.8	HSV-1 KOS; HSV-2 (A234)	Inhibition of HSV replication: HSV-1 DNA-polymerase in vitro; HSV-2 DNA-polymerase in silico.	[56]
35	Peptide	Griffithsin	*Griffithsia*	Plaque assay; CaSki	no cytotoxic effect	*n*/A	2.3 µg/mL (0.18 µM)	HSV-2 (333)	Inhibition of viral attachment (cell-to-cell spread).	[57]
36		Subtilosin	*Bacillus amyloliquefaciens*	Plaque assay; Vero cells	314 µg/mL (92.3 µM)	9.6 µg/mL (2.82 µM); 33	18.2 µg/mL (5.35 µM); 17.4	HSV-1 F; HSV-2 G	Late stages of the viral replicative cycle and intracellular glycoprotein transport.	[58,59]
37		Trichosanthin (TCS)	*Trichosanthes kirilowii*	ELISA; Vero cells	416.5 ± 34.5 µg/mL (15.42 ± 1.28 µM)	38.4 ± 17.5 µg/mL (1.42 ± 0.65 µM); 10.8	*n*/A	HSV-1 F	Suppression of p38 MAPK protein and Bcl-2 gene activity, replication (E and L), DNA expression and viral release.	[60–62]

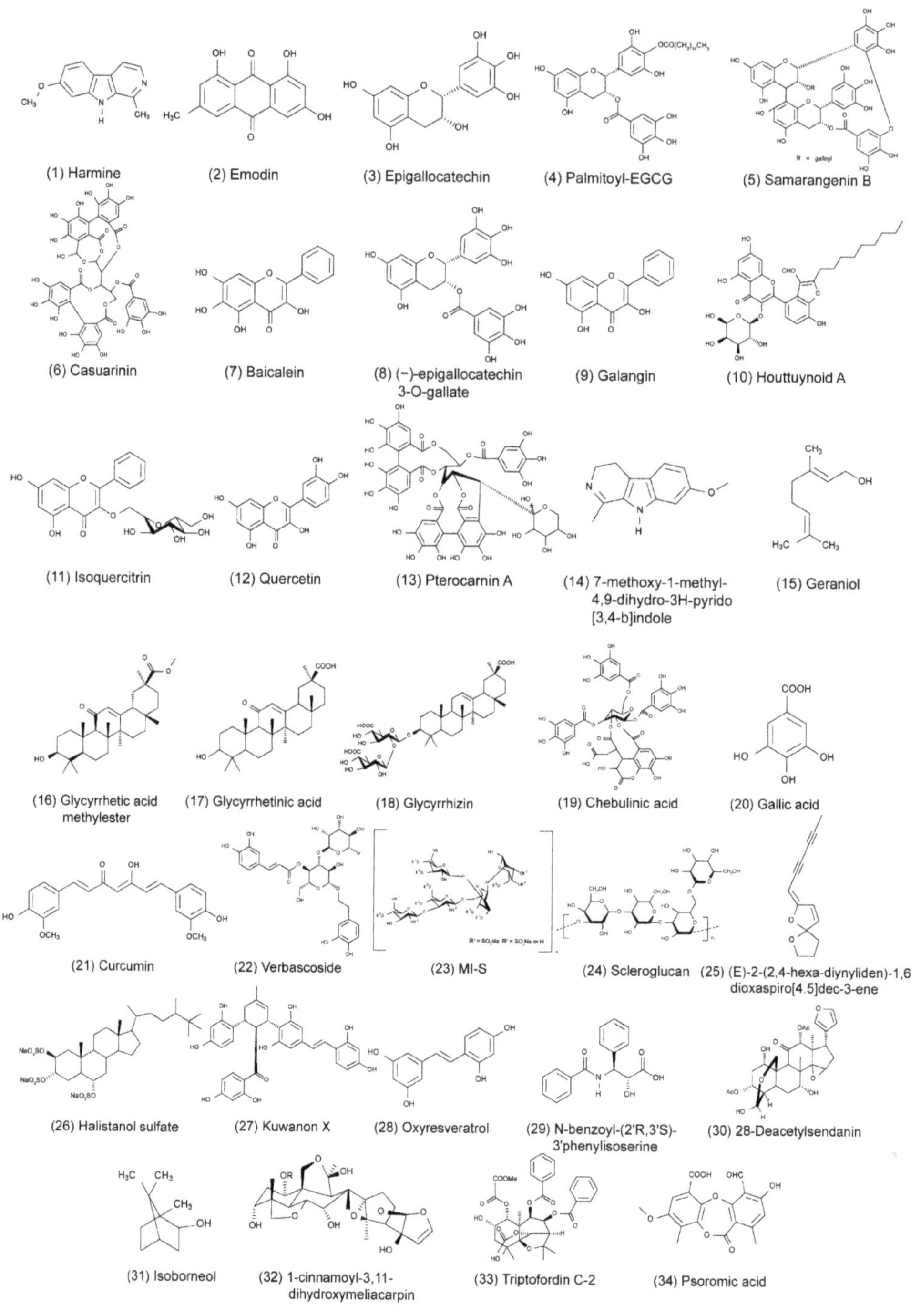

Figure 2. Chemical structures of distinct compounds with antiviral activity against herpes simplex viruses, which were isolated from natural sources. Enumeration is consistent with Table 1, where the characteristics of the compounds are summarized in greater detail.

2.1. Inhibition of Viral Replication

The major targets of substances inhibiting HSV replication are the viral enzymes DNA-polymerase and TK (Figure 3). Numerous compounds affecting HSV-TK or the viral DNA-polymerase could be isolated from plants and other natural sources. These include 28-deacetylsendanin (28-DAS), psoromic acid (PA), and samarangenin B (Sam B).

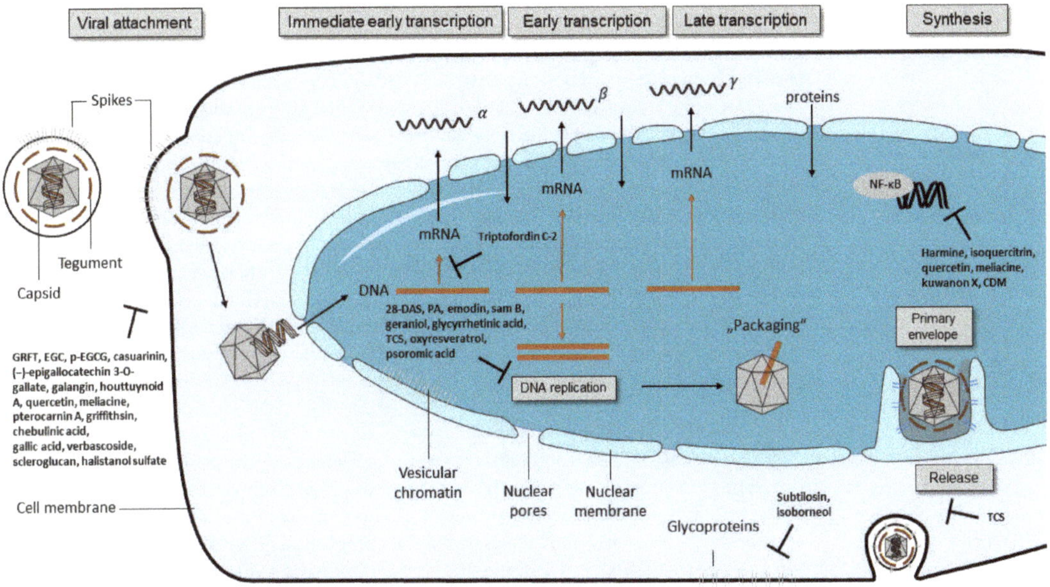

Figure 3. Replication cycle of herpes simplex viruses, including the targets of different natural antiviral compounds. During viral attachment, the viral glycoproteins B, D, and heterodimers of gH/gL bind to the host cell receptors. The transcription phase is divided into immediate-early, early, and late transcription where HSV genes are transcribed as α-, ß-, and γ-genes, respectively. These mRNAs are translated into immediate-early, early, and late proteins. Following DNA replication and the synthesis of the viral capsid, the primary envelopment of the capsid takes place. Subsequently, the capsids are released from the nucleus. Then, virions are released after secondary envelopment. Antiviral compounds may directly interfere with the distinct steps of the viral replication cycle or influence the cellular factors that are important for viral replication. Substances disturbing the viral replication cycle are 28-DAS, PA, emodin, sam B, geraniol, glycyrrhetinic acid, TCS, oxyresveratrol, and psoromic acid. Compounds such as harmine, isoquercitrin, quercetin, meliacine, kuwanon X, and CDM exhibit antiviral effects by addressing the primary essential cellular processes. The transcription factor NF-κB is activated by HSV-1 and HSV-2, which favors the infection. GRFT = griffithsin, EGC = epigallocatechin, *p*-EGCG = palmitoyl-EGCG, 28-DAS = 28-deacetylsendanin, PA = psoromic acid, TCS = trichosanthin, CDM = 1-cinnamoyl-3,11-dihydroxymeliacarpin.

28-DAS is a terpene that was isolated from *Melia azedarach*, the Persian lilac tree. Extracts from leaves have been used as antiviral agents in traditional medicine. 28-DAS showed good antiviral activity toward HSV-1 cell culture experiments. The 50% inhibitory concentration (IC_{50}) of 28-DAS was determined with 1.46 μg/mL. Subsequent analysis showed that there was a transient suppression of a 44 kDa marked viral protein, which is important for viral replication. 28-DAS affects TK (p44) levels, suggesting that 28-DAS has primary, secondary, or both effects on TK [50].

PA is a β-orcinol depsidone that was isolated from *Usnea fruticose* lichens. It was uncovered to inactivate HSV-1 DNA-polymerase, which catalyzes the synthesis of DNA during HSV replication. Moreover, it was demonstrated that PA inhibited the DNA-polymerase (IC_{50} = 0.7 μM; Ki = 0.3 μM) directly without any other prior activation or modification. In comparison, ACV (IC_{50} = 0.9 μM; Ki = 0.5 μM) is initially phosphorylated by the viral TK and modified by cellular enzymes before it can be processed by the HSV-DNA-polymerase. Based on an in silico study, PA was suggested to be a competitive inhibitor of HSV-2 DNA-polymerase. The antiviral activity was evaluated at an IC_{50} value of 1.9 ± 0.42 μM (SI: >163.2) against HSV-1 and 2.7 ± 0.43 μM (SI: >114.8) against HSV-2 using a plaque reduction assay. Combination treatment of ACV and PA remarkably improved the anti-HSV efficacy at EC_{50} (50% effective concentration) values of 1.1 ± 0.41 μM for HSV-1 and 1.8 ± 0.44 μM for HSV-2. Cytotoxicity was determined with a CC_{50} (50% cytotoxic concentration) of >310 μM [56].

Sam B is a catechin purified from *Limonium sinense*. Sam B (IC_{50} HSV-1: 11.4 ± 0.9 μM) showed higher antiviral activity than ACV (IC_{50} HSV-1: 55.4 ± 5.3 μM) in vitro, whereby cytotoxic effects could be excluded (CC_{50}: >100 μM) [22]. In addition, the neutralization efficacy of Sam B did not differ between pre- and co-treatment conditions, indicating that Sam B does not interfere with the viral adsorption or penetration process. This finding supports the perception that Sam B expresses its activity at the level of viral replication. Furthermore, a decreased ICP0 and ICP4 gene expression was reported. These genes play important roles regulating β and γ gene expression, which is needed for HSV-1 replication (Figure 3). Sam B disturbs DNA-polymerase transcripts, synthesis, and consequently blocks the production of gB, gC, gD, gG, and ICP5. Moreover, Sam B reduced the level of gB mRNA significantly. Kuo et al. concluded that Sam B might be more potent in the treatment of reactivations than nucleoside analogues due to the high impact on immediate-early transcripts [21].

2.2. *Compounds Targeting Viral Glycoproteins*

The process by which HSV attaches to the cell surface and enters the cell is mediated by different glycoproteins on the surface of the virus. The attachment of the virion is initiated by an interaction between glycoprotein C and heparan sulfate carbohydrates on the cell surfaces [63]. Glycoprotein D binds to cellular receptors such as Nectin-1 or HVEM (herpes virus entry mediator) and triggers the membrane fusion together with gB, gH, and gL. Drugs targeting highly conserved epitopes on viral glycoproteins could be more resistant to mutations because particular sequences seem to be crucial for viral infectivity and fitness [64]. Hereafter, the compounds griffithsin (GRFT), (−)-epigallocatechin 3-*O*-gallate (EGCG), and isoborneol with their different possibilities of targeting viral glycoproteins are described.

GRFT is a peptide produced by the red alge *Griffithsia*. The results of the in vitro studies indicated an effect on the viral glycoproteins B, D, and heterodimers of gH/gL. Those are indispensable for virus entry and the HSV spread directly between adjacent cells (cell-to-cell spread). However, understanding the exact mechanisms of how GRFT interferes with the viral entry and transmission is not yet completely resolved [57]. GRFT was shown to protect target cells from HSV infection when the cells were pre-treated with the compound, indicating an inhibitory effect of GRFT on viral entry. Furthermore, GRFT was effective in inhibiting viral transmission in already infected cells (post-entry conditions) at an EC_{50} of 2.3 μg/mL [57]. Moreover, GRFT showed antiviral effectivity in vivo and protected mice from genital herpes disease after an application of 20 μL 0.1% GRFT gel pre-infection [57]. GRFT neutralized the viral infection when the cells were pre-treated with concentrations of above 500 μg/mL [57]. The authors concluded that GRFT might affect the cell-to-cell transmission of the virus, thereby blocking viral infection [57].

Polyphenols isolated from tea plants such as *Camellia sinensis* from the family of *Camelliaceae* were shown to exceed antimicrobial and antiviral properties. One isolated component with anti-HSV-activity is EGCG. Isaacs et al. discussed that EGCG has the ability to interfere with the fusion process between the viral and cellular membranes by aggregating HSV glycoproteins B and D on the viral surface [25]. This finding was supported by the result that most virions pre-treated with EGCG were not infectious but appeared visually with an intact morphology [25].

Isoborneol from the *Salvia fruticosa* plant was shown to act dually as an antiviral agent against HSV-1. Firstly, the monoterpenoid alcohol inhibited HSV-1 protein glycosylation, resulting in an impairment of viral glycoprotein processing. Secondly, isoborneol directly inactivated HSV-1 at high concentrations, which was most probably by the interaction of its alcoholic moiety with lipids present on the viral envelope [51]. Infected Vero cells were treated with 0.06% isoborneol, and the viral loads decreased below the limit of analytical detection within 24 h [51].

2.3. Compounds Suppressing NF-κB Activity

NF-κB is a dimeric transcription factor, sequestered in the cytoplasm and, after its translocation into the nucleus, it mediates apoptotic, immune, or inflammatory responses. It was shown that NF-κB activation increases the efficiency of progeny HSV replication. In the early stages of HSV infection, gD–receptor interaction results in NF-κB nuclear translocation (early phase of infection) [65]. Furthermore, RNA-activated protein kinase also activates this process by the degradation of IκB in a later phase of infection [65]. Activated nuclear NF-κB participates in the synthesis of anti-apoptotic factors, which prevent a premature infection-induced cell death [66]. Based on these findings, compounds inhibiting NF-κB activation or translocation may disturb viral replication through programmed cell death (Figure 3).

Kuwanon X is a stilbene derivative from the mulberry tree (*Morus alba* L.). In addition to inhibitory effects against viral penetration and IE gene expression, kuwanon X therapy leads to NF-κB inactivation. Kuwanon X showed to be more efficient in simultaneous (IC_{50} HSV-1: 2.2 μg/mL) than in post-penetration treatment (IC_{50} HSV-1: 3.0 μg/mL). This difference might be caused by the blocking of viral adsorption and penetration by kuwanon X. Additionally, kuwanon X was shown to inhibit IE gene expression, which led to a reduced ICP4 and ICP27 protein synthesis. Those proteins are crucial for NF-κB nuclear translocation. The missing translocation results in an earlier programmed cell death [46].

Melia azedarach, more commonly known as Persian lilac tree or Chinaberry, contains the tetranortriterpenoid 1-cinnamoyl-3,11-dihydroxymeliacarpin (CDM) targeting the NF-κB nuclear translocation. CDM showed inhibitory effects against HSV-1 with an EC_{50} value of 0.78 μM. Cytotoxicity could not be determined up to a concentration of 100 μM on HCLE cells. The strong antiviral activity of CDM can be explained by multiple mechanisms. HSV glycoproteins B, C, and D are arrested into the Golgi complex by CDM causing an antiviral effect that is resilient against viral mutations. In addition, CDM blocks NF-κB translocation in conjunctival cells infected with HSV-1. Although it was not possible to identify the specific target in this pathway, an accumulation of p65 in the cytoplasm could be observed after CDM therapy. It was assumed that p65 is related to the downregulation of either ubiquitination processes or IK kinase complex, which are both possible causes of a NF-κB retention [52–54].

Quercetin and isoquercitrin are two major compounds of *Houttuynia cordata*, which were shown to suppress HSV replication by various mechanisms. Quercetin showed neutralizing activity at an EC_{50} value of 22.6 ± 4.2 μg/mL against HSV-1 and 86.7 ± 7.4 μg/mL HSV-2 and isoquercitrin at among 0.42 μg/mL against HSV-1. Both compounds are characterized by a similar chemical structure. They effectively locked HSV-induced NF-κB activation and NF-κB regulated IE genes transcription during the early phase of infection. Especially the ICP0 promoter was hindered by the downregulated NF-κB activation. ICP0 is meaningful for E and L gene expression. Quercetin and isoquercitrin blocked HSV-related NF-κB activation in the anti-apoptotic pathway in the late phase of infection [27]. However, only quercetin blocked the viral cell-attachment and inhibited plaque formation in pre-treated cell culture [27,67].

2.4. Compounds Affecting Viral Replication by Other Mechanisms

Another promising substance with antiviral activity against HSV is glycyrrhizin (Figure 3). Mainly found in the root of the licorice plant *Glycyrrhiza glabra*, it targets multiple viruses such as HSV, hepatitis B and C, HIV, and coronaviruses. The anti-HSV-1 activity was determined at an IC50 value of 225 ± 24.1 μM. The anti-inflammatory and immunoregulative properties of glycyrrhizin have been previously reported [34]. Glycyrrhizin inhibits HSV-1 entry into the cells via targeting adhesion molecules on the surface of the target cells [33,34].

Trichosanthin (TCS) is a protein derived from the roots of *Trichosanthes kirilowii* and known for its antiviral activity against HSV-1 and other viruses such as HIV-1. TCS neutralized HSV-1 at an EC_{50} of 38.4 μg/mL (subtoxic concentration). The drug synergy of combinatory treatment with TCS and ACV was observed, as the combination of TCS and small amounts of ACV showed a hundredfold higher neutralizing efficacy in vitro than TCS treatment alone [60–62]. The authors concluded that TCS uses a different mechanism of interfering with viral replication than ACV. Time-dependent cell culture experiments revealed an inhibitory effect of TCS against HSV-1 release, which leads to the conclusion that the virion maturation (protein synthesis and/or DNA replication) was inhibited by TCS [60–62]. Furthermore, an increased number of apoptotic cells in TCS treated and infected cultures was observed. HSV infections generally activate p38 Mitogen-Activated Protein Kinase (MAPK) and pro-survival protein Bcl-2. The latter blocks the mitochondrial release of cytochrome c, allowing the virus to replicate more efficiently. TCS was shown to decrease MAPK and Bcl-2 activity, most probably by inhibiting a step during viral replication [60–62]. However, uncovering the exact mechanism of how TCS interferes with the replication of HSV needs further investigation.

2.5. Efficacy of Natural Compounds In Vivo

Numerous natural compounds were shown to exhibit antiviral activity against HSV-1 and HSV-2 in vitro. To investigate whether these results can be extrapolated to living organisms, in vivo studies are necessary. However, only a few natural compounds that showed antiviral activity in cell culture experiments (Table 1) were further evaluated in animal studies. These compounds are discussed in the following section and summarized in Table 2.

The natural compound emodin contained in the plant *Rheum tanguticum* belongs to the anthraquinone family. Emodin reduced the replication of HSV-1 and HSV-2 on human laryngeal carcinoma (HEp-2) cells in vitro [17]. The antiviral efficacy of emodin was further investigated in mice. BALB/c mice were intracerebrally infected with a lethal dose of HSV-1 or HSV-2. Subsequently, the infected mice were orally treated with different amounts of emodin for seven days in 8 h intervals. The mice were observed for 40 days. Emodin protected the mice from a lethal outcome of infection in a dose-dependent manner. The survival was significantly higher in mice treated with emodin at 6.7 g/kg/day comparted to untreated control, in which all the mice died [17]. Notably, the treatment with emodin was even more effective than 0.1 mg/kg/day ACV orally in terms of increasing the survival rate and mean time to death of the infected mice [17].

Another compound that showed antiviral activity against HSV-1 in vitro and in vivo is the flavonoid baicalein, which is isolated from the roots of *Scutellaria baicalensis* [24]. Oral administration of baicalein at a dose of 200 mg/kg/day for seven days significantly increased the survival rate of mice that were intranasally infected with a lethal dose of HSV-1 [24]. However, the survival rate was higher in the ACV group (50 mg/kg/day) than in the baicalein group (200 mg/kg/day). The natural compound oxyresveratrol isolated from *Artocarpus lakoocha* exhibited an antiviral effect against HSV-1 and HSV-2 in vitro by inhibiting the early and late viral genes [47,48]. However, the administration of the compound only slightly increased the survival rate of mice with a cutaneous HSV-1 infection, and there was no significant difference compared to an untreated control [47].

Table 2. In vivo studies of anti-HSV chemical substances. P.O. = Per Os.

Group	Compound	Plant/Other	Animal	Virus	Way of Infection	Treatment; Dose	Survival under Treatment	Compared to Control/ACV	Refs.
Anthraquinone	Emodin	*Rheum tanguticum*	BALB/c mice	HSV-1F; HSV-2 (333)	Intracerebral	P.O.; 6.7 g/kg/day	HSV-1: 61.5% HSV-2: ≈70%	HSV-1: Untreated control: 0%/ACV: ≈20% ($p < 0.01$) HSV-2: Untreated control: 0%/ACV: ≈30% ($p < 0.01$)	[17]
Flavinoid	Baicalein	*Scutellaria baicalensis*	BALB/c mice	HSV-1 F	Intranasal	P.O.; 200 mg/kg/day	75%	Untreated control: 33.3% ($p < 0.05$)/ACV: ≈90%	[24]
Harmaline	7-methoxy-1-methyl-4,9-dihydro-3H-pyrido[3,4-b]indole	*Ophiorrhiza nicobarica Balkr*	BALB/c mice (female and male)	HSV-2 G	Genital	P.O.; 0.25 and 0.5 mg/kg 6 h after infection	0.25 mg/kg: 45% 0.5 mg/kg: 70%	Untreated control: 5% ($p < 0.05$)/ACV: 80%	[30]
Peptide	Griffithsin (GRFT)	*Griffithsia*	BALB/c mice (female)	HSV-2	Intravaginal	Intravaginal topically; 20 µL 0.1% GRFT gel pre-infection	≈80%	Untreated control: ≈20% ($p < 0.05$)	[57]
Phenolics	Curcumin	*The curry spice turmeric*	BALB/c mice (female)	HSV-2 (333)	Intravaginal	Intravaginal topically; 100 µg 6 h pre-infection	0%	0%	[68]
Polysaccharids	MI-S	*Agaricus brasiliensis*	BALB/c mice (female)	HSV-2 (333)	Intravaginal	Intravaginal topically; 20 mg/mL 20 min pre-infection	60%	Untreated control: 0% ($p < 0.0001$)	[69]
Stilbenoids and 2-arylbenzofurans	Oxyresveratrol	*Artocarpus lakoocha*	BALB/c mice (female)	HSV-1 (7401H)	Cutaneous	P.O.; 500 mg/kg 8 h pre-infection and 3x daily for 7 days after infection	25%	Untreated control: 0% (*n.s.*)/ACV: 100%	[47]
Terpene	Meliacine (CDM)	*Melia azedarach* L.	BALB/c mice (female)	HSV-2 MS and G	Intravaginal	Intravaginal topically; 1 mg 2x daily for 5 days	HSV-2 MS: 20% HSV-2 G: 86%	Untreated control: HSV-2 MS: 0%; HSV-2 G: 42%	[70]
			BALB/c mice (female and male)	HSV-1 (KOS)	Corneal	Corneal topically; 3x daily 1 day pre-infection and for 3 days after infection	Development of keratitis: 5%	Untreated control: 90% ($p < 0.001$)	[71]

Some compounds were also tested for their antiviral effectivity in treating genital HSV-2 infections, including curcumin, GRFT, meliacine, 7-methoxy-1-methyl-4,9-dihydro-3H-pyrido [3,4-b]indole (HM), and MI-S [30,57,68–71]. Intravaginal administration with 100 µg curcumin six hours before vaginal infection with HSV-2 significantly increased the survival time of mice compared to the untreated control [68]. However, prophylactic treatment with curcumin could only delay the lethal outcome of infection, and all mice died after 20 days post infection. Further in vivo studies with other natural compounds including the peptide GRFT isolated from the alga *Griffithsia*, the harmaline HM from the herb *Ophiorrhiza nicobarica Balkr*, as well as the polysaccharide MI-S isolated from the fungus *Agaricus brasiliensis* showed that these compounds significantly increased the survival rate of mice intravaginally infected with HSV-2 [30,57,69]. In the experiments, MI-S and GRFT were vaginally administered before infection, and HM was orally administered after infection with HSV-2. However, depending on the dose of HM administered, the survival rate of mice treated with ACV was at least 10% higher compared to HM treatment [30]. Furthermore, the terpene meliacine, from which CDM can be obtained, was shown to protect mice from developing severe genital HSV-2 infection. In this study, 50 mg of meliacine was vaginally administered as cream twice a day for five consecutive days [70]. In a further study, topical administration of meliciacie was also effective in preventing mice with a corneal HSV-1 infection from developing severe keratitis. Only 5% of treated mice showed signs of keratitis. The untreated group reached levels from 85 to 90% [71].

3. Summary and Additional Comments

The current standard therapy for HSV primary infection and reactivation includes ACV and valacyclovir. However, the emergence of drug resistances limits the available treatment options [5]. Therefore, there is a clear need for the development of new effective antiviral drugs. Plants traditionally used for medical purposes are a promising source of new antiviral compounds.

In the present review, we summarized compounds isolated from plants, bacteria, and fungi with different mechanisms inhibiting HSV, including the inhibition of viral attachment, penetration, and replication. The compounds belong to different groups such as catechins, flavonoids, phenolic acids, polysaccharides, terpenes, and peptides. With six compounds, flavonoids represent the largest group.

Some of the tested compounds showed a similar or even better antiviral activity against HSV-1 than ACV in vitro, including the anthraquinone emodin, the catechin epigallocatechin (EGC), the harmaline HM, and the β-orcinol depsidone PA as well as other promising compounds (Table 1 and Figure 1) [17,18,31,35,44,56]. Interestingly, when these compounds were supplemented with geraniol, they had a similar or better antiviral activity against HSV-2 [17,18,30,32,36,56]. These candidates might be good for further evaluation in the search for alternative treatments of ACV-resistant viruses. Additional studies are needed to investigate whether these compounds maintain their antiviral activity against HSV-1 and HSV-2 clinical isolates that are resistant to ACV. To date, only a few studies have included ACV-resistant strains in their experiments [4,47,69]. In the study of Luo et al. (2020), the antiviral effect of baicalein against an ACV-resistant HSV-1 strain (HSV-1 Blue) was comparable in its effect against the HSV-1 F strain without resistance [24]. As anticipated, ACV exhibited only a weak antiviral activity against the ACV-resistant virus. However, ACV showed a stronger inhibition against the HSV-1 F strain than baicalein. In a further in vitro study, the antiviral effect of MI-S was observed against HSV-1 KOS, an ACV-resistant HSV-1 strain (HSV-1 29R), and HSV-2 333 [69]. MI-S was similarly effective against HSV-1 KOS and HSV-1 29R when the compound was administered during or after infection. ACV showed no inhibitory activity against HSV-1 KOS when applied simultaneously with the virus, but it was more effective than MI-S under post-infection treatment conditions.

Only a few of those compounds were evaluated for their efficacy against HSV infections in in vivo studies. Of these compounds, emodin exhibited promising results, as it strongly increased the survival rate of mice infected with HSV-1 and HSV-2 [17]. The compound was even more effective than ACV in increasing the survival rate and mean time to death. Furthermore, HM significantly increased the survival rate of mice infected with HSV-2 [30]. Although standard therapy with ACV was more effective, the increase of survival through the compound was still striking. The results of these studies indicate that emodin and HM are promising candidates for future clinical trials. Clearly, there is a need for more elaborate in vivo studies as well as clinical trials that compare the compounds to the standard therapy of HSV.

4. Conclusions

To date, numerous herbal medicines and their main ingredients were investigated for their antiviral efficacy against HSV-1 and HSV-2 in cell culture and animal models. For instance, the anthraquinone emodin derived from the plant *Rheum tanguticum* as well as the harmaline HM isolated from the herb *Ophiorrhiza nicobarica Balkr* exhibited a strong antiviral effect against HSV in vitro and in vivo, which were comparable to or even better than ACV. Clinical studies are needed to determine the efficacy of these compounds in humans. Furthermore, natural compounds might be an effective substitute for drugs such as ACV in the treatment of ACV-resistant HSV infections. Taken together, herbal medicines represent a promising source to isolate novel compounds with antiviral activity against HSV-1 and HSV-2. Numerous compounds could be isolated and pre-clinically characterized thus far. Further clinical evaluation of the agents that are most promising in animal trials may lead to the development of novel therapy options in humans.

Author Contributions: Conceptualization, L.v.d.S., M.B., O.W. and A.K.; writing—original draft preparation, L.v.d.S., M.B., Y.S., C.S.H., O.W. and A.K.; writing—review and editing, C.S.H.; visualization, L.v.d.S. and M.B.; supervision, A.K.; funding acquisition, L.v.d.S., O.W. and A.K. All authors have read and agreed to the published version of the manuscript.

Funding: This study was supported by the Stiftung Universitätsmedizin Essen (awarded to A. Krawczyk), the Else-Kröner Promotionskolleg ELAN (awarded to L. van de Sand), and the Rudolf Ackermann Foundation (awarded to O. Witzke).

Institutional Review Board Statement: Not applicable.

Informed Consent Statement: Not applicable.

Acknowledgments: The authors thank Delia Cosgrove for proofreading of the manuscript.

Conflicts of Interest: The authors declare no conflict of interest.

References

1. Pebody, R.; Andrews, N.; Brown, D.; Gopal, R.; Melker, H.; François, G.; Gatcheva, N.; Hellenbrand, W.; Jokinen, S.; Klavs, I.; et al. The seroepidemiology of herpes simplex virus type 1 and 2 in Europe. *Sex. Transm. Infect.* **2004**, *80*, 185–191. [CrossRef] [PubMed]
2. Berrington, W.R.; Jerome, K.R.; Cook, L.; Wald, A.; Corey, L.; Casper, C. Clinical correlates of herpes simplex virus viremia among hospitalized adults. *Clin. Infect. Dis. Off. Publ. Infect. Dis. Soc. Am.* **2009**, *49*, 1295–1301. [CrossRef] [PubMed]
3. Kimberlin, D.W.; Lin, C.Y.; Jacobs, R.F.; Powell, D.A.; Corey, L.; Gruber, W.C.; Rathore, M.; Bradley, J.S.; Diaz, P.S.; Kumar, M.; et al. Safety and efficacy of high-dose intravenous acyclovir in the management of neonatal herpes simplex virus infections. *Pediatrics* **2001**, *108*, 230–238. [CrossRef]
4. Akinyi, B.; Odhiambo, C.; Otieno, F.; Inzaule, S.; Oswago, S.; Kerubo, E.; Ndivo, R.; Zeh, C. Prevalence, incidence and correlates of HSV-2 infection in an HIV incidence adolescent and adult cohort study in western Kenya. *PLoS ONE* **2017**, *12*, e0178907. [CrossRef] [PubMed]
5. Jiang, Y.-C.; Feng, H.; Lin, Y.-C.; Guo, X.-R. New strategies against drug resistance to herpes simplex virus. *Int. J. Oral Sci.* **2016**, *8*, 1–6. [CrossRef]
6. Baeten, J.M.; Strick, L.B.; Lucchetti, A.; Whittington, W.L.; Sanchez, J.; Coombs, R.W.; Magaret, A.; Wald, A.; Corey, L.; Celum, C. Herpes simplex virus (HSV)-suppressive therapy decreases plasma and genital HIV-1 levels in HSV-2/HIV-1 coinfected women: A randomized, placebo-controlled, cross-over trial. *J. Infect. Dis.* **2008**, *198*, 1804–1808. [CrossRef]
7. Delany, S.; Mlaba, N.; Clayton, T.; Akpomiemie, G.; Capovilla, A.; Legoff, J.; Belec, L.; Stevens, W.; Rees, H.; Mayaud, P. Impact of aciclovir on genital and plasma HIV-1 RNA in HSV-2/HIV-1 co-infected women: A randomized placebo-controlled trial in South Africa. *AIDS* **2009**, *23*, 461–469. [CrossRef]
8. Nagot, N.; Ouédraogo, A.; Foulongne, V.; Konaté, I.; Weiss, H.A.; Vergne, L.; Defer, M.C.; Djagbaré, D.; Sanon, A.; Andonaba, J.B.; et al. Reduction of HIV-1 RNA levels with therapy to suppress herpes simplex virus. *N. Engl. J. Med.* **2007**, *356*, 790–799. [CrossRef]
9. McMahon, M.A.; Siliciano, J.D.; Lai, J.; Liu, J.O.; Stivers, J.T.; Siliciano, R.F.; Kohli, R.M. The antiherpetic drug acyclovir inhibits HIV replication and selects the V75I reverse transcriptase multidrug resistance mutation. *J. Biol. Chem.* **2008**, *283*, 31289–31293. [CrossRef]
10. Matamoros, T.; Kim, B.; Menéndez-Arias, L. Mechanistic insights into the role of Val75 of HIV-1 reverse transcriptase in misinsertion and mispair extension fidelity of DNA synthesis. *J. Mol. Biol.* **2008**, *375*, 1234–1248. [CrossRef]
11. Farooq, A.V.; Shukla, D. Herpes simplex epithelial and stromal keratitis: An epidemiologic update. *Surv. Ophthalmol.* **2012**, *57*, 448–462. [CrossRef] [PubMed]
12. Stránská, R.; Schuurman, R.; Nienhuis, E.; Goedegebuure, I.W.; Polman, M.; Weel, J.F.; Wertheim-Van Dillen, P.M.; Berkhout, R.J.; van Loon, A.M. Survey of acyclovir-resistant herpes simplex virus in the Netherlands: Prevalence and characterization. *J. Clin. Virol.* **2005**, *32*, 7–18. [CrossRef] [PubMed]
13. Sauerbrei, A.; Bohn, K.; Heim, A.; Hofmann, J.; Weissbrich, B.; Schnitzler, P.; Hoffmann, D.; Zell, R.; Jahn, G.; Wutzler, P.H.; et al. Novel resistance-associated mutations of thymidine kinase and DNA polymerase genes of herpes simplex virus type 1 and type 2. *Antivir. Ther.* **2011**, *16*, 1297–1308. [CrossRef] [PubMed]
14. Blot, N.; Schneider, P.; Young, P.; Janvresse, C.; Dehesdin, D.; Tron, P.; Vannier, J.P. Treatment of an acyclovir and foscarnet-resistant herpes simplex virus infection with cidofovir in a child after an unrelated bone marrow transplant. *Bone Marrow Transpl.* **2000**, *26*, 903–905. [CrossRef] [PubMed]
15. Chen, D.; Su, A.; Fu, Y.; Wang, X.; Lv, X.; Xu, W.; Xu, S.; Wang, H.; Wu, Z. Harmine blocks herpes simplex virus infection through downregulating cellular NF-κB and MAPK pathways induced by oxidative stress. *Antivir. Res.* **2015**, *123*, 27–38. [CrossRef]

16. Hutterer, C.; Milbradt, J.; Hamilton, S.; Zaja, M.; Leban, J.; Henry, C.; Vitt, D.; Steingruber, M.; Sonntag, E.; Zeitträger, I.; et al. Inhibitors of dual-specificity tyrosine phosphorylation-regulated kinases (DYRK) exert a strong anti-herpesviral activity. *Antivir. Res.* **2017**, *143*, 113–121. [CrossRef]
17. Xiong, H.R.; Luo, J.; Hou, W.; Xiao, H.; Yang, Z.Q. The effect of emodin, an anthraquinone derivative extracted from the roots of *Rheum tanguticum*, against herpes simplex virus in vitro and in vivo. *J. Ethnopharmacol.* **2011**, *133*, 718–723. [CrossRef]
18. Lyu, S.Y.; Rhim, J.Y.; Park, W.B. Antiherpetic activities of flavonoids against herpes simplex virus type 1 (HSV-1) and type 2 (HSV-2) in vitro. *Arch. Pharm. Res.* **2005**, *28*, 1293–1301. [CrossRef]
19. Isaacs, C.E.; Wen, G.Y.; Xu, W.; Jia, J.H.; Rohan, L.; Corbo, C.; Di Maggio, V.; Jenkins, E.C., Jr.; Hillier, S. Epigallocatechin gallate inactivates clinical isolates of herpes simplex virus. *Antimicrob. Agents Chemother.* **2008**, *52*, 962–970. [CrossRef] [PubMed]
20. de Oliveira, A.; Adams, S.D.; Lee, L.H.; Murray, S.R.; Hsu, S.D.; Hammond, J.R.; Dickinson, D.; Chen, P.; Chu, T.C. Inhibition of herpes simplex virus type 1 with the modified green tea polyphenol palmitoyl-epigallocatechin gallate. *Food Chem. Toxicol.* **2013**, *52*, 207–215. [CrossRef] [PubMed]
21. Kuo, Y.C.; Lin, L.C.; Tsai, W.J.; Chou, C.J.; Kung, S.H.; Ho, Y.H. Samarangenin B from Limonium sinense suppresses herpes simplex virus type 1 replication in Vero cells by regulation of viral macromolecular synthesis. *Antimicrob. Agents Chemother.* **2002**, *46*, 2854–2864. [CrossRef]
22. Lin, L.C.; Kuo, Y.C.; Chou, C.J. Anti-herpes simplex virus type-1 flavonoids and a new flavanone from the root of *Limonium sinense*. *Planta Med.* **2000**, *66*, 333–336. [CrossRef] [PubMed]
23. Cheng, H.Y.; Lin, C.C.; Lin, T.C. Antiherpes simplex virus type 2 activity of casuarinin from the bark of *Terminalia arjuna* Linn. *Antivir. Res.* **2002**, *55*, 447–455. [CrossRef]
24. Luo, Z.; Kuang, X.P.; Zhou, Q.Q.; Yan, C.Y.; Li, W.; Gong, H.B.; Kurihara, H.; Li, W.X.; Li, Y.F.; He, R.R. Inhibitory effects of baicalein against herpes simplex virus type 1. *Acta Pharm. Sin. B* **2020**, *10*, 2323–2338. [CrossRef]
25. Isaacs, C.E.; Xu, W.; Merz, G.; Hillier, S.; Rohan, L.; Wen, G.Y. Digallate dimers of (-)-epigallocatechin gallate inactivate herpes simplex virus. *Antimicrob. Agents Chemother.* **2011**, *55*, 5646–5653. [CrossRef]
26. Li, T.; Liu, L.; Wu, H.; Chen, S.; Zhu, Q.; Gao, H.; Yu, X.; Wang, Y.; Su, W.; Yao, X.; et al. Anti-herpes simplex virus type 1 activity of Houttuynoid A, a flavonoid from *Houttuynia cordata* Thunb. *Antivir. Res.* **2017**, *144*, 273–280. [CrossRef]
27. Hung, P.Y.; Ho, B.C.; Lee, S.Y.; Chang, S.Y.; Kao, C.L.; Lee, S.S.; Lee, C.N. Houttuynia cordata targets the beginning stage of herpes simplex virus infection. *PLoS ONE* **2015**, *10*, e0115475. [CrossRef]
28. Chiang, L.C.; Chiang, W.; Liu, M.C.; Lin, C.C. In vitro antiviral activities of *Caesalpinia pulcherrima* and its related flavonoids. *J. Antimicrob. Chemother.* **2003**, *52*, 194–198. [CrossRef]
29. Cheng, H.Y.; Lin, T.C.; Yang, C.M.; Wang, K.C.; Lin, C.C. Mechanism of action of the suppression of herpes simplex virus type 2 replication by pterocarnin A. *Microbes Infect.* **2004**, *6*, 738–744. [CrossRef] [PubMed]
30. Bag, P.; Ojha, D.; Mukherjee, H.; Halder, U.C.; Mondal, S.; Chandra, N.S.; Nandi, S.; Sharon, A.; Sarkar, M.C.; Chakrabarti, S.; et al. An Indole Alkaloid from a Tribal Folklore Inhibits Immediate Early Event in HSV-2 Infected Cells with Therapeutic Efficacy in Vaginally Infected Mice. *PLoS ONE* **2013**, *8*, e77937. [CrossRef]
31. Bag, P.; Ojha, D.; Mukherjee, H.; Halder, U.C.; Mondal, S.; Biswas, A.; Sharon, A.; Van Kaer, L.; Chakrabarty, S.; Das, G.; et al. A dihydro-pyrido-indole potently inhibits HSV-1 infection by interfering the viral immediate early transcriptional events. *Antivir. Res.* **2014**, *105*, 126–134. [CrossRef]
32. Hassan, S.T.S.; Berchová-Bímová, K.; Šudomová, M.; Malaník, M.; Šmejkal, K.; Rengasamy, K.R.R. In Vitro Study of Multi-Therapeutic Properties of Thymus bovei Benth. Essential Oil and Its Main Component for Promoting Their Use in Clinical Practice. *J. Clin. Med.* **2018**, *7*, 283. [CrossRef]
33. Ikeda, T.; Yokomizo, K.; Okawa, M.; Tsuchihashi, R.; Kinjo, J.; Nohara, T.; Uyeda, M. Anti-herpes virus type 1 activity of oleanane-type triterpenoids. *Biol. Pharm. Bull.* **2005**, *28*, 1779–1781. [CrossRef]
34. Huang, W.; Chen, X.; Li, Q.; Li, P.; Zhao, G.; Xu, M.; Xie, P. Inhibition of intercellular adhesion in herpex simplex virus infection by glycyrrhizin. *Cell Biochem. Biophys.* **2012**, *62*, 137–140. [CrossRef] [PubMed]
35. Lin, L.T.; Chen, T.Y.; Chung, C.Y.; Noyce, R.S.; Grindley, T.B.; McCormick, C.; Lin, T.C.; Wang, G.H.; Lin, C.C.; Richardson, C.D. Hydrolyzable tannins (chebulagic acid and punicalagin) target viral glycoprotein-glycosaminoglycan interactions to inhibit herpes simplex virus 1 entry and cell-to-cell spread. *J. Virol.* **2011**, *85*, 4386–4398. [CrossRef]
36. Kesharwani, A.; Polachira, S.K.; Nair, R.; Agarwal, A.; Mishra, N.N.; Gupta, S.K. Anti-HSV-2 activity of *Terminalia chebula* Retz extract and its constituents, chebulagic and chebulinic acids. *BMC Complement. Altern. Med.* **2017**, *17*, 110. [CrossRef]
37. Kratz, J.M.; Andrighetti-Fröhner, C.R.; Kolling, D.J.; Leal, P.C.; Cirne-Santos, C.C.; Yunes, R.A.; Nunes, R.J.; Trybala, E.; Bergström, T.; Frugulhetti, I.C.; et al. Anti-HSV-1 and anti-HIV-1 activity of gallic acid and pentyl gallate. *Mem. Inst. Oswaldo Cruz.* **2008**, *103*, 437–442. [CrossRef]
38. Kratz, J.M.; Andrighetti-Fröhner, C.R.; Leal, P.C.; Nunes, R.J.; Yunes, R.A.; Trybala, E.; Bergström, T.; Barardi, C.R.; Simões, C.M. Evaluation of anti-HSV-2 activity of gallic acid and pentyl gallate. *Biol. Pharm. Bull.* **2008**, *31*, 903–907. [CrossRef]
39. El-Toumy, S.; Salib, J.; El-Kashak, W.; Marty, C.; Bedoux, G.; Bourgougnon, N. Antiviral effect of polyphenol rich plant extracts on herpes simplex virus type 1. *Food Sci. Hum. Wellness* **2018**, *7*, 91–101. [CrossRef]
40. Kutluay, S.B.; Doroghazi, J.; Roemer, M.E.; Triezenberg, S.J. Curcumin inhibits herpes simplex virus immediate-early gene expression by a mechanism independent of p300/CBP histone acetyltransferase activity. *Virology* **2008**, *373*, 239–247. [CrossRef]

41. Martins, F.O.; Esteves, P.F.; Mendes, G.S.; Barbi, N.S.; Menezes, F.S.; Romanos, M.T. Verbascoside isolated from *Lepechinia speciosa* has inhibitory activity against HSV-1 and HSV-2 in vitro. *Nat. Prod. Commun.* **2009**, *4*, 1693–1696. [CrossRef] [PubMed]
42. de Sousa Cardozo, F.T.G.; Camelini, C.M.; Mascarello, A.; José Rossi, M.; José Nunes, R.; Monte Barardi, C.R.; de Mendonça, M.M.; Simões, C.M.O. Antiherpetic activity of a sulfated polysaccharide from *Agaricus brasiliensis* mycelia. *Antivir. Res.* **2011**, *92*, 108–114. [CrossRef]
43. Marchetti, M.; Pisani, S.; Pietropaolo, V.; Seganti, L.; Nicoletti, R.; Degener, A.; Orsi, N. Antiviral effect of a polysaccharide from *Sclerotium glucanicum* towards herpes simplex virus type 1 infection. *Planta Med.* **1996**, *62*, 303–307. [CrossRef] [PubMed]
44. Álvarez, Á.; Habtemariam, S.L.; Abdel Moneim, A.E.; Melón, S.; Dalton, K.P.; Parra, F. A spiroketal-enol ether derivative from Tanacetum vulgare selectively inhibits HSV-1 and HSV-2 glycoprotein accumulation in Vero cells. *Antivir. Res.* **2015**, *119*, 8–18. [CrossRef]
45. da Rosa Guimarães, T.; Quiroz, C.G.; Borges, C.R.; de Oliveira, S.Q.; de Almeida, M.T.; Bianco, É.M.; Moritz, M.I.; Carraro, J.L.; Palermo, J.A.; Cabrera, G.; et al. Anti HSV-1 activity of halistanol sulfate and halistanol sulfate C isolated from *Brazilian marine* sponge *Petromica citrina* (Demospongiae). *Mar. Drugs* **2013**, *11*, 4176–4192. [CrossRef]
46. Ma, F.; Shen, W.; Zhang, X.; Li, M.; Wang, Y.; Zou, Y.; Li, Y.; Wang, H. Anti-HSV Activity of Kuwanon X from Mulberry Leaves with Genes Expression Inhibitory and HSV-1 Induced NF-κB Deactivated Properties. *Biol. Pharm. Bull.* **2016**, *39*, 1667–1674. [CrossRef]
47. Chuanasa, T.; Phromjai, J.; Lipipun, V.; Likhitwitayawuid, K.; Suzuki, M.; Pramyothin, P.; Hattori, M.; Shiraki, K. Anti-herpes simplex virus (HSV-1) activity of oxyresveratrol derived from Thai medicinal plant: Mechanism of action and therapeutic efficacy on cutaneous HSV-1 infection in mice. *Antivir. Res.* **2008**, *80*, 62–70. [CrossRef]
48. Likhitwitayawuid, K.; Sritularak, B.; Benchanak, K.; Lipipun, V.; Mathew, J.; Schinazi, R.F. Phenolics with antiviral activity from *Millettia erythrocalyx* and *Artocarpus lakoocha*. *Nat. Prod. Res.* **2005**, *19*, 177–182. [CrossRef]
49. Krawczyk, E.; Luczak, M.; Kniotek, M.; Nowaczyk, M. Cytotoxic, antiviral (in-vitro and in-vivo), immunomodulatory activity and influence on mitotic divisions of three taxol derivatives: 10-deacetyl-baccatin III, methyl (N-benzoyl-(2′R,3′S)-3′-phenylisoserinate) and N-benzoyl-(2′R,3′S)-3′-phenylisoserine. *J. Pharm. Pharm.* **2005**, *57*, 791–797. [CrossRef]
50. Kim, M.; Kim, S.K.; Park, B.N.; Lee, K.H.; Min, G.H.; Seoh, J.Y.; Park, C.G.; Hwang, E.S.; Cha, C.Y.; Kook, Y.H. Antiviral effects of 28-deacetylsendanin on herpes simplex virus-1 replication. *Antivir. Res.* **1999**, *43*, 103–112. [CrossRef]
51. Armaka, M.; Papanikolaou, E.; Sivropoulou, A.; Arsenakis, M. Antiviral properties of isoborneol, a potent inhibitor of herpes simplex virus type 1. *Antivir. Res.* **1999**, *43*, 79–92. [CrossRef]
52. Barquero, A.A.; Michelini, F.M.; Alché, L.E. 1-Cinnamoyl-3,11-dihydroxymeliacarpin is a natural bioactive compound with antiviral and nuclear factor-kappaB modulating properties. *Biochem. Biophys. Res. Commun.* **2006**, *344*, 955–962. [CrossRef]
53. Bueno, C.A.; Barquero, A.A.; Di Cónsoli, H.; Maier, M.S.; Alché, L.E. A natural tetranortriterpenoid with immunomodulating properties as a potential anti-HSV agent. *Virus Res.* **2009**, *141*, 47–54. [CrossRef]
54. Alché, L.E.; Assad Ferek, G.; Meo, M.; Coto, C.E.; Maier, M.S. An Antiviral Meliacarpin from Leaves of *Melia azedarach* L. *Z. Für. Nat. C* **2003**, *58*, 215–219. [CrossRef] [PubMed]
55. Hayashi, K.; Hayashi, T.; Ujita, K.; Takaishi, Y. Characterization of antiviral activity of a sesquiterpene, triptofordin C-2. *J. Antimicrob. Chemother.* **1996**, *37*, 759–768. [CrossRef] [PubMed]
56. Hassan, S.T.S.; Šudomová, M.; Berchová-Bímová, K.; Šmejkal, K.; Echeverría, J. Psoromic Acid, a Lichen-Derived Molecule, Inhibits the Replication of HSV-1 and HSV-2, and Inactivates HSV-1 DNA Polymerase: Shedding Light on Antiherpetic Properties. *Molecules* **2019**, *24*, 2912. [CrossRef] [PubMed]
57. Nixon, B.; Stefanidou, M.; Mesquita, P.M.; Fakioglu, E.; Segarra, T.; Rohan, L.; Halford, W.; Palmer, K.E.; Herold, B.C. Griffithsin protects mice from genital herpes by preventing cell-to-cell spread. *J. Virol.* **2013**, *87*, 6257–6269. [CrossRef]
58. Torres, N.I.; Noll, K.S.; Xu, S.; Li, J.; Huang, Q.; Sinko, P.J.; Wachsman, M.B.; Chikindas, M.L. Safety, formulation, and in vitro antiviral activity of the antimicrobial peptide subtilosin against herpes simplex virus type 1. *Probiotics Antimicrob. Proteins* **2013**, *5*, 26–35. [CrossRef]
59. Quintana, V.M.; Torres, N.I.; Wachsman, M.B.; Sinko, P.J.; Castilla, V.; Chikindas, M. Antiherpes simplex virus type 2 activity of the antimicrobial peptide subtilosin. *J. Appl. Microbiol.* **2014**, *117*, 1253–1259. [CrossRef] [PubMed]
60. Huang, H.; Chan, H.; Wang, Y.Y.; Ouyang, D.Y.; Zheng, Y.T.; Tam, S.C. Trichosanthin suppresses the elevation of p38 MAPK, and Bcl-2 induced by HSV-1 infection in Vero cells. *Life Sci.* **2006**, *79*, 1287–1292. [CrossRef]
61. He, D.X.; Tam, S.C. Trichosanthin affects HSV-1 replication in Hep-2 cells. *Biochem. Biophys. Res. Commun.* **2010**, *402*, 670–675. [CrossRef]
62. Zheng, Y.T.; Chan, W.L.; Chan, P.; Huang, H.; Tam, S.C. Enhancement of the anti-herpetic effect of trichosanthin by acyclovir and interferon. *FEBS Lett.* **2001**, *496*, 139–142. [CrossRef]
63. Spear, P.G. Herpes simplex virus: Receptors and ligands for cell entry. *Cell Microbiol.* **2004**, *6*, 401–410. [CrossRef] [PubMed]
64. Däumer, M.P.; Schneider, B.; Giesen, D.M.; Aziz, S.; Kaiser, R.; Kupfer, B.; Schneweis, K.E.; Schneider-Mergener, J.; Reineke, U.; Matz, B.; et al. Characterisation of the epitope for a herpes simplex virus glycoprotein B-specific monoclonal antibody with high protective capacity. *Med. Microbiol. Immunol.* **2011**, *200*, 85–97. [CrossRef] [PubMed]
65. Patel, A.; Hanson, J.; McLean, T.I.; Olgiate, J.; Hilton, M.; Miller, W.E.; Bachenheimer, S.L. Herpes Simplex Virus Type 1 Induction of Persistent NF-κB Nuclear Translocation Increases the Efficiency of Virus Replication. *Virology* **1998**, *247*, 212–222. [CrossRef]

66. Goodkin, M.L.; Ting, A.T.; Blaho, J.A. NF-κB Is Required for Apoptosis Prevention during Herpes Simplex Virus Type 1 Infection. *J. Virol.* **2003**, *77*, 7261–7280. [CrossRef] [PubMed]
67. Chiang, L.C.; Cheng, H.Y.; Liu, M.C.; Chiang, W.; Lin, C.C. In vitro anti-herpes simplex viruses and anti-adenoviruses activity of twelve traditionally used medicinal plants in Taiwan. *Biol. Pharm. Bull.* **2003**, *26*, 1600–1604. [CrossRef]
68. Vitali, D.; Bagri, P.; Wessels, J.M.; Arora, M.; Ganugula, R.; Parikh, A.; Mandur, T.; Felker, A.; Garg, S.; Kumar, M.N.V.R.; et al. Curcumin Can Decrease Tissue Inflammation and the Severity of HSV-2 Infection in the Female Reproductive Mucosa. *Int. J. Mol. Sci.* **2020**, *21*, 337. [CrossRef]
69. Cardozo, F.T.G.S.; Larsen, I.V.; Carballo, E.V.; Jose, G.; Stern, R.A.; Brummel, R.C.; Camelini, C.M.; Rossi, M.J.; Simões, C.M.O.; Brandt, C.R. In VivoAnti-Herpes Simplex Virus Activity of a Sulfated Derivative of *Agaricus brasiliensis* Mycelial Polysaccharide. *Antimicrob. Agents Chemother.* **2013**, *57*, 2541–2549. [CrossRef]
70. Petrera, E.; Coto, C.E. Therapeutic effect of meliacine, an antiviral derived from Melia azedarach L.; in mice genital herpetic infection. *Phytother. Res.* **2009**, *23*, 1771–1777. [CrossRef]
71. Alché, L.E.; Berra, A.; Veloso, M.J.; Coto, C.E. Treatment with meliacine, a plant derived antiviral, prevents the development of herpetic stromal keratitis in mice. *J. Med. Virol.* **2000**, *61*, 474–480. [CrossRef]

MDPI
St. Alban-Anlage 66
4052 Basel
Switzerland
Tel. +41 61 683 77 34
Fax +41 61 302 89 18
www.mdpi.com

Viruses Editorial Office
E-mail: viruses@mdpi.com
www.mdpi.com/journal/viruses

www.ingramcontent.com/pod-product-compliance
Lightning Source LLC
LaVergne TN
LVHW070650100526
838202LV00013B/930
* 9 7 8 3 0 3 6 5 4 0 3 7 5 *